Genetic Disorders Sourcebook,
1st Edition

Genetic Disorders Sourcebook,
2nd Edition

Head Trauma Sourcebook

Headache Sourcebook

Health Insurance Sourcebook

Health Reference Series Cumulative
Index 1999

Healthy Aging Sourcebook

Healthy Children Sourcebook

Healthy Heart Sourcebook for Women

Heart Diseases & Disorders
Sourcebook, 2nd Edition

Household Safety Sourcebook

Immune System Disorders Sourcebook

Infant & Toddler Health Sourcebook

Injury & Trauma Sourcebook

Kidney & Urinary Tract Diseases &
Disorders Sourcebook

Learning Disabilities Sourcebook,
1st Edition

Learning Disabilities Sourcebook,
2nd Edition

Liver Disorders Sourcebook

Lung Disorders Sourcebook

Medical Tests Sourcebook

Men's Health Concerns Sourcebook

Mental Health Disorders Sourcebook,
1st Edition

Mental Health Disorders Sourcebook,
2nd Edition

Mental Retardation Sourcebook

Movement Disorders Sourcebook

Obesity Sourcebook

Ophthalmic Disorders Sourcebook

Oral Health Sourcebook

Osteoporosis Sourcebook

Pain Sourcebook, 1st Edition

Pain Sourcebook, 2nd Edition

Pediatric Cancer Sourcebook

Physical & Mental Issues in Aging
Sourcebook

Podiatry Sourcebook

Pregnancy & Birth Sourcebook

Prostate Cancer

Public Health Sourcebook

Reconstructive & Cosmetic Surgery
Sourcebook

Rehabilitation Sourcebook

Respiratory Diseases & Disorders
Sourcebook

Sexually Transmitted Diseases
Sourcebook, 1st Edition

Sexually Transmitted Diseases
Sourcebook, 2nd Edition

Skin Disorders Sourcebook

Sleep Disorders Sourcebook

Sports Injuries Sourcebook, 1st Edition

Sports Injuries Sourcebook, 2nd Edition

Stress-Related Disorders Sourcebook

Substance Abuse Sourcebook

Surgery Sourcebook

Transplantation Sourcebook

Traveler's Health Sourcebook

Vegetarian Sourcebook

Women's Health Concerns Sourcebook

Workplace Health & Safety Sourcebook

Worldwide Health Sourcebook

Teen Health Series

Diet Information for Teens

Drug Information for Teens

Mental Health Information
for Teens

Sexual Health Information
for Teens

Sports
Injuries
SOURCEBOOK

Second Edition

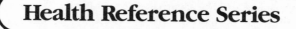

Health Reference Series

Second Edition

Sports Injuries SOURCEBOOK

Basic Consumer Health Information about the Diagnosis, Treatment, and Rehabilitation of Common Sports-Related Injuries in Children and Adults

Along with Suggestions for Conditioning and Training, Information and Prevention Tips for Injuries Frequently Associated with Specific Sports and Special Populations, a Glossary, and a Directory of Additional Resources

Edited by
Joyce Brennfleck Shannon

Omnigraphics

615 Griswold Street • Detroit, MI 48226

Bibliographic Note

Because this page cannot legibly accommodate all the copyright notices, the Bibliographic Note portion of the Preface constitutes an extension of the copyright notice.

Edited by Joyce Brennfleck Shannon

Health Reference Series

Karen Bellenir, *Managing Editor*
David A. Cooke, MD, *Medical Consultant*
Elizabeth Barbour, *Permissions Associate*
Dawn Matthews, *Verification Assistant*
Carol Munson, *Permissions Assistant*
Laura Pleva Nielsen, *Index Editor*
EdIndex, Services for Publishers, *Indexers*

* * *

Omnigraphics, Inc.

Matthew P. Barbour, *Senior Vice President*
Kay Gill, *Vice President—Directories*
Kevin Hayes, *Operations Manager*
Lief Gruenbert, *Development Manager*
David P. Bianco, *Marketing Consultant*

* * *

Peter E. Ruffner, *Publisher*

Frederick G. Ruffner, Jr., *Chairman*

Copyright © 2002 Omnigraphics, Inc.

ISBN 0-7808-0604-2

Library of Congress Cataloging-in-Publication Data

Sports injuries sourcebook : basic consumer health information about the diagnosis, treatment, and rehabilitation of common sports-related injuries in children and adults; along with suggestions for conditioning and training, information and prevention tips for injuries frequently associated with specific sports and special populations, a glossary, and a directory of additional resources / edited by Joyce Brennfleck Shannon.-- 2nd ed.
    p. cm. -- (Health reference series)
  Includes bibliographical references and index.
  ISBN 0-7808-0604-2 (lib. bdg. : alk. paper)
    1. Sports injuries. 2. Sports medicine. 3. Wounds and injuries. I. Shannon, Joyce Brennfleck. II. Health reference series (Unnumbered)

RD97 .S736 2002
617.1'027--dc21

               2002031196

∞

This book is printed on acid-free paper meeting the ANSI Z39.48 Standard. The infinity symbol that appears above indicates that the paper in this book meets that standard.

Printed in the United States

Table of Contents

v

Part III: Injuries Frequently Associated with Specific Sports

Part IV: Diagnosis, Treatment, and Rehabilitation of Sports Injuries

Part V: Conditioning and Training

Part VI: Preventing Common Sports Injuries

Part VII: Additional Help and Information

Preface

About This Book

Participation in sports and recreational activities should lead to better health and greater physical fitness, not a visit to the emergency department.

- According to the National Center for Health Statistics sports-related injuries result in 33.9 emergency visits per 1,000 persons 5-24 years old and account for almost one out of every four injury visits to emergency departments by this age group.

- The Consumer Product Safety Commission estimated there were a total of more than 1 million sports-related injuries to persons 35-54 in 1998.

- Baby boomers who rode bicycles died from head injuries at nearly twice the rate of children who rode bikes—69% of children wear helmets when bicycling compared to only 43% of baby boomers. Bicycle accidents accounted for 21% of all sports-related injuries to persons 65 and older.

This *Sourcebook* provides health information about sports-related injuries including common injuries and those associated with specific sports. The reader will learn about treatment and rehabilitation of sports injuries and how to prevent injuries through conditioning, training, and safety procedures. In addition, it provides information about developments that have occurred to improve medical treatment, rehabilitation, and prevention of sports-related injuries since the publication of the first edition of *Sports-Related Injuries Sourcebook*.

How to Use This Book

This book is divided into parts and chapters. Parts focus on broad areas of interest. Chapters are devoted to single topics within a part.

Part I: Sports-Related Injuries in the United States identifies physical activity trends and the sports-related injuries that occur with children, young adults, baby boomers, and senior adults.

Part II: Common Sports Injuries presents information on injuries to the head and brain, neck and spinal cord, face, knee, shoulder, and growth plates. Stress fractures, sprains and strains, overuse injuries, and a section on emotional abuse in youth sports are also included.

Part III: Injuries Frequently Associated with Specific Sports explains the risks associated with group sports and individual activities, including basketball, football, soccer, ice hockey, exercising, running, horseback riding, and winter and water sports. Information is also provided concerning risks associated with the use of bikes and scooters, inline skates and skateboards, BB guns, trampolines, and playgrounds.

Part IV: Diagnosis, Treatment, and Rehabilitation of Sports Injuries reviews clinical evaluations, medical treatments, and nuclear imaging procedures, gives guidelines for on-the-field management of injuries, and rehabilitation information for common injuries, concussions, and traumatic brain injury (TBI).

Part V: Conditioning and Training gives practical advice on sports nutrition, weight training, youth fitness, and the dangers of using steroids.

Part VI: Preventing Common Sports Injuries gives tips on safety gear and fitness recommendations, along with guidelines for preventing injuries in specific sports including baseball and softball, soccer, winter sports, water sports, and gymnastics.

Part VII: Additional Help and Information includes a glossary of important terms and directories of on-line resources and organizations that provide additional information.

Bibliographic Note

This volume contains documents and excerpts from publications issued by the following U.S. government agencies: Centers for Disease Control and Prevention (CDC); National Center for Health Statistics (NCHS); National Center for Injury Prevention and Control (NCIPC); National Institute of Arthritis and Musculoskeletal and Skin Diseases (NIAMS); National Institute of Child Health and Human Development (NICHD); National Institutes of Health (NIH); National Institutes of Health Osteoporosis and Related Bone Diseases; *Morbidity and Mortality Weekly Report* (MMWR); National Institute on Aging (NIA); National Institute on Drug Abuse (NIDA); National Safe Kids Campaign; SafeUSA; U.S. Coast Guard; U.S. Consumer Product Safety Commission (CPSC); and U.S. National Library of Medicine (NLM).

In addition, this volume contains copyrighted documents from the following organizations and individuals: A.D.A.M., Inc,; American Academy of Allergy, Asthma, and Immunology; American Academy of Family Physicians; American Academy of Otolaryngology; American Association of Neurological Surgeon/Congress of Neurological Surgeons; American Orthopaedic Society for Sports Medicine; American Physical Therapy Association; American Podiatric Medical Association; Massachusetts Governor's Committee of Physical Fitness and Sports; Medical College of Wisconsin Physicians & Clinics; National Athletic Trainers Association; National Center for Catastrophic Sport Injury Research; National Children's Center for Rural and Agricultural Health and Safety; National Safety Council; National Youth Sports Safety Foundation; Prevent Blindness America; Society for Academic Emergency Medicine; Society of Nuclear Medicine; Sports Medicine Performance Center of St. Francis Hospital; Sports Physical Therapy Section of the American Physical Therapy Association. Articles from the following journals are also included: *Academic Emergency Medicine*; *American Journal of Sports Medicine*; and *Physician and Sportsmedicine*.

Full citation information is provided on the first page of each chapter. Every effort has been made to secure all necessary rights to reprint the copyrighted material. If any omissions have been made, please contact Omnigraphics to make corrections for future editions.

Acknowledgements

Special thanks go to the many organizations, agencies, and individuals who have contributed materials for this *Sourcebook* and to the managing editor Karen Bellenir, medical consultant Dr. David Cooke, permissions specialists Liz Barbour and Carol Munson, verification assistant Dawn Matthews, indexer Edward J. Prucha, and document engineer Bruce Bellenir.

Note from the Editor

This book is part of Omnigraphics' *Health Reference Series*. The *Series* provides basic information about a broad range of medical concerns. It is not intended to serve as a tool for diagnosing illness, in prescribing treatments, or as a substitute for the physician/patient relationship. All persons concerned about medical symptoms or the possibility of disease are encouraged to seek professional care from an appropriate health care provider.

Our Advisory Board

The *Health Reference Series* is reviewed by an Advisory Board comprised of librarians from public, academic, and medical libraries. We would like to thank the following board members for providing guidance to the development of this series:

Dr. Lynda Baker,
Associate Professor of Library and Information Science,
Wayne State University, Detroit, MI

Nancy Bulgarelli,
William Beaumont Hospital Library, Royal Oak, MI

Karen Imarisio,
Bloomfield Township Public Library, Bloomfield Township, MI

Karen Morgan,
Mardigian Library, University of Michigan-Dearborn,
Dearborn, MI

Rosemary Orlando,
St. Clair Shores Public Library, St. Clair Shores, MI

Medical Consultant

Medical consultation services are provided to the *Health Reference Series* editors by David A. Cooke, MD. Dr. Cooke is a graduate of Brandeis University, and he received his M.D. degree from the University of Michigan. He completed residency training at the University of Wisconsin

Hospital and Clinics. He is board-certified in Internal Medicine. Dr. Cooke currently works as part of the University of Michigan Health System and practices in Brighton, MI. In his free time, he enjoys writing, science fiction, and spending time with his family.

Health Reference Series *Update Policy*

The inaugural book in the *Health Reference Series* was the first edition of *Cancer Sourcebook* published in 1989. Since then, the *Series* has been enthusiastically received by librarians and in the medical community. In order to maintain the standard of providing high-quality health information for the layperson the editorial staff at Omnigraphics felt it was necessary to implement a policy of updating volumes when warranted.

Medical researchers have been making tremendous strides, and it is the purpose of the *Health Reference Series* to stay current with the most recent advances. Each decision to update a volume will be made on an individual basis. Some of the considerations will include how much new information is available and the feedback we receive from people who use the books. If there is a topic you would like to see added to the update list, or an area of medical concern you feel has not been adequately addressed, please write to:

Editor
Health Reference Series
Omnigraphics, Inc.
615 Griswold Street
Detroit, MI 48226
E-mail: editorial@omnigraphics.com

The commitment to providing on-going coverage of important medical developments has also led to some format changes in the *Health Reference Series*. Each new volume on a topic is individually titled and called a "First Edition." Subsequent updates will carry sequential edition numbers. To help avoid confusion and to provide maximum flexibility in our ability to respond to informational needs, the practice of consecutively numbering each volume has been discontinued.

Part One

Sports-Related Injuries in the United States

Chapter 1

Physical Activity Trends in the United States

Physical activity is associated with numerous health benefits,[1] and increased participation in various types of leisure time physical activity had been encouraged during the 1990s.[2] To determine national estimates of leisure time physical activity during 1990–1998, data were obtained from the Behavioral Risk Factor Surveillance System (BRFSS). This report summarizes the results of that analysis, which indicate that leisure time physical activity trends have remained unchanged.

BRFSS is a population-based, random-digit-dialed telephone survey of the civilian, non-institutionalized U.S. population aged >18 years. Forty-three states and the District of Columbia collected data about physical activity for 1990, 1991, 1992, 1994, 1996, and 1998. Data were not collected by all states during 1993, 1995, and 1997. Respondents were asked about the two physical activities or exercises they engage in most often and about the frequency, duration, and distance (as appropriate) of each activity. Responses were then classified as one of 56 selected activities (Table 1.1). Moderate activity was defined as any of the 56 selected activities and vigorous activity was defined as aerobic physical activity classified as vigorous intensity based on estimated metabolic expenditure (MET) (Table 1.1). To classify an activity as vigorous, it must be aerobic with an assigned MET value[3] that is at least 60% of a person's maximal cardiorespiratory

"Physical Activity Trends—United States, 1990–1998," *MMWR Weekly*, March 09, 2001, 50(09);166-9, Centers for Disease Control and Prevention (CDC), 2001.

3

Table 1.1. Metabolic Expenditure Values Used for Calculating Intensity of Leisure-Time Physical Activity and Aerobic Classification of Activity, by Activity. Source: Behavioral Risk Factor Surveillance System, United States, 1990–1998. (Continued on next page)

Activity	Metabolic expenditure	Aerobic activity
Aerobic class	6.5	yes
Backpacking	7.0	yes
Badminton	4.5	yes
Basketball	6.0	yes
Bicycle machine	7.0	yes
Biking (pleasure)	6.0	yes
Boating (pleasure	6.0	no
Bowling	3.0	no
Boxing	9.0	yes
Calisthenics	3.5	yes
Canoeing (competitive)	3.5	yes
Carpentry	3.0	no
Dancing	4.5	yes
Fishing (bank or boat)	3.5	no
Gardening	4.0	no
Golf	4.5	no
Handball	10.0	yes
Health club exercise	5.5	yes
Hiking	6.0	yes
Home exercise	5.5	yes
Horseback riding	4.0	no
Hunting	5.0	yes
Jogging	7.0	yes
Judo, Karate	10.0	no
Mountain climbing	8.0	yes
Mowing lawn	5.5	yes
Other	4.5	no
Paddleball	6.0	yes

Table 1.1. (continued) Metabolic Expenditure Values Used for Calculating Intensity of Leisure-Time Physical Activity and Aerobic Classification of Activity, by Activity. Source: Behavioral Risk Factor Surveillance System, United States, 1990–1998.

Activity	Metabolic expenditure	Aerobic activity
Painting, papering	3.0	no
Racquetball	7.0	yes
Raking lawn	4.3	yes
Rope skipping	10.0	yes
Rowing machine	7.0	yes
Running	8.0	yes
Scuba diving	7.0	yes
Skating (any)	7.0	yes
Sledding	7.0	yes
Snorkeling	5.0	yes
Snowblowing	4.5	yes
Snowshoeing	8.0	yes
Snow shoveling	6.0	yes
Snow skiing	7.0	yes
Soccer	7.0	yes
Softball	5.0	no
Squash	12.0	yes
Stair climbing	8.0	yes
Stream fishing	6.0	no
Surfing	3.0	no
Swimming laps	6.0	yes
Table tennis	4.0	yes
Tennis	7.0	yes
Touch football	8.0	yes
Volleyball	4.0	no
Walking	3.5	yes
Water skiing	6.0	no
Weightlifting	3.0	no

capacity (MCC). MET values are determined using two regression equations for MCC:[4] one for men (METS 60% MCC = [0.6 x (60 - 0.55 x age)]/ 3.5) and one for women (METS 60% MCC = [0.6 x (48 - 0.37 x age)]/ 3.5).

To have achieved recommended levels of physical activity, a person must have reported engaging in moderate-intensity physical activity 5 times or more per week for 30 minutes or more each time, vigorous intensity physical activity 3 times or more per week for 20 minutes or more each time, or both during the preceding month. Persons reporting some activity during the preceding month but not enough to be classified as moderate or vigorous were classified as insufficient. Persons classified as inactive reported no physical activity outside of their occupation during the preceding month. Data were analyzed using SUDAAN to obtain prevalence estimates for recommended levels of physical activity. All data were age adjusted to the 2000 standard population.

The prevalence of those who engaged in recommended levels of activity increased slightly from 24.3% in 1990 to 25.4% in 1998, and the prevalence of those reporting insufficient activity increased from 45.0% in 1990 to 45.9% in 1998 (Figure 1.1). Those reporting no physical activity decreased from 30.7% in 1990 to 28.7% in 1998. The components of recommended activity remained relatively stable (Figure 1.2).

Reported by: Physical Activity and Health Board, Division of Nutrition and Physical Activity, and Cardiovascular Health Board, Division of Adult and Community Health, National Center for Chronic Disease Prevention and Health Promotion; and an EIS Officer, CDC.

Note: The findings in this report indicate that trends in physical activity remained stable during 1990–1998. Classifying persons according to their main pair of non-occupational activities during the preceding month suggests that only approximately one-fourth of U.S. adults meet recommended levels of physical activity.

During 1990–1998, the BRFSS formula for calculating vigorous intensity changed. In 1992, vigorous intensity was calculated as 50% of MCC; before 1992, it was calculated as 60% of MCC, the generally accepted threshold for vigorous activity. The data reported here vary from previous reports[1] because all years of data were calculated using the same formula for vigorous intensity (60% MCC). Therefore, the slight increase in vigorous physical activity that might have appeared after 1992 in previous reports was attributed to differences in calculating vigorous physical activity rather than an actual increase among the population.

The findings in this report are subject to at least four limitations. First, these data are self-reported and are subject to recall bias. Second, because these data do not include information on non-leisure time physical activities, total activity may be underestimated. Third, only the two most common activities the respondents engaged in during the preceding month are reported. Finally, these data are limited by coverage and non-response errors.

Moderate intensity physical activity has substantial health benefits.[1] Moderate-intensity activities include housework, childcare activities, occupational activity, or walking for transportation, which may be more prevalent among women and certain subgroups of the population. However, surveillance systems that primarily are based on

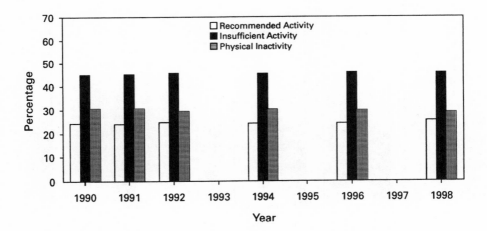

Figure 1.1. *Percentage of Persons Reporting Level* of Leisure-Time Physical Activity, by Year. Source: Behavioral Risk Factor Surveillance System, United States, 1990–1998.***

*Recommended level = moderate intensity activity 5 times or more per week for 30 minutes or more each time, vigorous intensity 3 times or more per week for 20 minutes or more each time, or both; insufficient = some activity but not enough to be classified as moderate or vigorous; inactive = no leisure time physical activity during the preceding month.

**Data were not collected by all states during 1993, 1995, and 1997.

sports-related vigorous activities may miss a substantial portion of this type of activity. Also, systems based on only two reported activities may miss less intense or moderate intensity activities. Public health programs usually encourage participation in moderate intensity rather than vigorous intensity activities for sedentary persons. Surveillance systems should be updated so that a broader range of physical activities can be measured. A more extensive measurement

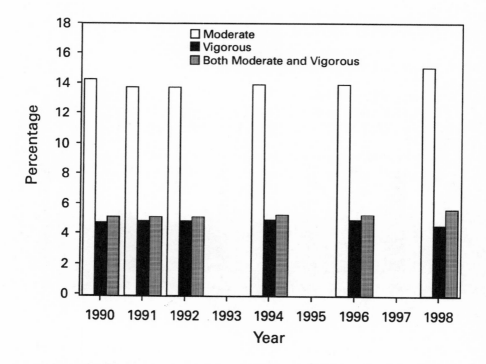

Figure 1.2. *Percentage of Persons Participating in Recommended Level of Leisure-Time Physical Activity, by Intensity* of Activity and Year. Source Behavioral Risk Factor Surveillance System, United States, 1990–1998.***

*Moderate = engaging in moderate intensity physical activity 5 or more times per week for 30 minutes or more each time; vigorous = engaging in vigorous intensity physical activity 3 or more times per week for 20 minutes or more each time.

**Data were not collected by all states during 1993, 1995, and 1997.

system would enable determination of whether the trends in this report are an accurate reflection of physical activity trends in the United States.

References

1. U.S. Department of Health and Human Services. *Physical activity and health: report of the Surgeon General.* Atlanta, Georgia: US Department of Health and Human Services, CDC, National Center for Chronic Disease Prevention and Health Promotion, 1996.

2. U.S. Department of Health and Human Services. *Healthy people 2000*–full report, with commentary. Washington, DC: U.S. Department of Health and Human Services, Public Health Service, 1991; DHHS publication no. (PHS) 91-50212.

3. Ainsworth BE, Haskell WL, Whitt MC, et al. Compendium of physical activities: an update of activity codes and MET intensities. *Med Sci Sports Exerc* 2000;9:S498–S516.

4. Pereria MA, Fitzgerald SJ, Gregg EW, et al. A collection of physical activity questionnaires for health-related research. *Med Sci Sports Exerc* 1997;29:S146–S52.

Chapter 2

How Do Children Spend Their Time?

Parents who have high expectations for their children and spend time with them have children who achieve at higher levels than other children, according to research supported by the National Institute of Child Health and Human Development.

After taking into account race, health, and other influences beyond parents' control, the researchers found that expecting a child to finish college was associated with an increase of six full points out of a total of 100 on a child's reading test score.

The researchers also examined 13 different types of parent-child activities including homework, housework, games, and sports. Children whose parents reported doing the most activities with them tended to have the highest scores on an applied math test. These findings suggest that home activities can prepare children for practical problem solving.

The study was based on a nationally representative sample of about 3,600 children under age 13, directed by Sandra Hofferth at the University of Michigan's Institute for Social Research. It identified a number of other factors linked to school achievement and emotional adjustment:

- **Warm relationships.** The researchers found that parents who had a warm relationship with their children—who hugged them

"How Do Children Spend Their Time? Children's Activities, School Achievement, and Well-Being," *Research on Today's Issues*, Issue No. 11, August 2000, The Population Reference Bureau for the Demographic and Behavioral Sciences Branch, Center for Population Research, National Institute of Child Health and Human Development (NICHD).

11

often, and told them they love them and were proud of them—reported that their children were happier, less withdrawn, and had fewer behavior problems than others. About 66 percent of parents reported behaving warmly toward their children, including hugging their children, telling the child "I love you," and joking or playing together several times a week. But the nature of the relationship appears to change as children age and spend more time with peers. Almost 80 percent of parents of preschoolers reported high levels of warmth in their relationships, compared with only 57 percent of parents of school-age children.

- **Reading vs. television.** While children spent little time reading—about 1.3 hours a week on average—those who read more achieved at higher levels than those who did not read at all or who read very little. In contrast, children spent 13 hours a week, on average, watching television, and those who watched more than this amount did worse on tests of verbal and math achievement than other children.

- **School involvement.** Parents who were more involved with their children's school had children who did better on achievement tests. About half the parents studied were involved in five or more different school activities in the year before they were interviewed. These activities included conferring with the teacher, principal, or counselor; presenting in the child's class or observing or volunteering in the class or school; attending a school event; and attending a PTA meeting. Almost 75 percent of parents reported having regular conversations with their children about school activities, subjects being studied, or school experiences.

- **School stability.** Children who did not change schools in the year before they were surveyed had scores on a scale of behavior problems six times lower than children who changed schools two or more times. After accounting for other factors that affect behavior problems, the findings suggest that changing schools more than once in one year was the single biggest predictor of school problems in children ages 12 and under.

Parent-Child Activities

Children whose parents reported doing the most activities with them tended to have the highest scores on an applied math test. Examples of these activities include:

- Washing or folding clothes
- Doing dishes
- Cleaning house
- Preparing food
- Looking at books or reading stories
- Talking about the family
- Working on homework together
- Building or repairing something
- Playing on the computer or video games
- Playing a board game or card game, or doing a puzzle
- Playing sports or outdoor activities
- Going shopping
- Doing arts and crafts.

Other Differences Examined

The study also analyzed how children's well-being and test scores are related to family characteristics and health:

- **Parents' education levels.** Children with the most-educated parents tended to achieve at higher levels than other children. Children in families with more-educated parents tended to spend more time reading and less time watching television than children of less-educated parents.

- **Family size and structure.** Children with two or fewer siblings tended to receive higher test scores than children from larger families. Children from single-parent families had lower achievement test scores and more behavior problems than other children. Children from two-parent families in which the household head was unemployed also tended to have more behavior problems than other children. Children in single-parent families spent less time reading than children of other types of households. On average, children in dual-income families spent more time in school, less time at home playing, and watched less television than children in families where the father was employed and the mother was not employed outside the home.

- **Health.** While 84 percent of the children studied were in excellent or very good health, according to their parents, 6 percent had fair or poor health or a health-related limitation on their activities. Health-related limitations on children's activities were linked to lower achievement test scores and more behavior problems.

Changes in How Children Spend Their Time

The study also provides the first look since 1981 at how U.S. children spend their time. The findings suggest that children are spending more time on average in day care and school, and more time accompanying their parents on errands and in household tasks, and they have less time for free play than they did in the early 1980s.

In 1997, when the data were collected, children spent about eight hours more per week in day care, preschool, or school programs than they did in 1981. They also spent three hours more per week doing household work, including shopping. Children also spent about three hours less per week in unstructured play and outdoor activities than they did in 1981.

The researchers report that many of the changes in how children spend their time are the result of widespread demographic changes in U.S. families, including increases in the number of households

Table 2.1. Children's Weekly Time Use, 1981 and 1997* (In hours and minutes)

Activity	1981	1997	Difference
School	21:22	29:22	+8:00
Playing	15:54	12:58	-2:56
TV viewing	15:12	13:09	-2:03
Eating	9:08	8:18	-0:50
Sports	2:20	5:17	+2:57
Studying	1:25	2:07	+0:42
Reading	0:57	1.16	+0:19
Household work	2:27	5:39	+3:12

*Children ages 3-11; selected activities.
Source: 1997 Panel Study of Income Dynamics, Child Development Supplement.

headed by single parents and in the number of women employed outside the home. On average, children whose mothers worked outside the home tended to spend the most time in school and day care and the least time in free play.

Less time spent eating is another indication that the work-family time crunch is affecting children, according to the researchers. Children spent about one hour less per week eating in 1997 than they did in 1981, a decrease of 10 percent. Altogether, free time—defined as time left over after eating, sleeping, personal care, and attending school, preschool or day care—decreased from 38 percent to 30 percent of a child's day. One-quarter of that free time was spent watching television (13 hours per week).

Time spent studying increased by almost 50 percent per week between 1981 and 1997. Total study time averaged more than 2 hours per week for all children; this figure appears low because it includes preschoolers who don't study at all. The time children spent in organized sports (standard team activities such as soccer, baseball, basketball, and swimming) more than doubled over the period to total more than 5 hours per week in 1997. Participation increased equally for girls and boys, but in 1997 boys spent twice as much time in sports activities as girls did. When other factors are held equal, black and Hispanic children spent less time in sports than non-Hispanic white children.

In the future, the researchers plan to examine the links among neighborhood, school, and family characteristics, and school achievement and emotional adjustment.

References

Sandra L. Hofferth, "Healthy Environments, Healthy Children: Children in Families" (Ann Arbor, MI: University of Michigan, 1997 Panel Study of Income Dynamics, Child Development Supplement, 1998).

Sandra L. Hofferth and John F. Sandberg, "How American Children Use Their Time," *Journal of Marriage and the Family*, 2001, Vol. 63, no. 2.

Additional Information

These findings come from the Child Development Supplement of the Panel Study of Income Dynamics, a new nationally representative, longitudinal study of children and families. Conducted at the

Survey Research Center, Institute for Social Research, the University of Michigan, this ongoing study is designed to allow researchers to examine the school achievement, social development, and health of all types of children. Website: www.isr.umich.edu/src/child-development/home.html.

Chapter 3

Sports-Related Injuries in Children

Patterns in Childhood Sports Injury

Objectives: To determine the relative frequency of sports-related injuries, compared to all musculoskeletal injuries, and to evaluate the sports-specific and anatomical site-specific nature of these injuries.

Methods: Patterns of injury in patients 5 to 21 years of age presenting to four pediatric emergency departments with musculoskeletal injuries in October 1999 and April 2000 were retrospectively reviewed. Information collected included age, gender, injury type, anatomical injury site, and cause of injury, sports-related or otherwise. Information about patient outcome and management was also obtained.

Results: There were a total of 1,421 injuries in 1,275 patients. Musculoskeletal injuries were more common in males (790/62%) than

Abstract of "Patterns in Childhood Sports Injury," by Dorothy T. Damore, Jordan D. Metzl, Maria Ramundo, Sharon Pan, and Robert van Amerongen, *Academic Emergency Medicine*, Volume 8, Number 5, 458, © 2001 Society for Academic Emergency Medicine, reprinted with permission; abstract of "Sports-Related Injuries in Children," by Bambi L. Taylor, MD and Magdy W. Attia, MD, *Academic Emergency Medicine*, Volume 7, Number 12 1376-1382, © Society for Academic Emergency Medicine, reprinted with permission; and "Childhood Sports Injuries and Their Prevention: A Guide for Parents with Ideas for Kids," National Institute of Arthritis and Musculoskeletal and Skin Diseases (NIAMS), NIH Pub. 00-4821, June 2000.

females. The mean age of the patients was 12.2 each accounting for 25% to 34% of injuries. The most common injury sites included the ankle and foot (285/20%), forearm and wrist (237/17%), and hand (235/17%). Sports injuries accounted for 41% (521) of all musculoskeletal injuries and were responsible for 8% (495/6,173) of all emergency department visits. Head, forearm, and wrist injuries were most commonly seen in biking, hand injuries in football and basketball, knee injuries in soccer, and ankle and foot injuries in basketball.

Conclusions: Sports injuries in children and adolescents were by far the most common cause of musculoskeletal injuries treated in the emergency department, accounting for 41% of all musculoskeletal injuries. This represents the highest percentage of sports-related musculoskeletal injuries per emergency department visit reported in children to date. As children and adolescents participate in sports in record numbers nationwide, sports injury research and prevention will become increasingly more important.

Sports-Related Injuries in Children

Objective: To describe the demographics and types of sports-related injuries (SRIs) in children. Methods: The authors performed a retrospective chart review of children 5-18 years of age diagnosed as having an SRI in a pediatric emergency department (ED) during a two-year period. Patients were identified by ICD-9 codes. Data collected were age, sex, sport, ED interventions, consultations, mechanism, location, and injury type. Pairwise comparisons were reported as odds ratios with 95% confidence intervals.

Results: Six hundred seventy-seven SRIs fit the inclusion criteria; 480 of the patients were male (71%). The mean ages of the males and females were 13.0 years (SD ± 3.0 yr) and 12.4 years (SD ± 2.9 yr), respectively. The six most common sports implicated were basketball (19.5%), football (17.1%), baseball/softball (14.9%), soccer (14.2%), in-line skating (Rollerblading)/skating (5.7%), and hockey (4.6%). Sprains/strains (32.0%), fractures (29.4%), contusions/abrasions (19.3%), and lacerations (9.7%) accounted for 90% of injury types. Pairwise comparison of the four injury types in the six sports listed showed significant associations for contusions/abrasions in baseball, sprains/strains in basketball, fractures in rollerblading/skating, and lacerations in hockey. Age variance, including all sports, of the younger group (5-11 yr) in fractures and the older group (12-18 yr) in sprains was significant. The most common injury location was wrist/hand (28%), followed by head/face (22%), and ankle/foot (18%). Each had significant sport-specific predilections. Contact with person or object was the mechanism for >50% of the SRIs. Sport-specific mechanisms followed lines drawn from the sport-specific injury types and locations.

Conclusions: The pediatric age group incurs a variety of injuries in numerous sports with diverse sex, age, mechanism, location, injury type, and sport-specific differences.

Preventing Childhood Sports Injuries

Childhood sports injuries may be inevitable, but there are some things you can do to help prevent them:

- Enroll your child in organized sports through schools, community clubs, and recreation areas where there may be adults who are certified athletic trainers (ATC). An ATC is also trained in the prevention, recognition, and immediate care of athletic injuries.[1]

- Make sure your child uses the proper protective gear for a particular sport. This may lessen the chances of being injured.

- Warm-up exercises, such as stretching and light jogging, can help minimize the chance of muscle strain or other soft tissue injury during sports. Warm-up exercises make the body's tissues warmer and more flexible. Cooling down exercises loosen the body's muscles that have tightened during exercise.[2] Make warm-ups and cool downs part of your child's routine before and after sports participation.

And don't forget to include sunscreen and a hat (where possible) to reduce the chance of sunburn, which is actually an injury to the skin. Sun protection may also decrease the chances of malignant melanoma—a potentially deadly skin cancer—or other skin cancers that can occur later in life. It is also very important that your child has access to water or a sports drink to stay properly hydrated while playing.

Treat Injuries with "RICE"

If your child receives a soft tissue injury, commonly known as a sprain or a strain, or a bone injury, the best immediate treatment is easy to remember. "RICE" (Rest, Ice, Compression, and Elevation) the injury. Get professional treatment if any injury is severe. A severe injury means having an obvious fracture or dislocation of a joint, prolonged swelling, or prolonged or severe pain.

- **Rest:** Reduce or stop using the injured area for 48 hours. If you have a leg injury, you may need to stay off of it completely.

- **Ice:** Put an ice pack on the injured area for 20 minutes at a time, 4 to 8 times per day. Use a cold pack, ice bag, or a plastic bag filled with crushed ice that has been wrapped in a towel.

- **Compression:** Compression of an injured ankle, knee, or wrist may help reduce the swelling. These include bandages such as elastic wraps, special boots, air casts, and splints. Ask your doctor which one is best.

- **Elevation:** Keep the injured area elevated above the level of the heart. Use a pillow to help elevate an injured limb.

Sprains and Strains

A sprain is an injury to a ligament—a stretching or a tearing. One or more ligaments can be injured during a sprain. A ligament is a band of tough, fibrous tissue that connects two or more bones at a joint and prevents excessive movement of the joint. Ankle sprains are the most common injury in the United States and often occur during sports or recreational activities. Approximately 1 million ankle injuries occur each year and 85 percent of these are sprains.

A strain is an injury to either a muscle or a tendon. A muscle is a tissue composed of bundles of specialized cells that, when stimulated by nerve impulses, contract and produce movement. A tendon is a tough, fibrous cord of tissue that connects muscle to bone.

Growth Plate Injuries

In some sports accidents and injuries, the growth plate may be injured. The growth plate is the area of developing tissues at the end of the long bones in growing children and adolescents. When growth is complete, sometime during adolescence, the growth plate is replaced by solid bone. The long bones in the body are the long bones of the fingers, the outer bone of the forearm, the collarbone, the hip, the bone of the upper leg, the lower leg bones, the ankle, and the foot. If any of these areas become injured, seek professional help from a doctor who specializes in bone injuries in children and adolescents (pediatric orthopaedist).

Repetitive Motion Injuries

Painful injuries such as stress fractures (where the ligament pulls off small pieces of bone) and tendinitis (inflammation of a tendon) can occur from overuse of muscles and tendons.[3] These injuries don't always show up on x-rays, but they do cause pain and discomfort. The injured area usually responds to rest. Other treatments include RICE, crutches, cast immobilization, or physical therapy.

Heat and Hydration—Playing It Safe Is Cool

Playing rigorous sports in the heat requires close monitoring of both body and weather conditions. Heat injuries are always dangerous and can be fatal. Children perspire less than adults and require a higher core body temperature to trigger sweating. Heat-related illnesses include dehydration (deficit in body fluids), heat exhaustion (nausea, dizziness, weakness, headache, pale and moist skin, heavy perspiration, normal or low body temperature, weak pulse, dilated pupils, disorientation, fainting spells), and heat stroke (headache, dizziness, confusion, and hot dry skin, possibly leading to vascular collapse, coma, and death).[4,5] These injuries can be prevented.

Exercise Is Beneficial

Exercise may reduce the chances of obesity, which is becoming more common in children. It may also lessen the risk of diabetes, a disease that is sometimes associated with a lack of exercise and poor eating habits.

As a parent, it is important for you to match your child to the sport, and not push him or her too hard into an activity that he or she may not like or be capable of doing. Sports also helps children build social skills and provides them with a general sense of well-being. Sports participation is an important part of learning how to build team skills.

The following "sports scorecard" shows winning ways to help prevent injuries from occurring.

Football

This popular sport "leads the pack" in the number of injuries, especially in boys, in organized sports.[6]

- *Common injuries and locations:* Bruises, sprains, strains, pulled muscles, soft tissue tears such as ligaments, broken bones, internal injuries (bruised or damaged organs), back injuries, and sunburn. Knees and ankles are the most common injury sites.

21

- *Safest playing with:* Helmet; mouth guard; shoulder pads; athletic supporters for males; chest/rib pads; forearm, elbow, and thigh pads; shin guards; proper shoes; sunscreen; and water.

- *Prevention:* Proper use of safety equipment, warm-up exercises, proper coaching, and conditioning.

Basketball

This popular sport has the highest rate of knee injuries requiring surgery among girls.[7]

- *Common injuries and locations:* Sprains, strains, bruises, fractures, scrapes, dislocation, cuts, and dental injuries. Ankles, knees (injury rates are higher in girls,[8] especially for the anterior cruciate ligament (ACL), the wide ligament that limits rotation and forward movement of the shin bone), and shoulder (rotator cuff strains and tears, where tendons at the end of muscles attach to the upper arm and shoulder bones).

- *Safest playing with:* Eye protection, elbow and knee pads, mouth guard, athletic supporters for males, proper shoes, and water. If playing outdoors, add a hat and sunscreen.

- *Prevention:* Strength training (particularly knees and shoulders), aerobics (exercises that develop the strength and endurance of heart and lungs), warm-up exercises, proper coaching, and use of safety equipment.

Soccer

This sport has dramatically increased in popularity in the past two decades in the U.S.

- *Common injuries:* Bruises, cuts and scrapes, headaches, and sunburn.

- *Safest playing with:* Shin guards, athletic supporters for males, cleats, sunscreen, and water.

- *Prevention:* Aerobic conditioning and warm-ups, and proper training in "heading" the ball. ("Heading" is using the head to strike or make a play with the ball.)

Baseball and Softball

Sometimes called "America's favorite pastime."

- *Common injuries:* Soft tissue strains, impact injuries that include fractures due to sliding and being hit by a ball, and sunburn.

- *Safest playing with:* Batting helmet, shin guards, elbow guards, athletic supporters for males, mouth guard, sunscreen, cleats, hat, and breakaway bases.

- *Prevention:* Proper conditioning and warm-ups.

Gymnastics

The performance of systematic exercises.[9]

- *Common injuries:* Sprains and strains of soft tissues.

- *Safest playing with:* Athletic supporters for males, safety harness, joint supports (such as neoprene wraps), and water.

- *Prevention:* Proper conditioning and warm-ups.

Track and Field

Competing at running, walking, jumping, throwing, or pushing events.[10]

- *Common injuries:* Strains, sprains, and scrapes from falls.

- *Safest playing with:* Proper shoes, athletic supporters for males, sunscreen, and water.

- *Prevention:* Proper conditioning and coaching.

Additional Information

National Institute of Arthritis and Musculoskeletal and Skin Diseases

NIAMS/National Institutes of Health
1 AMS Circle
Bethesda, MD 20892-3675
Toll-Free: 877-22-NIAMS (64267)
Tel: 301-495-4484
TTY: 301-565-2966
Fax: 301-718-6366
Website: www.nih.gov/niams
E-mail: NIAMSinfo@mail.nih.gov

American Academy of Orthopaedic Surgeons (AAOS)
6300 North River Road
Rosemont, IL 60018-4262
Toll-Free: 800-346-AAOS
Tel: 847-823-7186
Fax: 847-823-8125
AAOS Fax-on-Demand: 800-999-2939
Website: www.aaos.org
E-mail: custserv@aaos.org

American Academy of Pediatrics (AAP)
141 Northwest Point Boulevard
Elk Grove Village, IL 60007-1098
Tel: 847-434-4000
Fax: 847-434-8000
Website: www.aap.org
E-mail: kidsdocs@aap.org

American College of Rheumatology
1800 Century Place, Suite 250
Atlanta, GA 30345
Tel: 404-633-3777
Fax: 404-633-1870
Website: www.rheumatology.org
E-mail: acr@rheumatology.org

American Medical Society for Sports Medicine (AMSSM)
11639 Earnshaw
Overland Park, KS 66210
Tel: 913-327-1415
Fax: 913-327-1491
Website: www.amssm.org
E-mail: office@amssm.org

American Orthopaedic Society for Sports Medicine (AOSSM)
6300 N. River Road, Suite 200
Rosemont, IL 60018
Tel: 847-292-4900
Fax: 847-292-4905
Website: www.sportsmed.org

American Physical Therapy Association (APTA)
1111 North Fairfax Street
Alexandria, VA 22314-1488
Toll-Free: 800-999-2782
Tel: 703-684-2782
TDD: 703-683-6748
Fax: 703-684-7343
Website: www.apta.org

Arthritis Foundation
1330 West Peachtree Street
Atlanta, GA 30309
Toll-Free: 800-283-7800
Tel: 404-872-7100 or call your local chapter (listed in the local telephone directory)
Website: www.arthritis.org

National Athletic Trainers Association (NATA)
2952 Stemmons Freeway
Dallas, TX 75247-6916
Toll-Free: 800-879-6282
Tel: 214-637-6282
Fax: 214-637-2206
Website: www.nata.org
E-mail: natanews@nata.org

References

1. National Athletic Trainers Association. *What happens if your child is injured on the sports field?* Press release. 9/23/99.

2. O'Connor, Deborah. Preventing sports injuries in kids. *Patient Care*, 6/15/98, pp.60-83.

3. Powell, John W, Barber-Foss, Kim D. Injury Patterns in Selected High School Sports: A Review of the 1995-1997 Seasons. *Journal of Athletic Training* 1999;34:(3):277-284.

4. O'Connor, Deborah. Preventing sports injuries in kids. *Patient Care*, 6/15/98, pp.60-83.

5. American Academy of Family Physicians. *Heat-Related Illness: What You Can Do to Prevent It*. Brochure. 1994.

6. Requa, Ralph. The scope of the problem: the impact of sports-related injuries. In *Proceedings of Sports Injuries in Youth: Surveillance Strategies*, Bethesda, MD, 8-9 April 1991. National Institute of Arthritis and Musculoskeletal and Skin Diseases, National Institutes of Health, Bethesda, MD. 11/92, p.19.

7. Messina, DF; Farney, WC; DeLee, JC. The incidence of injury in Texas high school basketball. *The American Journal of Sports Medicine*. Vol. 27; No.3; 294-299; 1999.

8. Messina, DF; Farney, WC; DeLee, JC. The incidence of injury in Texas high school basketball. *The American Journal of Sports Medicine*. Vol. 27; No.3; 294-299; 1999.

9. Encyclopedia Britannica Online; http://members.eb.com

10. Encyclopedia Britannica Online; http://members.eb.com

Chapter 4

Statistics of Childhood: Young Adult Sports-Related Injuries

Sports-related injuries in children and young adults cause 2.6 million visits to the nation's hospital emergency departments for a cost of about $500 million annually, according to the National Hospital Ambulatory Medical Care Survey's data for 1997 and 1998. Results from the survey conducted by the Center for Disease Control and Prevention (CDC)'s National Center for Health Statistics were published in the March 2001 issue of the *Annals of Emergency Medicine*.

Sports-related injury visits to emergency departments were more frequent for persons five to 24 years of age. They represented over two-thirds of the total amount of sports injury visits (3.7 million for all ages). Sports injuries result in 33.9 emergency visits per 1,000 persons 5-24 years old, and account for almost one out of every four injury visits to emergency departments by this age group. The visit rate was twice as high for males as females.

"Protecting our children from injuries is the key," said CDC Director Jeffrey P. Koplan, MD, MPH. "Helmets, the right equipment, better safety practices, and instruction can all help reduce these preventable and oftentimes serious injuries. Participation in sports and recreation games and activities should lead to better health and greater physical fitness, not a visit to the emergency department," he said.

"Sports-Related Injuries Cause 2.6 Million Visits Annually by Children and Young Adults to Emergency Rooms," News Release, Monday, March 5, 2001, National Center for Health Statistics; and "Sports Injury Table," National Center for Health Statistics (NCHS), reviewed March 9, 2001.

Table 4.1. Average Annual Injury Visits to Hospital Emergency Departments by Persons between 5 and 24 Years of Age by Type of Activity Performed When Injury Occurred: United States, 1997-98

	Number of visits in thousands	Percent of visits in thousands	Percent of sports-related injury visits
All injury visits	11,904	100.0	
All sport-related activities[1]	2,616	22.0	100.0
—Group sport	1,170	9.8	44.7
Basketball	447	3.8	17.1
Football	271	2.3	10.3
Baseball/softball	245	2.1	9.4
Soccer	95	0.8	3.6
Other group sport[2]	112	0.9	4.3
—Individual sport	1,446	12.2	55.3
Pedal cycling	421	3.5	16.1
Ice- or roller skating/boarding	150	1.3	5.7
Gymnastics/cheerleading	146	1.2	5.6
Playground	137	1.2	5.2
Snow sport	111	0.9	4.2
Water sport	100	0.8	3.8
Exercising/track	94	0.8	3.6
Combative	61	0.5	2.3
Recreational	50	0.4	1.9
Other sport[3]	178	1.5	6.8
Non-sport activities[4]	7,947	66.8	
Visits without a specified cause[5]	1,340	11.3	

1. Includes all visits with a cause indicating an organized or unorganized sport, game, or recreational activity.
2. Includes other group sports such as volleyball, hockey, and lacrosse.
3. Includes all other categories such as games, all terrain vehicles, and unspecified sport/recreational activities.
4. Includes all visits with a specified activity not categorized under sports. This includes transport, household, personal, work, or maintenance activities. It also includes visits for any injuries caused by intentional behavior.
5. Includes any visits for which no cause was listed or the entry stated unknown causes.

Source: *National Hospital Ambulatory Medical Care Survey.*

For children and young adults, injuries associated with basketball and cycling—almost 900,000 a year—are the most frequent sports-related injuries seen in the nation's emergency departments. Football and baseball are associated with about one-quarter million visits each, and soccer injuries result in about 100,000 visits. These findings don't indicate that these sports are necessarily more dangerous, there just may be more people engaging in these activities.

In addition to pedal cycling, other sports that frequently result in emergency visits by persons 5-24 years of age include ice or roller skating and skate boarding (150,000 visits), gymnastics and cheer-leading (146,000 visits), and water and snow sports (100,000 visits each). Injuries on the playground account for about 137,000 emergency visits yearly.

Sports-related injuries are more likely than other injuries to be to the brain or skull and upper and lower extremities; more likely to be a fracture, strain or sprain; and more likely to have diagnostic and therapeutic services provided, especially orthopedic care.

The *National Hospital Ambulatory Medical Care Survey* is a national probability survey based on a sample of visits to a national representative sample of the nation's hospital emergency departments.

Additional Reading

Burt CW, Overpeck MD. Emergency visits for sports-related injuries. *Ann Emerg Med*. March 2001; 37:301-308.

Additional Information

Centers for Disease Control and Prevention
National Center for Health Statistics
Division of Data Services
6525 Belcrest Road
Hyattsville, MD 20782-2003
Tel: 301-458-4636
Website: www.cdc.gov/nchs

Chapter 5

Catastrophic Sport Injury Report of High School and College Sports

In 1931 the American Football Coaches Association initiated the *First Annual Survey of Football Fatalities* and this research has been conducted at the University of North Carolina at Chapel Hill since 1965. In 1977 the National Collegiate Athletic Association initiated a *National Survey of Catastrophic Football Injuries* which is also conducted at the University of North Carolina. As a result of these research projects important contributions to the sport of football have been made. Most notable have been the 1976 rule changes, the football helmet standard, improved medical care for the participants, and better coaching techniques.

Due to the success of these two football projects the research was expanded to all sports for both men and women, and a National Center for Catastrophic Sports Injury Research was established. The decision to expand the research was based on the following factors:

1. Research based on reliable data is essential if progress is to be made in sports safety.

2. The paucity of information on injuries in all sports.

3. The rapid expansion and lack of injury information in women's sports.

"Eighteenth Annual Report Fall 1982–Spring 2000," by Frederick O. Mueller, Ph.D. and Robert C. Cantu, M.D., © National Center for Catastrophic Sports Injury Research, updated July 19, 2001, reprinted with permission.

For the purpose of this research the term catastrophic is defined as any severe injury incurred during participation in a school/college sponsored sport. Catastrophic will be divided into the following three definitions:

1. Fatality

2. Non-Fatal—permanent severe functional disability.

3. Serious—no permanent functional disability but severe injury. An example would be a fractured cervical vertebra with no paralysis.

Sports injuries are also considered direct or indirect.

Direct: Those injuries which resulted directly from participation in the skills of the sport.

Indirect: Those injuries which were caused by systemic failure as a result of exertion while participating in a sport activity or by a complication which was secondary to a non-fatal injury.

Data Collection

Data were compiled with the assistance of coaches, athletic directors, executive officers of state and national athletic organizations, a national newspaper clipping service, and professional associates of the researchers. Data collection would not have been possible without the support of the National Collegiate Athletic Association, the National Federation of State High School Associations, and the American Football Coaches Association. Upon receiving information concerning a possible catastrophic sports injury, contact by telephone, personal letter, and questionnaire was made with the injured player's coach or athletic director. Data collected included background information on the athlete (age, height, weight, experience, previous injury, etc.), accident information, immediate and post-accident medical care, type injury, and equipment involved. Autopsy reports are used when available.

In 1987, a joint endeavor was initiated with the Section on Sports Medicine of the American Association of Neurological Surgeons. The purpose of this collaboration was to enhance the collection of medical data. Dr. Robert C. Cantu, Chairman, Department of Surgery and Chief, Neurosurgery Service, Emerson Hospital, in Concord, MA, has been responsible for contacting the physician involved in each case and for collecting the medical data. Dr. Cantu is also the Past-President of the American College of Sports Medicine.

Summary

Fall Sports

Football is associated with the greatest number of catastrophic injuries. For the 1999 football season there were a total of 21 high school direct catastrophic injuries, which is an decrease of seven from 1998 and a decrease of 13 when compared to the 1993 season. College football was associated with three direct catastrophic injuries in 1999, which is an increase of five when compared to 1998 and equals the 1982 and 1991 seasons low numbers.

In 1990 there were no fatalities directly related to football. The 1990 football report is historic in that it is the first year since the beginning of the research, 1931, that there has not been a direct fatality in football at any level of play. This clearly illustrates that this type of data collection and constant analysis of the data is important and plays a major role in injury prevention. The 1994 data shows zero fatalities at the high school level and one at the college level, with a slight rise in 1995 to four. These numbers are very low when one considers that there were 36 football direct fatalities in 1968.

In addition to the direct fatalities in 1999 there were also eleven indirect fatalities. All eleven of the indirect fatalities were at the high school level. Seven of the high school indirect fatalities were heart-related, two were heat-related, and one was associated with sickle cell and was listed as a natural death.

In addition to the fatalities there were seven permanent paralysis cervical spine injuries in 1999. This number is low when compared to the 25 to 30 cases every year in the early 1970s. Six of the injuries were at the high school level and one at the college. Football in 1999 was also associated with three cerebral injuries that resulted in permanent disability. All three of the injuries were at the high school level.

Serious football injuries with no permanent disability accounted for 9 injuries in 1999—eight in high school and one in college. High school athletes were associated with four cervical spine fractures, three brain injuries with full recovery, and one cervical spine contusion. College athletes were associated with one cervical spine contusion.

This decrease in catastrophic football injuries illustrates the importance of data collection and being sure that the information is passed on to those responsible for conducting football programs. A return to the injury levels of the 1960s and 1970s would be detrimental to the game and its participants.

Cross-country was not associated with any direct injuries in 1999. In the past eighteen years, cross-country was associated with one direct non-fatal injury and 12 indirect fatalities at the high school level and one indirect fatality at the college level. All thirteen of the indirect injuries were heart-related fatalities. Autopsy reports revealed congenital heart disease in three of these cases.

High school soccer had one direct death in 1999 and a total of 14 catastrophic injuries for the past eighteen seasons. The injury involved a participant with a fractured leg and a severed artery with partial disability. The three direct catastrophic injuries in 1992 were the highest number in the past eighteen years. There was one high school soccer indirect fatality in 1999 and it was related to a congenital heart problem. In 1999 college soccer was not associated with any direct or indirect catastrophic injuries. There were also two non-school injuries in 1998 that should be mentioned again in the 1999 report. A young boy was paralyzed after being hit when the soccer goal tipped and struck him in the head. The second case involved a 22-year-old soldier who was struck in the head by the soccer goal after attempting to move the goal with a group of players. Being struck by a soccer goal has been an on-going problem and precaution should be taken when it is being moved. In addition, concussion injuries as related to heading are a controversial area in soccer. There are helmet manufacturers that are now making soccer helmets to protect the participants from brain injuries while heading, even though the research indicates that concussion injuries during heading are related to head-to-head contact and not ball contact. The National Center will keep abreast of this controversial area.

In 1988 **field hockey** was associated with its first catastrophic injury since the study began in 1982. It was listed as a serious injury at the college level. The athlete was struck by the ball after a free hit. She received a fractured skull, had surgery, and has recovered from the injury. The 1996 data shows two field hockey direct injuries at the high school level. Both injuries involved being hit by the ball and resulted in a head and an eye injury. There were no direct or indirect field hockey injuries in 1998. The 1999 data show one non-fatal injury at the high school level and one serious injury at the college level.

The high school injury involved the loss of an eye after being hit with the stick during a drill, and the college injury resulted in a fractured skull after being hit by a ball.

In 1992-93 high school **water polo** was associated with its first indirect fatality and in 1988-89 college water polo had its first indirect fatality. There were no water polo injuries in 1999.

In summary, high school fall sports in 1999 were associated with 23 direct catastrophic injuries. Twenty-one were associated with football, one with field hockey, and one with soccer. There were five fatalities, ten involved permanent disability, and eight were considered serious. For the eighteen-year period 1982–1999, high school fall sports had 478 direct catastrophic injuries and 460, or 96.2%, were related to football participants. In 1999 high school fall sports were also associated with 11 football indirect fatalities, one in soccer for a total of 12 indirect fatalities. For the period from 1982–1999 there was a total of 147 indirect fall high school catastrophic injuries. One hundred and forty-six of the indirect injuries were fatalities and 112 were related to football. Four of the indirect fatalities involved females — three soccer players and a cross-country athlete.

During the 1999 college fall sports season there were a total of four direct catastrophic injuries, and three were in football. For the eighteen years, 1982–1999, there were a total of 108 college direct fall sport catastrophic injuries, and 105 were associated with football. There were no indirect college fatalities during the fall of 1999. From 1982 through the 1999 season there were a total of 31 college fall sport indirect catastrophic injuries. Twenty-five were associated with football.

High school football accounted for the greatest number of direct catastrophic injuries for the fall sports, but high school football was also associated with the greatest number of participants. There are approximately 1,500,000 high school and junior high school football players participating each year. The eighteen-year rate of direct injuries per 100,000 high school and junior high school football participants was 0.30 fatalities, 0.71 non-fatal injuries, and 0.76 serious injuries. These catastrophic injury rates for football are higher than those for both cross-country and soccer, but all three classifications of catastrophic football injuries have an injury rate of less than one per 100,000 participants. The indirect fatality rates for high school football, soccer, and cross-country are similar and are also less than one per 100,000 participants. Water polo rates are high, but are based on only seven years of data, and water polo has approximately 10,000 participants each year.

College football has approximately 75,000 participants each year and the direct injury rate per 100,000 participants is higher than college soccer and field hockey. The rate, for the eighteen-year period, for college football fatalities is less than one per 100,000 participants,

Table 5.1. Participation Figures Totals from Eighteen years, 1982/1983–1999/2000

Sport	High School		College	
	Men	**Women**	**Men**	**Women**
Football	25,800,000	4,654	1,350,000	0
Cross-country	2,931,328	2,117,997	178,369	147,902
Soccer	4,333,367	2,665,206	275,284	156,469
Basketball	9,429,806	7,401,102	244,537	209,913
Gymnastics	80,078	480,712	12,536	27,400
Ice Hockey	437,815	16,412	68,891	4,394
Swimming	1,442,275	1,765,510	142,200	145,967
Wrestling	4,255,373	12,263	126,943	0
Baseball	7,217,782	12,401	394,809	0
Softball	16,582	5,113,611	0	193,545
LaCrosse	387,821	221,480	92,076	59,900
Track	8,681,523	6,910,144	613,387	423,548
Tennis	2,420,807	2,418,769	139,337	135,792
Field Hockey	470	935,265	0	101,853
Skiing	65,978 (94-00)	53,845 (94-00)	12,716	11,011
Water Polo	92,793	49,213	18,324	1,407 (98-00)
Volleyball	199,474 (94-00)	2,205,677 (94-00)	6,010 (94-00)	73,392 (94-00)
Total	67,793,272	32,384,261	3,675,419	1,692,493

Updated: December 19, 2001

but the rate increases to 1.78 per 100,000 for non-fatal injuries and 5.41 per 100,000 participants for serious injuries.

Indirect fatality rates are similar in college cross-country and soccer, increase in football, with water polo being associated with the highest indirect fatality rate. Based on 12 years of data, water polo has approximately 1,500 participants each year. There were three college female athletes receiving a direct or indirect catastrophic injury in a fall sport for this eighteen-year period of time. Two were serious injuries in field hockey, and the other was an indirect death in soccer.

Incidence rates are based on eighteen-year participation figures received from the National Federation of State High School Associations and the National Collegiate Athletic Association.

Winter Sports

High school winter sports were associated with five direct catastrophic injuries in 1999–2000. One injury was related to basketball, two to ice hockey, and two to wrestling.

High school winter sports were also associated with five indirect injuries during the 1999–2000 school year. All of the injuries were fatalities, and four were associated with basketball and one with ice hockey. All of the fatalities were heart-related and all were males.

College winter sports had two direct basketball catastrophic injuries and one in ice hockey during the 1999–2000 school year. There were no indirect catastrophic injuries during that same time period.

A summary of high school winter sports, 1982–2000, shows a total of 92 direct catastrophic injuries (7 fatalities, 48 non-fatal, and 37 serious) and 102 indirect. Wrestling was associated with 42 or 45.6 percent of the direct injuries. Gymnastics were associated with 12, or 13.0%, of the direct injuries. Basketball was associated with 13 (14.1%), ice hockey was associated with 15 (16.3%), swimming was associated with nine (9.8%) direct injuries, and volleyball had one direct injury (1.1%). Basketball accounted for the greatest number of indirect fatalities with 78, or 76.5%, of the winter total.

College winter sports from 1982–2000 were associated with a total of 22 direct catastrophic injuries. Gymnastics was associated with six (27.3%), ice hockey eight (36.4%), basketball five (22.7%), swimming one (4.5%), skiing one (4.5%), and wrestling one (4.5%). There were also 25 indirect injuries during this time period. Fourteen, or 56%, were associated with basketball, three in wrestling, two in ice hockey, four in swimming, one in skiing, and one in volleyball.

High school wrestling accounted for the greatest number of winter sport direct injuries, but the injury rate per 100,000 participants was less than one for all three injury categories. High school wrestling has approximately 237,000 participants each year. High school basketball and swimming were also associated with low direct injury rates. Ice hockey and gymnastics were associated with the highest injury rates for the winter sports. Gymnastics has averaged approximately 4,500 male and 26,700 female participants during the past eighteen years. Ice hockey averages 25,000 participants each year. A high percentage of the ice hockey injuries involve a player being hit by an opposing player, usually from behind, and striking the skate rink boards with the top of his/her head.

Catastrophic direct injury rates for college winter sports are higher when compared to high school figures. Gymnastics had five non-fatal and one serious injury for the past eighteen years, but the injury rate is 23.93 per 100,000 participants for non-fatal male injuries and 7.30 per 100,000 for female non-fatal injuries. Participation figures show approximately 700 male and 1,500 female gymnastic participants each year.

College ice hockey was associated with four serious and four non-fatal injuries in eighteen years, but the injury rate is 5.81 per 100,000 participants for non-fatal and 4.35 for serious injuries. There are approximately 3,800 ice hockey participants each year. The first female college ice hockey player received a direct serious injury during the 1999–2000 season. The serious injury rate for female serious injuries was 22.76 injuries per 100,000 participants and averaged approximately 250 participants per year for the past 18 years. Swimming non-fatal incidence rates were not as high as gymnastics or ice hockey, but could be totally eliminated if swimmers would not use the racing dive into the shallow end of pools during practice or meets. In fact there has not been a direct injury in college swimming since the one non-fatal injury in 1982-1983.

College wrestling had only one direct catastrophic injury from the fall of 1982 to the spring of 2000. For this period of time there were 126,943 participants in college wrestling for an average of approximately 7,052 per year. The injury rate for this eighteen-year period of time was 0.79 per 100,000 participants. College skiing has approximately 1,000 female participants each year and the one fatality in 1989–1990 produced a ten-year injury rate of 9.08 per 100,000 participants. This was the only skiing direct fatality since the study was initiated.

Injury rates for college indirect fatalities were high when compared to the high school rates. Basketball had an injury rate of 5.32 fatalities per 100,000 male participants, skiing 7.86, ice hockey 1.45 and swimming 2.81. The year 1997–98 is the first year where there were any indirect fatalities in wrestling. There were three deaths due to heat stroke associated with the wrestlers trying to make weight for a match. The indirect injury rate for wrestling was 2.36 per 100,000 participants.

The female indirect injury rate for basketball was 0.48 per 100,000 participants, and 1.36 per 100,000 for volleyball.

Facts about Injuries

- Indirect high school catastrophic injury rates are all below one per 100,000 participants.

- College spring sports were not associated with any direct or indirect injuries in 2000.

Spring Sports

High school spring sports were associated with seven direct catastrophic injuries in 2000. Baseball was associated with two, lacrosse two, track two, and softball one. There were seven indirect fatalities in high school spring sports during the 1999–2000 school year.

From 1983 through 2000, high school spring sports were associated with 91 direct catastrophic injuries. Twenty-nine were listed as fatalities, 29 as catastrophic non-fatal, and 33 as serious. Baseball accounted for thirty-eight, track forty-six, lacrosse four, and softball three. Injury rates were less than one per 100,000 participants for each sport in all categories. There were four direct injuries to females in track and three in softball. There were also 37 indirect fatalities in high school spring sports during this time span. Twenty-three were related to track, nine in baseball, three in lacrosse, and two in tennis. Four of the indirect fatalities involved female track athletes.

College spring sports were associated with 18 direct catastrophic injuries from 1983 to 2000. Five of these injuries resulted in fatalities, seven were listed as non-fatal, and six were listed as serious. Baseball accounted for five injuries, lacrosse five, and track eight. There were also six indirect fatalities in college spring sports during this time. Two indirect fatalities were associated with tennis, one was associated with track, two in baseball, and one in lacrosse.

Injury rates for high school spring sports direct injuries were low. Baseball participation reveals approximately 400,000 players each year, track 480,000 males and 385,000 females, and tennis 135,000 males and 135,000 females. The baseball figures do not include the 280,000 softball participants each year. Lacrosse has approximately 21,000 male and 12,000 female participants each year. Injury rates for high school indirect injuries are also low.

College spring sports are related to low injury rates for direct injuries. Men's lacrosse had one fatality, one non-fatal and two serious injuries, and the injury rates were slightly higher than the other sports. Participation figures reveal approximately 5,000 men and 3,300 women lacrosse players each year. The 1991 injury was to a female lacrosse player.

Rates for indirect college fatalities in baseball, tennis, and track are low with lacrosse being slightly higher. There were two indirect tennis fatalities, one male and one female, but participation figures are low. Men average approximately 7,700 and women 7,500 participants each year.

Discussion

Football is associated with the greatest number of catastrophic injuries for all sports, but the incidence of injury per 100,000 participants is higher in both gymnastics and ice hockey. There have been dramatic reductions in the number of football fatalities and non-fatal catastrophic injuries since 1976 and the 1990 data illustrated a historic decrease in football fatalities to zero. This is a great accomplishment when compared to the 36 fatalities in 1968. This dramatic reduction can be directly related to data collected by the American Football Coaches Association Committee on Football Injuries (1931–2000) and the recommendations that were based on that data. Non-fatal football injuries, permanent disability, decreased to one for college football in 1995. There was a dramatic reduction in high school football from 13 in 1990 to four in 1991. There was an increase to ten in 1992 and 13 in 1993, but a reduction to five in 1994. The 1997 data show an increase to fourteen and the 1999 numbers a decrease to ten. Permanent disability injuries in football have seen dramatic reductions when compared to the data from the late 1960s and early 1970s, but a continued effort must be made to eliminate these injuries. In addition, there were nine serious injuries in football in 1999—eight in high school and one in college. All of the serious cases involved head or neck injuries and in a number of these cases excellent medical care saved the athlete from permanent disability or death.

Football catastrophic injuries may never be totally eliminated, but progress has been made. Emphasis should again be focused on the preventive measures that received credit for the initial reduction of injuries.

1. The 1976 rule change which prohibited initial contact with the head in blocking and tackling. There must be continued emphasis in this area by coaches and officials.

2. The NOCSAE football helmet standard that went into effect at the college level in 1978 and at the high school level in 1980. There should be continued research in helmet safety.

3. Improved medical care of the injured athlete. An emphasis on placing athletic trainers in all high schools and colleges. There should be a written emergency plan for catastrophic injuries both at the high school and college levels.

4. Improved coaching technique when teaching the fundamental skills of blocking and tackling. Keeping the head out of football!

It should be noted that since 1979, according to the Consumer Product Safety Commission, there have been at least 23 deaths and 38 serious injuries to children when movable soccer goals have fallen on them. The most recent cases involved a 10-year-old male in May 1998. A soccer goal frame fell on his head while he was helping move it. The injury left him paralyzed. In August of 1999 a 22-year-old soldier was killed when a soccer goal fell and hit him in the head. He and his friends were trying to move the metal goals. There has been one fatality in this study, which involved a college athlete hanging on a soccer goal and the goal falling and striking the victim's head.

On May 4, 1999, the Consumer Product Safety Commission and the soccer goal industry announced the development of a new safety standard that will reduce the risk of soccer goal tip-over. The "Provisional Safety Standard and Performance Specification for Soccer Goals" (ASTM-PS-75-99) requires that movable soccer goals, except very lightweight goals, not tip over when the goal is weighted in a downward or horizontal direction. The standard also specifies warning labels must be attached to the goal, such as: "Warning: Always anchor goal. Unsecured goal can fall over causing serious injury or death."

A *Loss Control Bulletin* from K & K Insurance Group, Inc., Fort Wayne, IN, suggests the following safeguards:

1. Keep soccer goals supervised and anchored.

2. Never permit hanging or climbing on a soccer goal.

3. Always stand to the rear or side of the goal when moving it— never to the front.

4. Stabilize the goal as best suits the playing surface, but in a manner that does not create other hazards to players.

5. Develop and follow a plan for periodic inspection and mainte- nance (e.g., dry rot, joints, and hooks).

6. Advise all field maintenance persons to re-anchor the goal if moved for mowing the grass or other purposes.

7. Remove goals from fields no longer in use for the soccer pro- gram as the season progresses.

8. Secure goals well from unauthorized access when stored.

9. Educate and remind all players and adult supervisors about the past tragedies of soccer goal fatalities.

High school wrestling, gymnastics, ice hockey, baseball, and track should receive close attention. Wrestling has been associated with 42 direct catastrophic injuries during the past eighteen years, but the injury rate per 100,000 participants is lower than both gymnastics and ice hockey. Due to the fact that college wrestling was only associ- ated with one catastrophic injury during this same time period, contin- ued research should be focused on the high school level. High school wrestling coaches should be experienced in the teaching of the proper skills of wrestling and should attend coaching clinics to keep updated on new teaching techniques and safety measures. They should also have experience and training in the proper conditioning of their ath- letes. These measures are important in all sports, but there are a number of contact sports, like wrestling, where the experience and training of the coach is of the utmost importance. Full speed wres- tling in physical education classes is a questionable practice unless there is proper time for conditioning and the teaching of skills. The physical education teacher should also have expertise in the teach- ing of wrestling skills. It should also be emphasized that wrestling coaches need to be aware of the dangers associated with athletes making weight. Improper weight reduction can lead to serious inju- ries and death. During the 1997–1998 academic year there were three college students that died while trying to make weight for a match—

all three died of heat stroke complications. These were the first wrestling deaths associated with weight reduction, but there is no information on the number of wrestlers who had medical problems associated with weight loss, but recovered. All three of these wrestlers were trying to lose large amounts of weight in a short period of time. All three were also working out in areas of high heat, and were all wearing sweat clothes or rubber suits. Making weight has always been a part of the wrestling culture, but it is dangerous and life threatening. New rule changes went into effect for the 1998–1999 high school and college seasons, and hopefully, making weight will be a thing of the past and will never again result in the deaths of young high school and college athletes.

Men and women gymnastics were associated with high injury rates at both the high school and college levels. Gymnastics needs additional study at both levels of competition. Both levels have seen a dramatic participation reduction and this trend may continue with the major emphasis being in private clubs.

Ice hockey injuries are low in numbers but the injury rate per 100,000 participants is high when compared to other sports. Ice hockey catastrophic injuries usually occur when an athlete is struck from behind by an opponent and makes contact with the crown of his/her head and the boards surrounding the rink. The results are usually fractured cervical vertebrae with paralysis. Research in Canada has revealed high catastrophic injury rates with similar results. After an in-depth study of ice hockey catastrophic injuries in Canada, Dr. Charles Tator has made the following recommendations concerning prevention:

1. Enforce current rules and consider new rules against pushing or checking from behind.

2. Improve strength of neck muscles.

3. Educate players concerning risk of neck injuries.

4. Continued epidemiological research.

Catastrophic injuries in swimming were all directly related to the racing dive in the shallow ends of pools. There has been a major effort by both schools and colleges to make the racing dive safer and the catastrophic injury data support that effort. There has not been a college injury for the past 17 years, but in 1997–98 a high school swimmer was paralyzed after diving into the shallow end of a pool while practicing a racing dive. It is a fact that since the swimming community was made aware of this fact, and along with rule changes and coach's awareness, the number of direct catastrophic injuries in swimming has been reduced. The competitive racing start has changed and now involves the swimmer getting more depth when entering the water. Practicing or starting competition in the deep end of the pool or being extremely cautious could eliminate catastrophic injuries caused by the swimmer striking his/her head on the bottom of the pool. The National Federation of State High School Associations Swimming and Diving Rules Committee voted that in pools with water depth less than three and one-half feet at the starting end, swimmers will have to start the race in the water. This rule change is a refinement of a 1991–1992 rule change and took effect in the 1992–1993 season. The new rules read that in four feet or more of water, swimmers may use a starting platform up to a maximum of 30 inches above the water. Between three and one-half and four feet, swimmers may start no higher than 18 inches above the water. Less than that, it's in the pool. In April 1995 the National Federation revised rule 2-7-2, which now states that starting platforms shall be securely attached to the deck/wall. If they are not, they shall not be used and deck or in-water starts will be required. These new rules point out the importance of constant data collection and analysis. Rules and equipment changes for safety reasons must be based on reliable injury data.

High school spring sports have been associated with low incidence rates during the past eighteen years, but baseball was associated with thirty-eight direct catastrophic injuries and track with forty-six. A majority of the baseball injuries have been caused by the head first slide or by being struck with a thrown or batted ball. The 2000 data show one player being hit in the chest with a ball causing death, and one player being struck in the head with a batted ball resulting in disability. If the head first slide is going to be used, proper instruction should be involved. Proper protection for batting practice should be provided for the batting practice pitcher and he/she should always wear a helmet. This should also be true for the batting practice coach. During the 1999 baseball season three high school pitchers were struck by a batted ball. There are always a number of non-school baseball injuries and the cause of injury is usually the same.

The pole vault was associated with a majority of the fatal track injuries. There have been fifteen high school fatal pole vaulting injuries from 1983 to 2000. This does not include the coach who was demonstrating in 1998, bounced out of the pit, struck his head on concrete, and died. In addition to the fatalities there were also seven permanent disability and six serious injuries. All 28 of these accidents involved the vaulter bouncing out of or landing out of the pit area. The three pole vaulting deaths in 1983 were a major concern and immediate measures were taken by the National Federation of State High School Associations. Beginning with the 1987 season all individual units in the pole vault landing area had to include a common cover or pad extending over all sections of the pit.

Every time there is a pole vaulting death there are more proponents of eliminating the event. The crux of the opposition to the event appears to be the potential liability and also the lack of qualified coaches to teach the pole vault. Additional recommendations in the 1991 rule book: stabilize the pole vault standards so they cannot fall into the pit, pad the standards, remove all hazards from around the pit area, and control traffic along the approach. Obvious hazards like concrete or other hard materials around the pit should be eliminated. The state of Ohio has developed a program to teach proper techniques to coaches. It has been estimated that there are approximately 25,000 high school pole vaulters. If this number is correct, the catastrophic injury rate for high school pole vaulters would be higher than any of the sports included in the research.

There have also been 15 accidents in high school track involving participants being struck by a thrown discus, shot put, or javelin. In 1992, a female athlete was struck by a thrown discus in practice and died. In 1993, a track manager was struck in the neck by a javelin, but he was lucky and completely recovered from the accident. In 1994, a female track athlete was struck in the face by a javelin and will recover. In 1995, a male athlete was struck in the head by a shot put during warm-ups and had a fractured skull. In 1997, a male athlete was struck by a discus and died. In 1998 a female athlete was struck by a discus and died, and a male athlete was struck in the head by a shot put but recovered. In 1999 a male athlete was struck by a javelin and a discus struck a female athlete. In 2000 a junior high school athlete was struck in the head by a discus and has permanent disability. There have also been spectators struck by the discus during high school meets. Safety precautions must be stressed for these events in both practice and competitive meets with the result being the elimination of this type of accident. The National Federation of State High School Associations put a new rule in for the 1993 track season that fenced off the back and sides of the discus circle to help eliminate this type of accident. Good risk management should eliminate these types of accidents. *These types of injuries are not acceptable and should never happen.*

The one fatality in high school lacrosse during the 1987 season was associated with a player using his head to strike the opponent. He struck the opponent with the top or crown of his helmet. This technique is prohibited by the lacrosse rules and should be strictly enforced. Lacrosse has been a safe sport when considering the fact that high school lacrosse has only been involved with four catastrophic injuries in eighteen years. A possible new area of concern are the recent lacrosse deaths being associated with players being struck in the chest with the ball and causing death (commotio cordis). There have been four cases, two high schools and two colleges, in the past three years. The lacrosse community will have to keep a close watch on these types of deaths and possibly carry out in-depth evaluations of these injuries.

College spring sports are also associated with a low injury incidence. Injury rates are slightly higher in lacrosse but the participation figures are so low that even one injury will increase the incidence rate dramatically. It is important to point out that there have been five college male lacrosse catastrophic injuries during the past eighteen years. The college death in 1999 involved a male player being struck in the chest by a ball. There was a paralyzing injury to a summer league lacrosse player in 1999.

For the eighteen-year period from the fall of 1982 through the spring of 2000 there have been 809 direct catastrophic injuries in high school and college sports. High school sports were associated with 120 fatalities, 268 non-fatal, and 273 serious injuries for a total of 661. College sports accounted for 15 fatalities, 43 non-fatal, and 90 serious injuries for a total of 148. During this same eighteen-year period of time there have been a total of 348 indirect injuries and all but five resulted in death. Two hundred and sixty-six of the indirect injuries were at the high school level and 62 were at the college level. It should be noted that high school annual athletic participation for 1999–2000 includes approximately 6,537,623 athletes (3,861,749 males and 2,675,874 females). National Collegiate Athletic Association participation for 1998-1999 was 360,076 athletes. There were 211,273 males and 148,803 females.

During the eighteen-year period from the fall of 1982 through the spring of 2000 there have been 100,177,533 high school athletes participating in the sports covered by this report. Using these participation numbers would give a high school direct catastrophic injury rate of 0.66 per 100,000 participants. The indirect injury rate is 0.28 per 100,000 participants. If both direct and indirect injuries were combined the injury rate would be 0.94 per 100,000. This means that approximately one high school athlete out of every 100,000 participating would receive some type of catastrophic injury. The combined fatality rate would be 0.40 per 100,000, the non-fatal rate 0.27, and the serious rate 0.28.

During this same time period there were approximately 5,367,912 college participants with a total direct catastrophic injury rate of 2.76 per 100,000 participants. The indirect injury rate is 1.15 per 100,000 participants. If both indirect and direct injuries were combined the injury rate would be 3.91. The combined fatality rate would be 1.40, the non-fatal rate 0.84, and the serious rate 1.68.

Female Catastrophic Injuries

There have been a total of 74 direct and 30 indirect catastrophic injuries to high school and college female athletes from 1982/83–1999/00, which includes cheerleading. Fifty of these were direct injuries at the high school level and 24 at the college level. The 50 high school direct injuries included nine in gymnastics, 25 in cheerleading, two in swimming, two in basketball, four in track, three in softball, three in field hockey, one in ice hockey, and one in volleyball. The 26 high school indirect fatalities included nine in basketball, five in swimming, four in track, three in soccer, one in cross-country, one in volleyball, and three in cheerleading. The 24 college direct injuries were associated with cheerleading (17), gymnastics (2), field hockey (2), skiing (1), ice hockey (1), and lacrosse (1). The four college indirect fatalities included one in tennis, one in basketball, one in soccer, and one in volleyball. Catastrophic injuries to female athletes have increased over the years. As an example, in 1982–83 there was one female catastrophic injury and during the past 17 years there has been an average of 6.1 per year. A major factor in this increase has been the change in cheerleading activity, which now involves gymnastic type stunts. If these cheerleading activities are not taught by a competent coach and keep increasing in difficulty, catastrophic injuries will continue to be a part of cheerleading. High school cheerleading accounted for 50.0% of all high school direct catastrophic injuries to female athletes and 70.8% at the college level. Of the 74 direct catastrophic injuries to high school and college female athletes from 1982/83–1999/2000, cheerleading was related to 42 or 56.8%. The cheerleading numbers have been updated from previous reports. Read the special section on cheerleading.

Athletic administrators and coaches should place equal emphasis on injury prevention in both female and male athletics. Injury prevention recommendations are made for both male and female athletes.

Athletic catastrophic injuries may never be totally eliminated, but with reliable injury data collection systems and constant analysis of the data these injuries can be dramatically reduced.

Recommendations for Prevention

1. Mandatory medical examinations and a medical history taken before allowing an athlete to participate.

2. All personnel concerned with training athletes should emphasize proper, gradual, and complete physical conditioning in order to provide the athlete with optimal readiness for the rigors of the sport.

3. Every school should strive to have a team trainer who is a regular member of the faculty and is adequately prepared and qualified.

4. There should be a written emergency procedure plan to deal with the possibility of catastrophic injuries.

5. There should be an emphasis on employing well-trained athletic personnel, providing excellent facilities, and securing the safest and best equipment available. There should be strict enforcement of game rules and administrative regulations should be enforced to protect the health of the athlete.

6. Coaches and school officials must support the game officials in their conduct of the athletic contests. Coaches should know and have the ability to teach the proper fundamental skills of the sport. This recommendation includes all sports and not only football. The proper fundamentals of blocking and tackling should be emphasized to help reduce head and neck injuries in football. Keep the head out of football.

7. There should be continued safety research in athletics (rules, facilities, and equipment).

8. Strict enforcement of the rules of the game by both coaches and game officials will help reduce serious injuries.

9. When an athlete has experienced or shown signs of head trauma (loss of consciousness, visual disturbance, headache, inability to walk correctly, obvious disorientation, or memory loss), he/she should receive immediate medical attention and

should not be allowed to return to practice or the game without permission from the proper medical authorities. It is important for a physician to observe the head injured athlete for several days following the injury.

10. Athletes and their parents should be warned of the risks of injuries.

11. Coaches should not be hired if they do not have the training and experience needed to teach the skills of the sport and to properly train and develop the athletes for competition.

12. Weight loss in wrestling to make weight for a match can be dangerous and cause serious injury or death. Coaches should be aware of safety precautions and rules associated with this practice.

Special Note

All of the data in this report meet the stated definition of injury for high school and college sports. It is important to note that information is constantly being updated due to the fact that catastrophic injury information may not always reach the center in time to be included in the current final report.

References

1. Tator CH, Edmonds VE: *National Survey of Spinal Injuries in Hockey Players*, Canada Medical Association 1984; 130: 875-880.

Case Studies

Football

High School

A 16-year-old high school football player died on September 15, 2000 after making a tackle in a game. The player received a blow to the chest and cause of death was listed as commotio cordis or cardiac concussion. The athlete was 6' 1" tall and weighed 245 pounds. He was pronounced dead at the hospital.

A 17-year-old high school football player received a brain injury on September 15, 2000 and died on September 17, 2000. The exact activity at the time of the injury was unknown. The neurosurgeon involved treating the athlete said the player died of a medium grade brain injury which he believes was complicated by abnormal structured arteries at the base of the brain that resulted in malignant brain swelling.

A 17-year-old high school football player was injured in a game on September 8, 2000. The athlete was playing defense on an eight-man football team and was tackling the ball carrier. The helmet of the ball carrier hit into the chest of the tackler. The athlete collapsed on the field and never regained consciousness. Cause of death was commotio cordis or cardiac concussion.

A 17-year-old high school football player collapsed during a team practice on September 4, 2000 and died the following day September 5, 2000. Cause of death was heat stroke. The athlete was 6' 4" tall and weighed 305 pounds. The temperature was 77 degrees, but there was very high humidity.

A 15-year-old high school football player collapsed at practice after a 1½ mile run in hot and humid weather. The accident happened on August 9, 2000 and the athlete died on August 16, 2000. He was 6 feet tall and weighed 250 pounds. Cause of death was heat stroke.

A 17-year-old high school football player collapsed during a preseason football practice on June 7, 2000. Coaching staff and nurses tried to resuscitate him without success. He was transported to the hospital where he was pronounced dead. Cause of death was a congenital heart problem.

A 17-year-old high school football player was working out with the team having just finished lifting weights and was running laps when he collapsed. He was pronounced dead at the hospital. Cause of death was heart-related. Autopsy results revealed that he had a birth defect that caused his right coronary artery to bend at an awkward angle, creating a blockage of blood. He died on July 18, 2000.

A 15-year-old high school football player died on October 27, 2000. The player collapsed on the sideline during a game and died at the hospital. Cause of death was heart-related.

A 14-year-old high school football player was running a warm-up lap at practice on October 4, 2000 when he complained of chest pain to a teammate. His coach administered CPR and the athlete was transported to the hospital where he died. Cause of death was heart-related.

A 15-year-old high school football player died while participating in a game on October 13, 2000. It was reported initially that he fractured his neck while tackling, but the autopsy showed that he died of a heart attack, which resulted from hypertrophic cardiomyopathy.

A 16-year-old high school football player collapsed and died at the end of a practice in September 2000. The coroner stated that the athlete had an enlarged heart.

A 16-year-old high school football player collapsed during the opening kickoff of a game on September 22, 2000. The coroner stated that the athlete died of a heart-related problem.

A 15-year-old high school football player collapsed after a light workout at a team meeting on October 3, 2000. Cause of death was undetermined but the autopsy showed hypertrophic cardiomyopathy.

College

A 20-year-old college football player died after complaining of exhaustion following practice on August 8, 2000. Practice lasted two hours and the athlete was dressed in a helmet, T-shirt, and shorts on a muggy day with temperatures in the 80s. He was 6' 4" tall and weighed 309 pounds. He was pronounced dead at the hospital. There was also the possibility of a cardiac condition. Cause of death was heat stroke.

An 18-year-old college football player collapsed during a fitness test and was pronounced dead at the hospital. The event happened on the first full day of practice. The athlete was 5' 11" tall and weighed 190 pounds. Cause of death was heat stroke. The temperature was in the 80s and the athlete had a physical exam one hour earlier.

Soccer

High School

A 17-year-old male high school junior soccer player was injured on October 16, 1999, while performing a leg check to obtain the ball from his opponent. He received three fractures in his leg and a ruptured artery. At the present time he has partial disability.

A 14-year-old female high school soccer player collapsed during a soccer match on April 5, 2000. Despite receiving medical attention quickly, she died about an hour later at the hospital. The athlete had a congenital heart problem that she was not aware of.

Ice Hockey

High School

A 15-year-old high school ice hockey player was skating off the ice when a player from the opposing team charged him from behind. The injured athlete slid across the ice and crashed headfirst into the boards severing his spinal column. The athlete is quadriplegic. The case went to court and the other athlete was charged with two felony counts of aggravated battery and received two years of probation.

A 17-year-old female high school ice hockey player received a serious brain and vertebra injury on January 22, 2000. She was knocked to the ice twice during the game hitting her head on the ice. She suffered a fractured cervical vertebra and a concussion. At the present time she has some memory loss and weakness on the right side of her body. She is not allowed to play contact sports for one year, but all signs point to a full recovery.

A 16-year-old male high school ice hockey player suffered a heart attack during the first junior varsity game of the season. The heart attack was the result of a rare, undiagnosed congenital heart condition according to the Chief Deputy coroner.

College

A 22-year-old female college ice hockey player was injured on January 15, 2000. She received a compression fracture of L2 and L3. There was no permanent disability and she returned to playing ice hockey in 30 days. At the time of the injury she was hit by an opponent and was thrown into the boards back first. She was off her feet when she hit the boards.

Basketball

High School

An 18-year-old male high school basketball player was injured in a game on February 22, 2000. The player was undercut by an opponent and hit the floor with his shoulder and neck. He spent one night in the hospital and did not return to play basketball that season due to a lengthy recovery period. There was a full recovery.

A 16-year-old male high school basketball player was injured on January 28, 2000, and died the same day. He collapsed at halftime of the game and died. Cause of death was listed as sudden cardiac death.

A high school senior collapsed at practice on November 1, 1999, and died later at the hospital. Cause of death was unknown but was believed to be heart-related.

A 16-year-old male high school basketball player collapsed and died during a junior varsity basketball game on January 12, 2000. Cause of death was an irregular heartbeat caused by a congenital heart abnormality.

A 17-year-old male high school basketball player collapsed at the end of a light practice on November 29, 1999. He was doing wind sprints at the time. He died later that day at the hospital. Death was believed to be heart-related.

College

A 25-year-old male college basketball player was injured in a game on February 22, 2000. An opposing player accidentally slammed an elbow into the throat of the injured player. The player was taken to the hospital where it was determined that he had a fractured larynx. After two surgeries the player is able to speak again and there was a full recovery.

A 20-year-old male college basketball player died on October 11, 1999, while running sprints during practice in the gymnasium. He lost his footing and hit headfirst into the wall. He suffered a fractured cervical vertebra.

Wrestling

High School

A male high school wrestler received a spinal cord injury on January 29, 2000. His opponent who weighed about 210 pounds slammed the injured wrestler, who weighed about 200 pounds, on his back to the mat. The injured wrestler was being held in a V-position, which put the other wrestler's weight on the spine. The injured wrestler could not move and felt tingling in his legs. He had a full recovery.

A male high school wrestler was injured trying to escape from a hold during a match. The injured wrestler's head hit the mat and his opponent, who weighed 275 pounds, landed on him causing the injured wrestler's head to roll under his shoulders. He had surgery to fuse C-5 and C-6. The athlete is quadriplegic.

LaCrosse

High School

A 14-year-old male high school lacrosse player died from a blow to the chest during a game on March 25, 2000. The athlete was a goalie and stopped a shot with his chest. Cause of death was commotio cordis.

A male high school lacrosse player was struck in the chest by a shot during a game on April 10, 2000. He was playing goalie at the time. He collapsed and stopped breathing, but pulse and breathing were restored after the coach and trainer performed CPR. He has recovered, but there are still some questions about memory functions.

A 17-year-old high school lacrosse player died on March 1, 2000, after collapsing while running sprints during the first practice of the season. The trainer administered CPR until the ambulance arrived, but he died later at the hospital. Cause of death was believed to be heart-related.

Baseball

High School

A 15-year-old male high school baseball player died on March 28, 2000, after being hit in the chest with a thrown ball while running from first to second base. Cause of death was commotio cordis.

A male high school baseball player was struck on the right side of the head by a line drive off of an aluminum bat during a game on May 3, 1999. The player was knocked unconscious for about three minutes and briefly went into convulsions. Three months after the accident the player still has not regained all the strength in his left hand.

A 17-year-old male high school baseball player collapsed after running the bases and sliding into home plate during practice. He was taken to the hospital where he died. Cause of death was heart-related.

A 17-year-old male high school baseball player collapsed after a game on April 14, 2000, after running a cooling down lap. He had been previously diagnosed with aortic stenosis, but decide to play anyway. Cause of death was heart-related.

Track

High School

A 15-year-old male junior high school track athlete received a serious head injury when he was struck in the head by a thrown discus. The injury happened on March 7, 2000. The injury was an open depressed skull fracture, with brain lacerations. The athlete now has learning problems, seizures, and personality differences.

An 18-year-old male high school track athlete died after a pole vaulting accident on March 27, 2000. He vaulted onto a 16-foot pit, landed on the back of the mat, and flew off of the mat and hit his head on the asphalt behind the mat. He was hospitalized with a skull fracture and a blood clot.

A 14-year-old male high school track athlete had just finished a cool down run of one mile when he collapsed. He died in the ambulance on the way to the hospital. Death was believed to be heart-related.

An 18-year-old male high school track athlete collapsed and died moments after placing second in a one-mile race. Cause of death was listed as cardiac arrest.

Field Hockey

High School

A female high school field hockey player lost an eye during a field hockey drill before a game when she was struck in the eye by a teammate stick. The player's parents sued the school for not directing players to wear protective goggles.

College

A 19-year-old female college field hockey player was struck in the head by a field hockey ball. She was standing three feet away from the player who hit the ball. The athlete received a fracture temporal bone and had a full recovery.

Softball

High School

A 14-year-old female softball player was pitching a baseball to two male baseball players after practice and was struck in the head by a batted ball. It was not thought to be a serious injury, but later at home the athlete complained of dizziness and nausea. She had surgery for a fractured skull and a hematoma. The athlete died.

Tennis

High School

A 17-year-old male high school tennis player was jogging a few warm-up laps before practice when he collapsed. CPR was administered and he was transported to the hospital where he died. Cause of death was cardiac arrhythmia.

Special Section on Cheerleading

The Consumer Product Safety Commission reported an estimated 4,954 hospital emergency room visits in 1980 caused by cheerleading injuries. By 1986 the number had increased to 6,911 and in 1994 the number increased to approximately 16,000. Granted, the number of cheerleaders has also increased dramatically during this time frame. It is important to stress that catastrophic injuries have been a part of cheerleading during the last 18 years, and coaches and administrators should be aware of the situation.

The National Center for Catastrophic Sports Injury Research has been collecting cheerleading catastrophic injury data during the past eighteen years, 1982/83–1999/2000. There were three serious injuries during the 1998–1999 school year.

Cheerleading has changed dramatically in the past eighteen years and now has two distinctive purposes; 1) of a service-oriented leader of cheers on the sideline; and 2) as a highly skilled competing athlete. A number of schools, both high schools and colleges, across the country have limited the types of stunts that can be attempted by their cheerleaders. The Illinois State High School Association has banned the basket toss. The rule states, "cheerleaders cannot toss another squad member into the air during any part of a cheer, performance, routine, or other activity. Illinois has already banned pyramid formations higher than two levels. As already stated in this report, high school and college cheerleaders account for almost one-half of the catastrophic injuries to female athletes.

The basic question that has to be asked is what is the role of the cheerleader? Fourteen states consider cheering a sport, and organize state championship competition. Nine more organize cheerleading championships as a school activity. Over 74,000 girls are participating in competitive competitions. Is cheering an activity that leads the spectators in cheers or is it a sport? If the answer is to entertain the crowd and to be in competition with other cheerleading squads, then there must be safety guidelines initiated. Following are a list of sample guidelines that may help prevent cheerleading injuries:

1. Cheerleaders should have medical examinations before they are allowed to participate. Included would be a complete medical history.

2. Cheerleaders should be trained by a qualified coach with training in gymnastics and partner stunting. This person

should also be trained in the proper methods for spotting and other safety factors.

3. Cheerleaders should be exposed to proper conditioning programs and trained in proper spotting techniques.

4. Cheerleaders should receive proper training before attempting gymnastic type stunts and should not attempt stunts they are not capable of completing. A qualification system demonstrating mastery of stunts is recommended.

5. Coaches should supervise all practice sessions in a safe facility. Mini-trampolines and flips or falls off of pyramids and shoulders should be prohibited.

7. Pyramids over two high should not be performed. Two high pyramids should not be performed without mats and other safety precautions.

8. If it is not possible to have a physician or athletic trainer at games and practice sessions, emergency procedures must be provided. The emergency procedure should be in writing and available to staff and athletes.

9. There should be continued research concerning safety in cheerleading.

10. When a cheerleader has experienced or shown signs of head trauma (loss of consciousness, visual disturbances, headache, inability to walk correctly, obvious disorientation, or memory loss) she/he should receive immediate medical attention and should not be allowed to practice or cheer without permission from the proper medical authorities.

11. Cheerleading coaches should have some type of safety certification. The American Association of Cheerleading Coaches and Advisors offers this certification.

The Michigan High School Athletic Association is the second state to recognize cheerleading as a sport. West Virginia incorporated cheerleading into athletics seven years ago. Michigan will have a committee define the sport and will have a state Cheerleading Tournament. Rules and regulations will now govern cheerleading and this is an important move toward a safer activity. Also, the American Association of Cheerleading Coaches and Advisors Safety Certification Program has been implemented and over 500 coaches have participated in safety certification programs. The state of Vermont has adopted the safety certification program as their standard of care and the following NCAA Athletic Conferences have also adopted the program: the Big Ten, Southwest, Southeast, and the Western Athletic Conferences.

According to the National Federation of State High School Associations, the primary purpose of spirit groups (cheerleaders) is to serve as support groups for the interscholastic athletic programs within the school. In January of 1993, 18 rule revisions were adopted for spirit groups. One of the major rules prohibits tumbling over, under, or through anything (people or equipment). All of the other rules were adopted to enhance the safety of the participants.

Additional Information

Consumer Product Safety Commission
Washington, DC 20207
Website: http://cpsc.gov

Write for a free copy of "Guidelines for Moveable Soccer Goal Safety."

The Coalition to Promote Soccer Goal Safety
c/o Soccer Industry Council of America
200 Castlewood Drive
North Palm Beach, FL 33408
Tel: 561-840-1171
Fax: 561-863-8984
Website: www.wylie1.com/socyel/sica.html

National Federation of State High School Associations
P.O. Box 690
Indianapolis, IN 46206
Tel: 317-972-6900
Fax: 317-822-5700
Website: www.nfsh.org

Write for information about new cheerleading rules and updates.

Chapter 6

Baby Boomer Sports Injuries Report

Sports-related injuries among those ages 35 to 54—today's baby boomers—increased about 33% from 1991 to 1998. There were just under 276,000 hospital emergency room treated injuries to persons 35 to 54 in 1991 compared to slightly more than 365,000 sports injuries to persons of these ages in 1998. This increase in injuries, which occurred in 16 popular sports activities, was due primarily to baby boomers' increased numbers participating in these sports.

When all medically attended injuries in these popular sports were included, CPSC estimated there were a total of more than 1 million injuries to baby boomers in 1998 (compared to 778,000 such injuries to persons 35 to 54 in 1991). These sports injuries to baby boomers cost the nation over $18.7 billion in 1998.

Bicycling and basketball were associated with the largest number of 1998 baby boomer sports injuries treated in hospital emergency rooms. Of special note, baby boomers suffered a relatively high number of head injury-related deaths while bicycling.

Baby boomers represented almost one-third of all Americans who participated in sports in 1998. These 79.1 million people comprised over 29 percent of the total U.S. population. In 1998, there were 14 million more Americans in the 35 to 54 age group than in 1991.

"Baby Boomer Sports Injuries," U.S. Consumer Product Safety Commission, April 2000.

Sports Injuries and Deaths

Seven sports showed significant increasing trends in the number of emergency room treated injuries in the 35 to 54 age group in 1998. These were: bicycling, golf, soccer, basketball, exercise and running, weightlifting, and in-line skating. Participation data showed increases in baby boomers' sports participation for most of these sports. (Participation data was not available for weightlifting, and exercise and running.)

Three sports showed significant decreasing trends in the number of emergency room treated injuries and decreasing trends in the number of participants. These were: skiing, tennis, and volleyball.

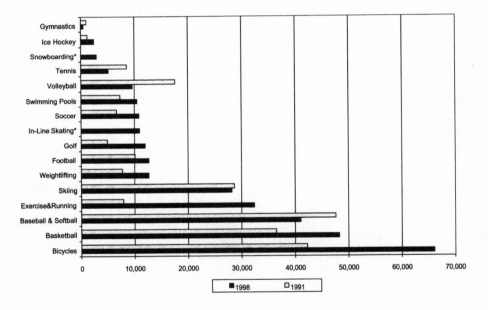

Figure 6.1. Estimated Number of Emergency Room Treated Injuries Among Persons 35 – 54 Years of Age Associated with 16 Popular Sports Categories, 1991 and 1998.

*In-line skating and snowboarding were new sports in the 1990s. Injury data were first collected for in-line skating in 1993 (4,310 estimated injuries) and snowboarding in 1994 (1,520 estimated injuries).

Source: U.S. Consumer Product Safety Commission, Directorate for Epidemiology, National Electronic Injury Surveillance System (NEISS).

For three sports, there were large numbers of deaths reported to CPSC. These were: bicycling (290 deaths a year, all but 35 motor vehicle-related); swimming (67 deaths a year associated with swimming pools); and skiing (7 deaths a year).

Safety Equipment-Related Issues

Baby boomers who rode bicycles died from head injuries at nearly twice the rate as children who rode bikes. This difference is likely the result of greater helmet usage among children. According to CPSC, 69% of children wear helmets when bicycling compared to only 43% of baby boomers.

Baby boomer in-line skaters, however, were injured less frequently than other skaters. In 1998, about 3.2 out of every 1,000 baby boomer in-line skaters were treated in an emergency room for a skating injury. Among children under 18, this number was 4.6 out of every 1,000. For the population as a whole, it was 4.1 per 1,000 skaters. Baby boomers suffered a much smaller proportion of arm and hand injuries than other age groups, which may be an indication they are wearing appropriate protective equipment such as gloves, wrist guards, and elbow pads.

Conclusion

It is important for baby boomers to stay active and to participate in sports. But safety is an essential consideration. For example, baby boomers can reduce serious head injuries by wearing bike helmets when bike riding. Other sports-related injuries can be avoided or reduced by following such precautions as wearing other appropriate sports safety equipment, warming up before vigorous exercise, and increasing one's amount of exercise gradually.

Chapter 7

Sports-Related Injuries to Persons 65 Years of Age and Older

- From 1990 to 1996, sports-related injuries to persons 65 years of age and older increased significantly, from 34,000 to 53,000. This is an increase of 54% in that 7-year period.

- The increased incidence of injury occurred not only among the youngest of the 65 and over population, but also among those 75 years and older. Sports-related injuries to persons 75 and older increased by 29%.

- Sports-related injuries increased much more to persons 65 and over than to any other age group. By contrast, they increased 18% to persons age 25-64 (vs. 54% for 65 and older).

- Sports-related injuries have increased more than other consumer product related injuries treated in hospital emergency rooms for persons 65 and over.

- The increase in sports-related injuries is greater than the increase in the population 65 and over, so it cannot be explained solely by the increase in population of this age group. From 1990 to 1996, the population 65 and over increased by just over 8%, whereas sports-related injuries to this age group increased 54%.

"Sports-Related Injuries to Persons 65 Years of Age and Older," by George W. Rutherford, Jr., M.S. Thomas J. Schroeder, M.S., U.S. Consumer Product Safety Commission, April 1998.

- Injuries to older persons have increased the most in connection with more active sports, such as bicycling, exercise activity (with and without equipment), weight training, and skiing.

- The highest number of sports injuries to persons 65 and older were associated with bicycles and bicycling. Bicycling injuries increased 75% from 1990 to 1996. Of bicycling injuries to older persons, 30% were to persons 75 years of age and older. Most injuries resulted from falls, and head injuries were 21% of the total. Virtually none of the fall victims was wearing a bike helmet.

- The number of injuries related to exercise activity (with and without equipment) increased 173% from 1990 to 1996. The 75 and older group accounted for 40% of those injured in 1996 in this category. The most common injuries were falls, tripping, and strains in normal exercise activity.

- Injuries from less active sports, such as fishing, golf, bowling, and shuffleboard increased only moderately or not at all from 1990 to 1996. For example, fishing injuries increased 6%.

- For the first time in 1996 we find a small number of injuries among the 65 and over population in very active and physically challenging sports such as snowboarding and in-line skating.

- In both 1990 and 1996, about 60% of the 65 and older victims of sports injuries were males. In both of these years, males were about 40% of the population 65 and older.

- The hospitalization rate for persons 65 and over with sports-related injuries is 10%. This is lower than the 18% hospitalization rate for injuries with all consumer products for persons in this age group.

- The average cost per injury for sports-related injuries treated in emergency rooms has declined since 1990. While more injuries are occurring, they appear, on the average, to be less costly and severe.

Conclusions

- The increase in injuries is most likely attributable to increasingly active lifestyles and to increased participation in sports activities by older Americans.

- Especially notable is the increased participation by people 65 and over in more active sports, such as bicycling, exercise (with and without equipment), weight training, and skiing.

- Americans are remaining physically active into their 70's, 80's and even into their 90's.

- The lower hospitalization rate for sports-related injuries suggests that the population participating in sports activities is healthier overall than those who are not participating in sports.

- Persons involved in activities such as bicycling can reduce their risk of injury by using bike helmets. Bicycle helmets reduce the risk of serious head injury.

- Individuals should use safety gear and take appropriate safety precautions, especially in active sports such as inline skating and use of exercise equipment and weights.

- All forms of exercise, from walking and gardening to swimming, tennis and biking, contribute to improved health and well-being. By getting regular exercise—and doing it safely—older Americans can enjoy a healthier life.

Introduction

Since 1990, the U.S. population 65 years of age and older has increased by approximately 2.63 million people.[1] Such a population increase could be expected to have an impact on the overall injury frequency in this age cohort, including injuries related to consumer products. Consumer product related injuries to persons aged 65 years and older were examined using the National Electronic Injury Surveillance System (NEISS), an injury surveillance network operated by the U.S. Consumer Product Safety Commission, which tracks consumer product related injuries from a national statistical sample of hospital emergency rooms. NEISS data for the years 1990 through 1996 were reviewed and injury estimates for the 65 and older age group calculated for each year. These estimates show an increase in consumer product related injuries for each year during this time period.

In 1990, there were an estimated 979,000 consumer product related emergency room (ER) treated injuries to persons 65 years of age and older. This estimate increased in 1996 to 1,322,200 consumer product related injuries. By comparison, overall frequencies of emergency room treated consumer product related injuries to those under 65 years old declined between 1990 and 1996.

Between 1990 and 1996, population based injury rates also declined in every age group except the population 65 years and older.

The rate of emergency room treated injuries per 1,000 population in the age 65 and older group increased from 31.34 in 1990 to 39.04 in 1996. In 1996, the injury rate in this age group was higher than that for persons 25-44 years of age or persons 45-64 years of age. By contrast, data from analyses performed in the late 1980s[2] indicated that the population age 65 and older at that time had a lower overall injury rate than other segments of the population.

One possible explanation for this increase in consumer product related injuries is that those over age 65 are maintaining increasingly active lifestyles, resulting in greater exposures to the risk of injury. This paper looks at NEISS data on sports-related injuries as a potential indicator of activity level in the population age 65 and older and describes sports-related injuries seen in this growing population.

Methodology

This analysis was prepared using data from the National Electronic Injury Surveillance System (NEISS), which consists of a national probability sample of 101 hospitals, drawn from the over 5,000 hospitals with 24-hour emergency departments, nationwide. The sample includes hospitals of differing sizes and locations, as well as children's hospitals and trauma centers.

The sampling frame is divided into four size strata based on the annual number of emergency department visits reported by each hospital, and a stratum for children's hospitals. Since its inception in the 1970s, the NEISS sample has been updated several times to maintain its statistical validity.

For in-scope cases, the coder at each NEISS hospital abstracts information on as many as fourteen different variables. These variables include date of treatment, case record number, age, sex, injury diagnosis, body part injured, consumer products involved (up to two products may be specified), indicator for third product involved, disposition of the case (i.e. treated and released, hospitalized, dead on arrival) accident locale, whether fire or a motor vehicle was involved, and up to two lines of narrative to provide a brief description of the incident.

Because of the statistical design of the NEISS, sampling errors associated with NEISS estimates can be calculated.[3] A variance computation program that accounts for the stratified sample design was used to calculate variances of estimates and the associated covariance between estimates across annual time periods. To determine if the difference in annual estimates was statistically significant, student "t" tests (adjusting for the covariance between years) were performed.[4]

Because activities such as skiing (limited to a few hospitals), and bicycling (in the 65 and older age group, reported mostly from warm weather hospitals), had high variances associated with the recent injury estimates, the "t" test did not indicate significant change. A nonparametric test based on Spearman's rank correlation coefficient was used to test for trends in these sports, for which the consistency of the year-to-year increases, over the seven year period, led us to believe that there may in fact have been an increase.[5] A significance level of 0.05 was used for all statistical testing.

Injury cost estimates were based on the Injury Cost Model developed by the U.S. Consumer Product Safety Commission, Directorate for Economic Analysis. The Injury Cost Model is structured to measure eleven different types of costs separately, one component at a time, and then to add them together to establish the total cost of an injury. A variety of techniques are used to estimate the eleven cost components including regression analysis, sample means from large databases, and direct analytic solution. The cost components include: medical costs, the costs of insurance, foregone earnings, pain and suffering caused by the injury, and disability costs.

Results

NEISS data on product related injuries from 1990 were compared with those from 1996. There was an increase in the total estimated consumer product related injuries between 1990 and 1996 for the population 65 years of age and older, from 979,000 (1990) to 1,322,200 (1996), a 35% increase.

There was an even greater increase in sports-related injuries over that same time period. Figure 7.1 illustrates that in 1990, there were an estimated 34,400 sports-related injuries to persons 65 years of age and over, while in 1996, the estimate increased by 54% to 53,000 injuries (p <.05). The rate of injury associated with sports activities in this population also increased from 1.10 per 1,000 population in 1990, to 1.57 per 1,000 population in 1996. The injury rate seen with all consumer products increased from 31.34 in 1990 to 39.04 in 1996.

While there is scant data on the number of older adults participating in sports activities, one can speculate from the rising injury rate, that the increase in sports-related injuries in the age 65 and older group is more likely to be due to an increased participation level than an increase in the risk of any of the sports activities themselves.

To further explore sports-related injuries in the over 65 population, incidence of injury was analyzed for two subgroups comprising

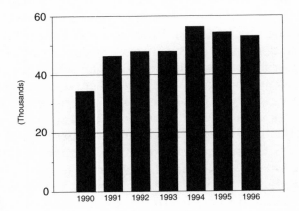

Figure 7.1. *Estimated Sports-Related Injuries to Persons 65 Years of Age and Older, Treated in Hospital Emergency Departments, 1990-1996*

Table 7.1. Estimated Sports-Related Injuries to Persons 65 and Older. Estimated U.S. Population Ages 65 and Older, in (000s) by Year and Age Group.

1990

Age Group	1990 Injuries	1990 Pop. (1,000s)	1990 Percent Injuries	1990 Percent Pop.
Total	34,400	31,237	100.0%	100.0%
65-74 Years	25,899	18,098	75.3%	57.9%
75+ Years	8,501	13,138	24.7%	42.1%

1996

Age Group	1996 Injuries	1996 Pop. (1,000s)	1996 Percent Injuries	1996 Percent Pop.
Total	53,000	33,867	100.0%	100.0%
65-74 Years	37,566	18,673	70.9%	55.1%
75+ Years	15,434	15,195	29.1%	44.9%

Note: Population estimates are rounded and may not add to total.

that population: 65-74 years of age; 75 years and older. Table 7.1 shows that within the 65 and older population, the age distribution shifted between 1990 and 1996. In 1996, there were relatively fewer injuries in the age 65-74 group than in 1990 (75.3% in 1990, 70.9% in 1996), and relatively more injuries in the 75 and older group than in 1990 (24.7% in 1990, 29.1% in 1996). The proportion of the population in the age 75 and older group also increased between the two time periods from 42.1% in 1990 to 44.9% in 1996, but not enough to account for the increase in injuries. This finding suggests that sports participation is not limited to the youngest seniors, and that as the over age 65 cohort ages, they may remain active into their 70s, 80s, and perhaps even 90s.

The types of sports activities in which seniors were injured changed somewhat between 1990 and 1996. The number of emergency room treated injuries related to active sports such as bicycling, exercise activity, and snow skiing increased significantly between 1990 and 1996, while injuries from less active sports, such as golf and fishing increased less or not at all over that time period. It is interesting to note that there were a small number of injuries seen for the first time in 1996 involving "extreme" or more physically challenging sports such as snowboarding and in-line skating.

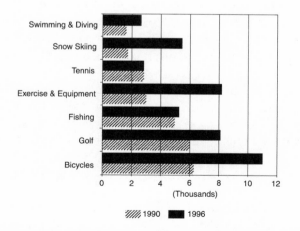

Figure 7.2. Estimated Emergency Room Treated Injuries to Persons 65 Years of Age and Older, Top Sports Activities, 1990-1996

The leading groups of sports were examined for distribution by sex of victim. It was found that almost 60% of the injuries were to males in both 1990 and 1996. Males represented about 40% of the 65 and older population in both of these years.

Highlights of Specific Sport-Related Injury Hazards

Figure 7.2 illustrates the distribution of sports activities associated with the highest number of injuries to the population 65 and older in 1996, and the change in distribution of injuries between 1990 and 1996. The sports activities with the largest increases in injuries in 1996 from 1990 were bicycling, exercise activity/exercise equipment/weightlifting, and snow skiing. Golf injuries also increased between 1990 and 1996, but not significantly. The smallest change in the number of injuries between 1990 and 1996 was seen in tennis and fishing. Table 7.2 presents 1996 data which summarizes those sports activities in which persons age 65 and older are most often injured. The injuries are broken out for the four age groups comprising the age 65 and older population. A more detailed description of the injuries associated with the top sports activities follows.

Bicycles/Bicycling

The highest number of injuries to the age 65 and older population were associated with bicycles and bicycling, with an estimated 11,000 emergency room treated injuries in 1996. The estimated number of injuries increased significantly between 1990 and 1996—by 75% or approximately 4,700 injuries. Thirty percent of the injuries in 1996 occurred in persons over 75 years of age. Approximately 13% of the injured persons 65 and over were hospitalized for their bicycle-related injuries.

Falls from the bike were the most frequent pattern of injury, about 60% of the total. Head injuries from either falls or motor vehicle collisions were 21% of the total injuries, and when helmet use was mentioned, virtually none of the victims were wearing helmets.

Exercise Activity with or without Equipment/Weightlifting

Estimated injuries associated with these activities increased 173% from 3,007 in 1990 to 8,197 in 1996. (p = .0001). Forty percent of those injured in 1996 were 75 years of age or older, with nine percent of all those injured being hospitalized.

70

The most frequent patterns of injury associated with these activities were falling, or strains from normal exercise activity. Smaller numbers of injuries resulted from falls against the equipment and from product-related problems such as sharp parts or equipment failures.

Snow Skiing

Skiing injuries to persons 65 and older increased by 217% from 1,716 in 1990 to 5,432 in 1996. This difference was not significant

Table 7.2. Estimated Sports Activity Related Injuries to Persons 65 Years of Age and Older. Specific Activities by 10 Year Age Groups, 1996

Sport	Total	65-74	75-84	85-94	95+
Total	53,033*	37,566	12,818	2,288	361
Bicycles	11,002	7,747	2,359	586	**
Exercise Activity/ Equipment/ Weightlifting	8,197	4,926	2,577	677	**
Golf & Golf Carts	8,127	5,983	2,093	**	0
Snow Skiing	5,432	4,372	1,026	**	**
Fishing	5,268	3,648	1,552	**	0
Tennis	2,818	2,252	566	0	0
Swimming/Diving Swimming Pools	2,623	1,342	860	**	**
Bowling	2,326	1,478	702	**	0
Skating	1,460	1,325	**	**	0
Baseball & Softball	1,364	1,056	**	**	0
All Terrain Vehicles	818	818	0	0	0
Horseback Riding	731	529	**	0	0
Basketball	532	**	**	**	0

*   Several additional products were also reported, and are included in the total, for which the total 1996 estimate was less than 500. These products were: snowmobiles, personal watercraft, squash/racketball, volleyball, soccer, minibikes/trailbikes, ball sports not elsewhere classified, gymnastics, go carts, football, billiards, shuffleboard, water skiing, handball, and sleds.

**   Estimate less than 500. Sample size too small to include estimate.

between the 1990 and 1996 estimates. Because variance of NEISS estimates is strongly influenced by the number of hospitals reporting, and because the skiing cases are reported mostly from just a few hospitals, this is not an unexpected finding. When the non-parametric test for consistency of year to year changes was applied the pattern for skiing was statistically significant. Persons 65 and over who were injured while skiing were hospitalized for their injuries in 8% of the cases. The most frequent pattern of skiing injury was a fall.

Golf

The estimated number of golf-related injuries to persons 65 and older increased by 2,139, about 36%, from 1990 to 1996. However, this change was not found to be significant at the .05 level. Golf injuries were virtually all to persons under 85 years old; 26% were to persons between 75 and 84 years of age. Just under 6% of golf injury victims 65 and over were hospitalized. Golf-related injuries were most frequently strains and sprains and other minor injuries. However, there were some fractures, primarily to ankles, mostly from falls.

Other Sports Injuries

In addition to the four sports activities which were associated with the highest number of injuries to the over age 65 cohort, Table 7.3 also shows a number of other sports activities and the injury incidence associated with them. There was an unexpectedly high proportion of hospitalization cases with bowling (about 20%—not shown in table). Broken hips or femurs were the most frequent reason given for these hospitalizations.

Costs Associated with Sports-Related Injuries

The costs associated with sports-related injuries to persons 65 years of age and over also were examined. In 1990, sports-related emergency room treated injuries for the population 65 years and older, cost society about $364 million; in 1996, they cost about $516 million, an increase of about 42% (both expressed in 1996 dollars). When the increase in sports injuries and the increase in the cost of those injuries are considered together, the average cost per injury declined from 1990 to 1996. That is, while there are more injuries occurring, on the average, they appear to be less costly and possibly less severe. The hospitalization rate for sports injuries in this population also declined from about 13% in 1990 to about 10% in 1996. Because of the changes in the health care system and the increasing emphasis on cost cutting measures and reduced hospital stays, however, it is difficult to draw any firm conclusions about the changes since 1990 in the cost and severity of these sports-related injuries.

When the sports injury hospitalization rates of the age 65 and older population are compared with hospitalization rates for all consumer product related injuries for that same age group, it is apparent that the sports hospitalization rate is lower. When all product related injuries are considered for 1996, members of this population were hospitalized on average about 18% of the time for their injuries, while for sports activities, they were hospitalized approximately 10% of the time. This data hints that the population participating in sports activities might be healthier overall that the rest of the same age cohort, a subject that deserves further study.

Discussion

Estimates of sports-related injuries to persons 65 years of age and older have increased from 1990 to 1996. They have increased more than other product related injuries treated in hospital emergency rooms, and more than can be explained solely by the increase in population. These increases are most likely explained by greater activity and participation in sports activities among seniors. The increased incidence of sports-related injuries is occurring not only among the youngest of the 65 and older population, but among the 75-84 year old and 85-94 year old age groups.

There is some indication in the data that there may also be a tendency toward increased participation in more active sports. The size of the population in the 65 and over age group has increased. However, less active sports such as fishing and golf, had only small increases in the injury estimates, while injuries associated with more active sports like bicycling, exercise equipment, and snow skiing, increased, not only in frequency, but in their share of the total of sports-related injuries to this age group.

Persons age 65 and over that suffered sports-related injuries were hospitalized about 10% of the time. However, when all product related injuries are considered, this group is hospitalized about 18% of the time. From this finding, it appears that, in general, sports injuries may be less severe than many other product related injuries. This may be because the activities themselves are less dangerous, or because the population participating is healthier than those injured in other ways.

Table 7.3. Summary of Findings. Sports Injuries to Persons 65 and Older. Estimated Emergency Room Treated Injuries, 1996 for Top Seven Sporting Activities

Sports Activity	Difference 90 to 96	Significance (p = <.05) Adjusted "t" test / Non-parametric test	1996 Age 75+	Most Frequent Body Part Injured	Most Frequent Diagnosis	Most Frequent Pattern	Percent Hospitalized 1996
Overall	+18,664 +54%	Yes / Yes	15,433 29%	n/a	n/a	n/a	10%
Bicycles	+4,713 +75%	no / yes	3,255 30%	shoulder & trunk	fractures	falls	13%
Exercise Activity & Equip. Weightlifting	+5,190 +173%	yes / yes	3,271 40%	leg & foot shoulder and trunk	fractures and dislocations	falls, tripping, strains in normal activity	9%

Sports-Related Injuries to Persons 65 Years of Age and Older

Sport							
Golf & Golf Carts	+2,139 +36%	no no	2,144 26%	leg & foot mostly ankle	strains and sprains	normal play of the game	6%
Snow Skiing	+3,716 +217%	no yes	1,060 20%	shoulder and trunk	strains and sprains	falls	8%
Fishing	+285 +6%	no no	1,620 31%	fingers	punctures	hooks in	12% fingers
Tennis	-3	no no	566 20%	evenly distributed, except head & face are very low	strains and sprains	falls, strains and strains in normal play	
Swimming/ Diving/ Swimming Pools	+1,003 +62%	no no	1,281 49%	shoulder and trunk	fractures and dislocations	falls on pool decks	8%

Valid data is needed on participation in sports activities by the age 65 and over population. Based on day to day observations and discussions with seniors, it appears that this population is more active and is likely to participate more in sports activities. Examined in combination with the injury data, sports participation data could help explain better the reason for the increase in these injuries.

Individuals should use the appropriate protective gear for the activity, such as bicycle helmets for bicycling and helmets and wrist guards for skating. It is very important to read and understand the instructions that come with any complex piece of equipment, and to maintain the equipment which you use for the activity in good operating condition.

References

1. U.S. Bureau of the Census, U.S. Population Estimates by Age, Sex, Race, and Hispanic Origin: 1990 to 1996, March 1997.

2. U.S. Consumer Product Safety Commission. Products Associated with Injuries and Deaths to Persons 65 Years of Age and Older. Unpublished Report. Rutherford, George W. Jr. M.S., Meadows, Susan, Brown, Victoria.

3. U.S. Consumer Product Safety Commission. The NEISS Sample (Design and Implementation), Washington, D.C., U.S. Consumer Product Safety Commission; July 1997.

4. Kish, Leslie, *Survey Sampling*, John Wiley and Sons, Inc., Section 12.4 "Correlations from Overlaps in Repeated Surveys."

5. Blalock, Hubert M, Jr. *Social Statistics, Second Edition*, McGraw-Hill Book Company, Chapter 18, pp 415-418.

6. Office of the Surgeon General of the United States, *Physical Activity and Health: A Report of the Surgeon General*, 1997.

Part Two

Common Sports Injuries

Chapter 8

Head and Brain Injury

Head Injury

What is the significance of sports-related injuries?

Each year, more than 750,000 Americans report injuries sustained during recreational sports, with 82,000 involving brain injuries. In fact, brain injuries cause more deaths than any other sports injury.

Football

Football is responsible for more than 250,000 head injuries in the United States. In any given season, 10 percent of all college players and 20 percent of all high school players sustain brain injuries.

Boxing

Nearly 90 percent of professional boxers have sustained a brain injury.

"Head Injury," reprinted with permission of Neurosurgery://ON-CALL® at www.neurosurgery.org, © 1998 American Association of Neurological Surgeons/Congress of Neurological Surgeons; "Facts about Concussion and Brain Injury, Version 2," National Center for Injury Prevention and Control (NCIPC); and "New Study Links Head Injury, Severity of Injury, with Alzheimer's Disease," Press Release: October 23, 2000, National Institute on Aging (NIA).

Soccer

Approximately 5 percent of soccer players sustain brain injury as a result of head-to-head contact, falls, or being struck on the head by the ball. Heading or hitting the ball with the head is the most risky activity; when done repeatedly, it can cause a concussion.

Horseback Riding

Brain injuries account for 60 percent of equestrian-related fatalities, and 17 percent of all equestrian injuries are brain injuries.

Baseball and Softball, In-line Skating, Roller-skating, and Skateboarding

Brain injuries occur when skaters fall and hit their heads on the pavement. The leading cause of injury and death in baseball is being hit by the ball; the second leading cause is collision.

Gymnastics

Gymnastics has one of the highest injury rates among girls' sports and the risk of injury increases with the level of competition.

What is a brain injury?

When an individual sustains an injury to the brain, there may be a brief loss of consciousness (concussion) or a prolonged period of unconsciousness (coma), depending on the severity of the injury.

What is a concussion?

Cerebral concussions are a type of head injury that frequently occur among athletes. Cerebral concussions are considered diffuse brain injuries and can be defined as traumatically induced alterations of mental status. A concussion results from shaking the brain within the skull and often causes shearing injuries to nerve fibers and neurons.

Grading the concussion is a helpful tool in the management of the injury and depends on the number of previous concussions, duration of post-traumatic amnesia, loss of consciousness, and persistence of symptoms.

According to the Cantu Guidelines, Grade I concussions usually are not associated with loss of consciousness and athletes may return to play if no symptoms appear for one week.

Players who sustain a Grade II concussion usually lose consciousness for less than five minutes, and may return to play after one week of being asymptomatic.

Grade III concussions usually involve memory loss for more than 24 hours and unconsciousness for more than five minutes. Players who sustain this grade of brain injury should be sidelined for at least one month.

Following repeated concussions, a player should be sidelined for longer periods of time and possibly not allowed to play for the remainder of the season.

What is a coma?

The word coma refers to a state of unconsciousness. This unconsciousness may be very deep, where no amount of stimulation will cause the person to respond. In other cases, however, a person who is in a coma may move, make noise, or respond to pain but is unable to obey simple, one step commands, such as "hold up two fingers," or "stick out your tongue." The process of recovery from coma is a continuum along which a person gradually regains consciousness.

For people who sustain severe injury to the brain and are comatose, it usually takes longer to recover and sometimes result in permanent impairments.

How is a coma patient evaluated?

Ongoing evaluations of a person in a coma are important to access the person's status, identify and prevent complications, and to determine the appropriate medical treatment needed. The Glasgow Coma Scale is usually administered upon admission to determine depth of coma and, periodically thereafter, to help determine duration of coma more accurately.

Brain imaging technologies, particularly computerized topography scans (CT-Scans) and magnetic resonance imaging (MRI) can offer important information about an individual's status over time. The purpose of performing an emergency CT scan is to rule out a large mass lesion that requires immediate surgical evacuation.

For patients with an abnormal admission CT scan, intracranial pressure monitoring is appropriate. The main objective of intensive monitoring is to help the physician maintain adequate cerebral perfusion and oxygenation and avoid medical and surgical complications while the brain recovers.

What are the symptoms of a brain injury?

Physical Effects

- Pain: Constant or reoccurring pain, especially headache

- Paralysis: Loss of feeling and/or ability to control or coordinate motor functions (walking, talking, grasping)

- Sensory: Changes in ability to speak, hear, taste, or see; dizziness; disturbance in balance; hypersensitivity to light or sound

Effects on Cognition / Thinking

- Concentration: Shortened attention span; easily distracted; overstimulated by environment; difficulty staying focused on a task, following directions, or understanding information; feeling of disorientation and confusion

- Language: Difficulty finding the "right" word; difficulty expressing thoughts

Who is at greatest risk for sports-related injuries?

Children ages 5 to 14 account for nearly 40 percent of sports-related injuries and, of those, 75 percent are to boys. The majority of sports-related injuries among girls are associated with participation in softball, gymnastics, volleyball, and field hockey. The majority of sports-related injuries among boys are associated with participation in football, basketball, baseball, soccer, wrestling, and ice hockey.

Head and Brain Injuries

A blow or jolt to the head can disrupt the normal function of the brain. Doctors often call this type of brain injury a "concussion" or a "closed head injury." Doctors may describe these injuries as "mild" because concussions are usually not life threatening. Even so, the effects of a concussion can be serious.

After a concussion, some people lose consciousness or are "knocked out" for a short time, but not always—you can have a brain injury without losing consciousness. Some people are simply dazed or confused. Sometimes whiplash can cause a concussion.

Because the brain is very complex, every brain injury is different. Some symptoms may appear right away, while others may not show up for days or weeks after the concussion. Sometimes the injury makes it hard for people to recognize or to admit that they are having problems.

The signs of concussion can be subtle. Early on, problems may be missed by patients, family members, and doctors. People may look fine even though they're acting or feeling differently.

Because all brain injuries are different, so is recovery. Most people with mild injuries recover fully, but it can take time. Some symptoms can last for days, weeks, or longer.

In general, recovery is slower in older persons. Also, persons who have had a concussion in the past may find that it takes longer to recover from their current injury.

This section explains what can happen after a concussion, how to get better, and where to go for more information and help when needed.

Medical Help

People with a concussion need to be seen by a doctor. Most people with concussions are treated in an emergency department or a doctor's office. Some people must stay in the hospital overnight for further treatment.

Sometimes the doctors may do a CT scan of the brain or do other tests to help diagnose your injuries. Even if the brain injury doesn't show up on these tests, you may still have a concussion.

Your doctor will send you home with important instructions to follow. For example, your doctor may ask someone to wake you up every few hours during the first night and day after your injury. Be sure to carefully follow all your doctor's instructions. If you are already taking any medicines—prescription, over-the-counter, or "natural remedies"—or if you are drinking alcohol or taking illicit drugs, tell your doctor. Also, talk with your doctor if you are taking "blood thinners" (anticoagulant drugs) or aspirin, because these drugs may increase your chances of complications. If it's all right with your doctor, you may take acetaminophen (for example, Tylenol® or Panadol®) for headache or neck pain. Use of trade names is for identification only and does not imply endorsement by the U.S. Department of Health and Human Services.

Danger Signs—Adults

In rare cases, along with a concussion, a dangerous blood clot may form on the brain and crowd the brain against the skull. Contact your doctor or emergency department right away if, after a blow or jolt to the head, you have any of these danger signs:

- Headaches that get worse

- Weakness, numbness, or decreased coordination

- Repeated vomiting

The people checking on you should take you to an emergency department right away if you:

- Cannot be awakened

- Have one pupil—the black part in the middle of the eye—larger than the other

- Have convulsions or seizures

- Have slurred speech

- Are getting more and more confused, restless, or agitated

Danger Signs—Children

Take your child to the emergency department right away if the child has received a blow or jolt to the head and:

- Has any of the danger signs listed for adults

- Won't stop crying

- Can't be consoled

- Won't nurse or eat

Although you should contact your child's doctor if your child vomits more than once or twice, vomiting is more common in younger children and is less likely to be an urgent sign of danger than it is in an adult.

Symptoms of Brain Injury

Persons of All Ages

"I just don't feel like myself."

The type of brain injury called a concussion has many symptoms. These symptoms are usually temporary, but may last for days, weeks, or even longer. Generally, if you feel that "something is not quite right," or if you're "feeling foggy," you should talk with your doctor. Here are some of the symptoms of a concussion:

- Low-grade headaches that won't go away
- Having more trouble than usual:
  - Remembering things
  - Paying attention or concentrating
  - Organizing daily tasks
  - Making decisions and solving problems
- Slowness in thinking, acting, speaking, or reading
- Getting lost or easily confused
- Neck pain
- Feeling tired all the time, lack of energy
- Change in sleeping pattern:
  - Sleeping for much longer periods of time than before
  - Trouble sleeping or insomnia
- Loss of balance, feeling light-headed or dizzy
- Increased sensitivity to:
  - Sounds
  - Lights
  - Distractions
- Blurred vision or eyes that tire easily
- Loss of sense of taste or smell
- Ringing in the ears
- Change in sexual drive
- Mood changes:
  - Feeling sad, anxious, or listless
  - Becoming easily irritated or angry for little or no reason
  - Lack of motivation

Young Children

Although children can have the same symptoms of brain injury as adults, it is harder for young children to let others know how they are feeling. Call your child's doctor if your child seems to be getting worse or if you notice any of the following:

- Listlessness, tiring easily

- Irritability, crankiness

- Change in eating or sleeping patterns

- Change in the way they play

- Change in the way they perform or act at school

- Lack of interest in favorite toys

- Loss of new skills, such as toilet training

- Loss of balance, unsteady walking

Older Adults

Older adults with a brain injury may have a higher risk of serious complications such as a blood clot on the brain. Headaches that get worse or an increase in confusion are signs of this complication. If these signs occur, see a doctor right away.

Getting Better

"Sometimes the best thing you can do is just rest and then try again later."

How fast people recover from brain injury varies from person to person. Although most people have a good recovery, how quickly they improve depends on many factors. These factors include how severe their concussion was, what part of the brain was injured, their age, and how healthy they were before the concussion.

Rest is very important after a concussion because it helps the brain to heal. You'll need to be patient because healing takes time. Return to your daily activities, such as work or school, at your own pace. As the days go by, you can expect to gradually feel better.

If you already had a medical problem at the time of your concussion, it may take longer for you to recover from your brain injury. Anxiety and depression may also make it harder to adjust to the symptoms of brain injury.

While you are healing, you should be very careful to avoid doing anything that could cause a blow or jolt to your head. On rare occasions, receiving another concussion before a brain injury has healed can be fatal.

Even after your brain injury has healed, you should protect yourself from having another concussion. People who have had repeated brain injuries, such as boxers or football players, may have serious problems later in life. These problems include difficulty with concentration and memory and sometimes with physical coordination.

Tips for Healing—Adults

Here are a few tips to help you get better:

- Get plenty of sleep at night, and rest during the day.

- Return to your normal activities gradually, not all at once.

- Avoid activities that could lead to a second brain injury, such as contact or recreational sports, until your doctor says you are well enough to take part in these activities.

- Ask your doctor when you can drive a car, ride a bike, or operate heavy equipment because your ability to react may be slower after a brain injury.

- Talk with your doctor about when you can return to work or school. Ask your doctor about ways to help your employer or teacher understand what has happened to you.

- Consider talking with your employer about returning to work gradually and changing your work activities until you recover.

- Take only those drugs that your doctor has approved.

- Don't drink alcoholic beverages until your doctor says you are well enough to do so. Alcohol and certain other drugs may slow your recovery and can put you at risk of further injury.

- If it's harder than usual to remember things, write them down.

- If you're easily distracted, try to do one thing at a time. For example, don't try to watch TV while fixing dinner.

- Consult with family members or close friends when making important decisions.

- Don't neglect your basic needs such as eating well and getting enough rest.

Tips for Healing—Children

Parents and caretakers of children who have had a concussion can help them heal by:

87

- Having the child get plenty of rest.

- Making sure the child avoids activities that could result in a second blow or jolt to the head—such as riding a bicycle, playing sports, or climbing playground equipment—until the doctor says the child is well enough to take part in these activities.

- Giving the child only those drugs that the doctor has approved.

- Talking with the doctor about when the child should return to school and other activities and how to deal with the challenges the child may face.

- Sharing information about concussion with teachers, counselors, babysitters, coaches, and others who interact with the child so they can understand what has happened and help meet the child's needs.

Help for People with Brain Injuries

"It was the first time in my life that I couldn't depend on myself."

There are many people who can help you and your family as you recover from your brain injury. You don't have to do it alone.

Show this information to your doctor or health care provider and talk with them about your concerns. Ask your doctor whether you need specialized treatment and about the availability of rehabilitation programs.

Your doctor may be able to help you find a health care provider who has special training in the treatment of concussion. Early treatment of symptoms by professionals who specialize in brain injury may speed recovery. Your doctor may refer you to a neurologist, neuropsychologist, neurosurgeon, or specialist in rehabilitation.

Keep talking with your doctor, family members, and loved ones about how you are feeling, both physically and emotionally. If you do not think you are getting better, tell your doctor.

Help for Families and Caregivers

"My husband used to be so calm. But after his injury, he started to explode over the littlest things. He didn't even know that he had changed."

When someone close to you has a brain injury, it can be hard to know how best to help. They may say that they are "fine" but you can tell from how they are acting that something has changed.

If you notice that your family member or friend has symptoms of brain injury that are getting worse or are not getting better, talk to them and their doctor about getting help. They may also need help if you can answer "yes" to any of the following questions:

- Has their personality changed?
- Do they get angry for no reason?
- Do they get lost or easily confused?
- Do they have more trouble than usual making decisions?

You might also want to talk with people who have experienced what you are going through. The Brain Injury Association can put you in contact with people who can help.

New Study Links Head Injury, Severity of Injury, with Alzheimer's Disease

A new analysis of head injuries among World War II veterans links serious head injury in early adulthood with Alzheimer's disease (AD) in later life. The study, by researchers at Duke University and the National Institute on Aging (NIA), also suggests that the more severe the head injury, the greater the risk of developing AD.

For some time, scientists have been examining the association between head injury and AD. Studies in recent years have gone back and forth, some finding a relationship and others not. This new finding, by Brenda L. Plassman, Ph.D., of Duke University, Richard J. Havlik, M.D., M.P.H., of NIA, and colleagues is of great interest not only for its conclusions, but also for how the research was conducted. By looking at documented evidence of head injury from medical records of the veterans, scientists were able to move away from information solely based on a participant's or family member's recall about injuries that may have occurred decades—in this case 50 years—earlier.

The study appeared in the Oct. 24, 2000, issue of the journal *Neurology*. The work by Plassman and colleagues at Duke and Johns Hopkins University was supported by NIA. Dr. Havlik heads the NIA's Epidemiology, Demography, and Biometry program.

Havlik cautions that the new findings do not demonstrate a direct cause-and-effect relationship between head injury in early life and the development of dementia, but rather show an association between the two that needs to be studied further. "This study made a great effort to address some of the limitations of previous epidemiologic research in this area. We now need to hone in on what's behind these findings, especially what may be happening biologically, " says Havlik. "While we may not fully understand what's going on, as a practical matter, it may be one more reason to wear that bike helmet instead of keeping it in a closet," Havlik adds. Havlik cautions, however, that the findings from the veterans study may not be applied to today's common exposures to head injury, such as in sports, where helmets are used or where injuries may not be as serious as those examined among veterans who were hospitalized for head trauma.

The researchers began the study by looking at military medical records of male Navy and Marine World War II veterans who were hospitalized during their period of service with a diagnosis of head injury or an unrelated condition. The use of records instead of recall, the scientists said, allowed them to avoid the problem of "recall error," with which, they estimated, probably fewer than 70 percent of people with a true head injury in prior studies would have recalled their injuries many years later.

A specially trained team evaluated the records according to agreed-upon criteria for defining head injury and its severity. (Mild injury involved loss of consciousness or post-traumatic amnesia for less than 30 minutes with no skull fracture, moderate involved loss of consciousness or post-traumatic amnesia for more than 30 minutes but less than 24 hours, and/or a skull fracture, and severe injury was loss of consciousness or post-traumatic amnesia for 24 or more hours.) Veterans were located in 1996-1997 and most contacted agreed to participate in the study. Eventually, 548 veterans who had suffered a head injury and 1,228 veterans without a history of head injury, who comprised the control group for the study, took part.

Using a three-stage screening and assessment process, including home visits in some cases, the scientists then identified the aged veterans with dementia. They also determined whether the veterans had Alzheimer's disease specifically or another type of dementia.

The researchers then compared the number of veterans with AD or other dementia in the group who had suffered a head injury to those in the group with no head injury. The risk of AD and dementia was increased about two-fold among all those with moderate head injury. And risk increased with the severity of the injury. Those with head injuries categorized as severe—who had been hospitalized and who remained unconscious or amnesic for 24 hours or more—had a four-fold greater risk.

Why head injury may be involved in AD and dementia is still unknown. The researchers, in one attempt to help address that question, also looked for a possible interaction effect between head injury and genetic factors associated with AD. Among study participants, they looked at apolipoprotein E, or APOE, an important gene in AD. APOE has various forms, or alleles, and its e4 allele has been associated with increased risk of AD. The scientists wanted to see if increased risk of AD associated with head injury was only present in those men with an APOE e4 allele. The analysis did not find a statistically significant interaction.

The analyses also looked at other factors that possibly could influence the development of dementia among the veterans, including education, positive family history of dementia, and a history of alcohol or tobacco use, but none was involved in the association between head injury and dementia found in this study.

Plassman and her colleagues note more generally that the findings are consistent with current thinking on the etiology, or course, of AD. The increased risk of dementia, some 50 years after the head injuries had occurred, is one more indication that AD is a chronic disease that unfolds over many decades, she points out. "Understanding how head injury and other AD risk factors begin their destructive work early in life may ultimately lead to finding ways to interrupt the disease process early on," says Plassman.

An estimated 1.5 to 2 million individuals per year suffer a significant head injury in the U.S. It is estimated that up to 4 million Americans currently have AD.

The NIA leads the federal effort supporting and conducting basic and clinical research on Alzheimer's disease and on its caregiving aspects. The Institute, a component of the National Institutes of Health, operates the Alzheimer's Disease Education & Referral Center (ADEAR), which provides information to health professionals and the public on AD and memory impairment.

Resources for Getting Help

Several groups help people with brain injury and their families. They provide information and put people in touch with local resources, such as support groups, rehabilitation services, and a variety of health care professionals.

Among these groups, the Brain Injury Association (BIA) has a national office that gathers scientific and educational information and works on a national level to help people with brain injury. In addition, 44 affiliated state Brain Injury Associations provide help locally.

Brain Injury Association (BIA)
105 North Alfred Street
Alexandria, VA 22314
Toll-Free: 800-444-6443
Tel: 703-236-6000
Fax: 703-236-6001
Website: www.biausa.org
E-mail: familyhelpline@biausa.org

Brain Trauma Foundation
523 72nd St., 8th floor
New York, NY 10021
Tel: 212-772-0608
Fax: 212-772-0357
Website: www.braintrauma.org
E-mail: info@braintrauma.org

Centers for Disease Control and Prevention (CDC)
4770 Buford Highway, NE
Atlanta, GA 30341-3724
Tel: 770-488-4031
Fax: 770-488-4338
Website: www.cdc.gov/ncipc/didop/tbi.htm
E-mail: DARDINFO@cdc.gov

National Rehabilitation Information Center (NARIC)
4200 Forbes Boulevard
Suite 202
Lanham, MD 20706
Toll-Free: 800-346-2742
Tel: 301-459-5900
Website: www.naric.com
E-mail: naricinfo@heitechservices.com

National Stroke Association
9707 East Easter Lane
Englewood, CO 80112-3747

Toll-Free: 800-787-6537
Tel: 303-649-9299
Fax: 303-649-1328
Website: www.stroke.org
E-mail: info@stroke.org

Alzheimer's Disease Education & Referral Center (ADEAR)

P.O. Box 8250
Silver Spring, MD 20907-8250
Toll-Free: 800-438-4380
Website: www.alzheimers.org
E-mail: adear@alzheimers.org

Chapter 9

Neck and Spinal Cord Injuries

Spinal/Neck Injury

Definition: Injury to the neck or spinal cord.

Important Information about Neck and Spinal Injuries

When someone has a spinal injury, additional movement may cause further damage to the spine. The purpose of first aid is to prevent further harm to the victim until you can obtain medical help.

- If in doubt about whether a person has received a spinal injury, assume he or she has.

- A spinal cord injury is very serious because it can mean the loss of sensation and function in the parts of the body below the site of the injury.

Causes

- awkward positioning of the body
- bullet or stab wound
- direct trauma to the face, neck, head, or back

This chapter includes "Spinal/Neck Injury," © 2001 A.D.A.M., Inc., reprinted with permission; "Whiplash Information Page," National Institute of Neurological Disorders and Stroke (NINDS), reviewed 07-1-2001; and "Burners," reprinted with permission from http://www.familydoctor.org/handouts/478.html. Copyright © American Academy of Family Physicians. All Rights Reserved.

- diving accident
- electric shock
- exertion
- twisting of the trunk

Symptoms

- stiff neck
- head held in unusual position
- weakness
- difficulty walking
- shock (with pale, clammy skin; bluish lip and fingernails; and decreased consciousness)
- paralysis of extremities
- headache, neck pain, abdominal pain, or back pain
- numbness or tingling that radiates down an arm or leg
- loss of bladder or bowel control

Do not

- bend, twist, or lift the victim's head or body
- attempt to move the victim before medical help arrives unless it is absolutely necessary
- remove a helmet if a spinal injury is suspected.

Call your healthcare provider if

- there has been any injury to the neck or spinal cord. Keep the victim absolutely immobile. Unless there is urgent danger, keep the victim in the position where he or she was found.

First Aid

1. Check the victim's airway, breathing, and circulation. If necessary, begin rescue breathing and CPR. If you think the victim might have a head, neck, or spinal injury; lift the chin rather than tilt the head back when attempting to open the airway. Keep the victim's head, neck, and back in line and roll him or her as a unit.

2. Immobilize the victim's head and torso in the position in which they were found. Do not attempt to reposition the neck.

3. If the victim must be moved, get several people to help. Use a sturdy support (such as a plank) as a stretcher. Together, roll the victim's entire body as a unit—keeping the head, neck, and back in a straight line—onto the stretcher.

4. Immobilize the victim's head and torso in the position found. Place rolled-up towels, clothing, or blankets around the victim's head and torso. Use ropes, belts, tape, or strips of cloth to hold the victim in place on the stretcher. Carry the stretcher as horizontally as possible.

5. If a stretcher is not available and the injured person must be turned over, use the logrolling technique. One rescuer stationed at the victim's head keeps the head and shoulders in a fixed position while the second rescuer extends the victim's arm (the one on the side the victim will be rolled toward) above his head. Then the first rescuer takes this arm and uses it as additional support for the head. Both rescuers gently roll the victim without moving his neck.

6. If you are the only rescuer and the victim must be moved, use the clothes drag technique with victim lying face up or face down (however he or she was found).

7. If the victim vomits or is choking on blood, carefully roll him or her on one side. Vomiting can signal internal injuries.

8. Keep the victim warm to help prevent shock.

9. Give first aid for obvious injuries, but keep the victim in the position found.

Prevention

*   Regular exercise, good posture, and lifting heavy objects correctly (letting your leg muscles do most of the work) all help prevent back problems.

*   Wear seat belts.

*   Avoid alcohol with driving.

*   Avoid diving into lakes, rivers, and surf.

- Avoid motorcycles and all-terrain vehicles.
- Avoid football.
- Back pain, if it occurs, should be discussed with the doctor.

What Is Whiplash?

Whiplash—a soft tissue injury to the neck—is also called neck sprain or neck strain. It is characterized by a collection of symptoms that occur following damage to the neck, usually because of sudden extension and flexion. The disorder commonly occurs as the result of an automobile accident and may include injury to intervertebral joints, discs, and ligaments; cervical muscles; and nerve roots. Symptoms such as neck pain may be present directly after the injury or may be delayed for several days. In addition to neck pain, other symptoms may include neck stiffness, injuries to the muscles and ligaments (myofascial injuries), headache, dizziness, abnormal sensations such as burning or prickling (paresthesias), or shoulder or back pain. In addition, some people experience cognitive, somatic, or psychological conditions such as memory loss, concentration impairment, nervousness/irritability, sleep disturbances, fatigue, or depression.

Is There Any Treatment?

Treatment for individuals with whiplash may include pain medications, nonsteroidal anti-inflammatory drugs, antidepressants, muscle relaxants, and a cervical collar (usually worn for 2 to 3 weeks). Range of motion exercises, physical therapy, and cervical traction may also be prescribed. Supplemental heat application may relieve muscle tension.

What Is the Prognosis?

Generally, prognosis for individuals with whiplash is good. The neck and head pain clears within a few days or weeks. Most patients recover within 3 months after the injury, however, some may continue to have residual neck pain and headaches.

Burners

A *burner* is an injury to one or more nerves between your neck and shoulder. It is also called a *stinger*. It usually happens in sports like football. It's not a serious neck injury.

What Causes a Burner?

If you play football, you can get a burner when you tackle or block another player. One of 3 things happens:

- Your shoulder is pushed down at the same time that your head is forced to the opposite side. This stretches nerves between your neck and shoulder.

- Your head is quickly moved to one side. This pinches nerves on that side.

- The area above your collarbone is hit directly. This bruises nerves.

How Do I Know if I Have a Burner?

You'll have a burning or stinging feeling between your neck and shoulder, and probably in your arm. Your shoulder and arm may feel numb, tingly, or weak.

Your doctor will ask questions and examine you. Burners happen in only one arm at a time. If both of your arms or one arm and a leg are hurt, you may have a serious neck injury, not a burner. Your doctor will then protect your neck and get x-rays.

How Are Burners Treated?

Burners get better on their own. You may need physical therapy to stretch and strengthen your muscles.

Some burners last a few minutes. Others take several days or weeks to heal. If your burner lasts more than a few weeks, you may have a test called an electromyogram (EMG). This test can show that you have a burner and give an idea about how long it will last.

When Can I Return to My Sport?

Before you go back to playing, you must have no pain, numbness, or tingling. You must be able to move your neck in all directions. Your strength must be back to normal. You must be able to play your sport without problems from the injury.

Can I Get Another Burner?

Yes, but daily stretching exercises can help prevent burners. Tilt your head up, down, left, and right. Turn your head left and right to look over your shoulders. Hold each stretch for 20 seconds. If you play football, wear extra neck protection.

An Important Point!

Don't just assume that you have a burner. You might have a serious neck injury. If you have burning, stinging, numbness, or tingling in your arms or legs, stop what you're doing. Slowly lie down on the ground and wait for a trainer or a doctor to examine you.

This information provides a general overview on this topic and may not apply to everyone. To find out if this applies to you and to get more information on this subject, talk to your family doctor. Visit familydoctor.org for information on this and many other health-related topics.

Additional Information

American Chronic Pain Association (ACPA)
P.O. Box 850
Rocklin, CA 95677-0850
Tel: 916-632-0922
Fax: 916-632-3208
Website: www.theacpa.org
E-mail: ACPA@pacbell.net

National Chronic Pain Outreach Association (NCPOA)
7979 Old Georgetown Road, Suite 100
Bethesda, MD 20814-2429
Tel: 301-652-4948
Fax: 301-907-0745
E-mail: ncpoa@cfw.com

National Headache Foundation
428 W. St. James Pl., 2nd Floor
Chicago IL 60614-2750
Toll-Free: 888-NHF-5552 (643-5552)
Tel: 773-388-6399
Fax: 773-525-7357
Website: www.headaches.org
E-mail: info@headaches.org

Chapter 10

Know the Score on Facial Sports Injuries

Playing catch, shooting hoops, bicycling on a scenic path, or just kicking around a soccer ball have more in common than you may think. On the upside, these activities are good exercise and are enjoyed by thousands of Americans. On the downside, they can result in a variety of injuries to the face.

Many injuries are preventable by wearing the proper protective gear, and your attitude toward safety can make a big difference. However, even the most careful person can get hurt. When an accident happens, it's your response that can make the difference between a temporary inconvenience and permanent injury.

When Someone Gets Hurt

- Ask "Are you all right?" Determine whether the injured person is breathing and knows who and where they are.

- Be certain the person can see, hear, and maintain balance. Watch for subtle changes in behavior or speech, such as slurring or stuttering. Any abnormal response requires medical attention.

This chapter includes "Know the Score on Facial Sports Injuries," reprinted with permission of the American Academy of Otolaryngology–Head and Neck Surgery Foundation, www.entnet.org. Copyright © 2002. All rights reserved. The section titled "Additional Nose Fracture Information," is from "Nose Fractures," updated 8/21/01 by Ashutosh Kacker, M.D., © 2001 A.D.A.M., Inc., reprinted with permission.

- Note weakness or loss of movement in the forehead, eyelids, cheeks, and mouth.

- Look at the eyes to make sure they move in the same direction and that both pupils are the same size.

- If any doubts exist, seek immediate medical attention.

When Medical Attention Is Required, What Can You Do?

- Call for medical assistance (911).

- Do not move the victim, or remove helmets or protective gear.

- Do not give food, drink, or medication until the extent of the injury has been determined.

- Remember HIV—be very careful around body fluids. In an emergency protect your hands with plastic bags.

- Apply pressure to bleeding wounds with a clean cloth or pad, unless the eye or eyelid is affected or a loose bone can be felt in a head injury. In these cases, do not apply pressure but gently cover the wound with a clean cloth.

- Apply ice or a cold pack to areas that have suffered a blow (such as a bump on the head) to help control swelling and pain.

What First Aid Supplies Should You Have on Hand in Case of an Emergency?

- sterile cloth or pads
- scissors
- ice pack
- tape
- sterile bandages
- cotton tipped swabs
- hydrogen peroxide
- nose drops
- antibiotic ointment
- eye pads
- cotton balls
- butterfly bandages

Facial Fractures

Sports injuries can cause potentially serious broken bones or fractures of the face.

Common symptoms of facial fractures include:

- swelling and bruising, such as a black eye

- pain or numbness in the face, cheeks or lips
- double or blurred vision
- nosebleeds
- changes in teeth structure or ability to close mouth properly

It is important to pay attention to swelling because it may be masking a more serious injury. Applying ice packs and keeping the head elevated may reduce early swelling.

If any of these symptoms occur, be sure to visit the emergency room or the office of a facial plastic surgeon. (such as an otolaryngologist—a head and neck surgeon) where x-rays may be taken to determine if there is a fracture.

Upper Face

When you are hit in the upper face (by a ball for example) it can fracture the delicate bones around the sinuses, eye sockets, bridge of the nose, or cheek bones. A direct blow to the eye may cause a fracture, as well as blurred or double vision. All eye injuries should be examined by an eye specialist (ophthalmologist).

Lower Face

When your jaw or lower face is injured, it may change the way your teeth fit together. To restore a normal bite, surgeries often can be performed from inside the mouth to prevent visible scarring of the face; and broken jaws often can be repaired without being wired shut for long periods. Your doctor will explain your treatment options and the latest treatment techniques.

Soft Tissue Injuries

Bruises, cuts, and scrapes often result from high speed or contact sports, such as boxing, football, soccer, ice hockey, bicycling, skiing, and snowmobiling. Most can be treated at home, but some require medical attention. You should get immediate medical care when you have:

- deep skin cuts
- obvious deformity or fracture
- loss of facial movement
- persistent bleeding

- change in vision
- problems breathing and/or swallowing
- alterations in consciousness or facial movement

Bruises

Also called contusions, bruises result from bleeding underneath the skin. Applying pressure, elevating the bruised area above the heart and using an ice pack for the first 24 to 48 hours minimizes discoloration and swelling. After two days, a heat pack or hot water bottle may help more. Most of the swelling and bruising should disappear in one to two weeks.

Cuts and Scrapes

The external bleeding that results from cuts and scrapes can be stopped by immediately applying pressure with gauze or a clean cloth. When the bleeding is uncontrollable, you should go to the emergency room.

Scrapes should be washed with soap and water to remove any foreign material that could cause infection and discoloration of the skin. Scrapes or abrasions can be treated at home by cleaning with 3% hydrogen peroxide and covering with an antibiotic ointment or cream until the skin is healed. Cuts or lacerations, unless very small, should be examined by a physician. Stitches may be necessary, and deeper cuts may have serious effects. Following stitches, cuts should be kept clean and free of scabs with hydrogen peroxide and antibiotic ointment. Bandages may be needed to protect the area from pressure or irritation from clothes. You may experience numbness around the cut for several months. Healing will continue for 6 to 12 months. Scars that look too obvious after this time should be seen by a facial plastic surgeon.

Nasal Injuries

Perhaps because it protrudes, the nose is one of the most injured areas on the face. Early treatment of a nose injury consists of applying a cold compress and keeping the head higher than the rest of the body. You should seek medical attention in the case of:

- breathing difficulties
- deformity of the nose

- persistent bleeding
- cuts

Bleeding

Nosebleeds are common and usually short-lived. Often they can be controlled by squeezing the nose with constant pressure for 5 to 10 minutes. If bleeding persists, seek medical attention.

Bleeding also can occur underneath the surface of the nose. An otolaryngologist/facial plastic surgeon will examine the nose to determine if there is a clot or collection of blood beneath the mucus membrane of the septum (a septal hematoma) or any fracture. Hematomas should be drained so the pressure does not cause nose damage or infection.

Fractures

Some otolaryngologists—head and neck specialists—set fractured bones right away before swelling develops, while others prefer to wait until the swelling is gone. These fractures can be repaired under local or general anesthesia, even weeks later.

Ultimately, treatment decisions will be made to restore proper function of the nasal air passages and normal appearance and structural support of the nose. Swelling and bruising of the nose will last for 10 days or more.

Neck Injuries

Whether seemingly minor or severe, all neck injuries should be thoroughly evaluated by an otolaryngologist. Injuries may involve specific structures within the neck, such as the larynx (voicebox), esophagus (food passage), or major blood vessels and nerves.

Throat Injuries

The larynx is a complex organ consisting of cartilage, nerves, and muscles with a mucous membrane lining all encased in a protective tissue (cartilage) framework.

The cartilage can be fractured or dislocated; either is serious because of the possibility of injuring the airway and obstructing breathing. Hoarseness or difficulty breathing after a blow to the neck are warning signs of a serious injury and the injured person should receive immediate medical attention.

Prevention

The best way to treat facial sports injuries is to prevent them. To insure a safe athletic environment, the following guidelines are suggested:

- Be sure the playing areas are large enough that players will not run into walls or other obstructions.

- Cover fixed goal posts and other structures with thick, protective padding.

- Carefully check equipment to be sure it is functioning properly.

- Require protective equipment—such as helmets and padding for football, bicycling, and in-line skating; face masks, head and mouth guards for baseball; ear protectors for wrestlers; and eyeglass guards or goggles for racquetball and snowmobiling are just a few.

- Prepare athletes with warm-up exercises before engaging in intense team activity.

- In the case of sports involving fast-moving vehicles, for example, snowmobiles or dirt bikes—check the path of travel, making sure there are no obstructing fences, wires, or other obstacles.

- Enlist adequate adult supervision for all children's competitive sports.

Additional Information

American Academy of Otolaryngology—Head and Neck Surgery
One Prince St.
Alexandria, VA 22314-3357
Tel: 703-836-4444
Website: www.entnet.org

Additional Nose Fracture Information

A fractured nose is a break in the bone over the bridge of the nose. It is the most common facial fracture. It usually results from a blunt injury and is often associated with other facial fractures. The bruised appearance usually disappears after 2 weeks.

Sometimes, as a result of a blunt injury, the septum (wall dividing the nostrils) can separate. The symptoms may be the same as a fractured nose.

Nose injuries and neck injuries are often seen together because a blow that is forceful enough to injure the nose may be hard enough to injure the neck.

Serious nose injuries cause problems that require immediate professional attention. However, for minor nose injuries, the doctor may prefer to see the victim after the swelling subsides.

Occasionally, plastic surgery may be necessary to correct a deformity of the nose or nasal septum caused by a trauma.

Symptoms

- pain
- blood coming from the nose
- bruising around the eyes
- misshapen appearance (may not be obvious until swelling subsides)
- signs of trauma
- swelling
- difficulty breathing through the nose

Do Not

- try to straighten a broken nose.
- move the victim if there is reason to suspect a head or neck injury.

Call Your Healthcare Provider

- if you suspect a neck or head injury
- you are unable to stop the bleeding
- there is clear fluid draining continuously from the nose
- the victim is having difficulty breathing

First Aid

1. Reassure the victim and try to keep the victim calm.

2. Have the victim breathe through the mouth and lean forward in a sitting position in order to keep blood from going down the back of the throat.

3. Apply cold compresses to the nose to reduce swelling. If possible, the victim should hold the compress so that excessive pressure is not applied.

4. To help relieve pain, acetaminophen taken orally is recommended.

Prevention

- Protective headgear should be worn while playing contact sports, riding bicycles, skateboards, roller skates, or roller blades.

- Seatbelts and appropriate car seats should be used.

Chapter 11

Stress Fractures

What Is a Stress Fracture?

Each day, the body makes new bone to replace the bone that is broken down by the stress of everyday living. Usually, this process is balanced, with the body replacing the equal amount of bone lost. However, this balance may become upset. The body, due to several factors, may not produce sufficient bone. As a result, micro cracks, called stress fractures, can occur in the bone.

Factors that may affect the building process are too little sleep, a diet with inadequate calcium, a rapid increase in activity. Sometimes stress fractures may result from minor trauma, like accidentally kicking one leg when running.

How Will I Know if I Have a Stress Fracture?

Stress fractures produce pain in a limited area directly over the point of the bone where the fracture has occurred. The pain is made worse by activity and is improved with rest.

On physical examination, there is pain when pressure is applied to the injured area. Hopping or jumping on a leg with a stress fracture will cause increased pain. Frequently, but not always, there is swelling around the injured area.

X-rays are not usually helpful in diagnosing an early stress fracture because the bones will look normal and the micro cracks are not visible. After several weeks of rest to allow the bone to repair itself, a healing reaction callus can be seen on an X-ray.

The diagnosis of an early stress fracture can usually be confirmed by a bone scan. In this procedure, a substance normally used by the bone for repair is injected into the patient's bloodstream. After 2 or 3 hours, the patient is placed under a scanner to detect the amount of the substance distributed throughout the bones. All of the bones will absorb some of the substance, but if a bone is repairing a stress fracture, it will absorb more of it at the fracture site, and will appear darker than the other bones. A MRI may also be used to confirm the diagnosis.

How Is a Stress Fracture Treated?

A cast is usually not required for a stress fracture. Unlike a fracture caused by a blow to the body which injures the skin, muscle, and bone, a stress fracture involves only the bone. Therefore the skin and muscles provide protection for the injured bone.

If pain occurs while walking, crutches or a cane should be used to keep weight off the injured extremity. Returning to activity will be a gradual process. Swimming or biking, both non-weight bearing activities can be done to maintain cardiovascular and muscle conditioning in the early period after the stress fracture.

Gradually, impact activities like walking can be added. When the patient can walk rapidly without pain, running can be started. Jumping should only be done when running does not cause any pain. A gradual increase of stress to the bone is the key. Each increase in activity should be done slowly and for short amounts of time. After a while, the activity can be done at a higher intensity and a longer duration. Eventually, the level of activity can be increased (see charts 1 and 2).

If, when advancing to the next level of intensity, pain occurs, the patient should return to the lower level for several day before trying again. The physician will guide the patient through these steps and can monitor the degree of fracture healing with X-rays.

It should be noted that while the normal amount of calcium required for bone repair is 1500 milligrams in postmenopausal women and 1000 milligrams for all other adults, increasing calcium intake above this level will not help the stress fracture heal more rapidly.

Chart 1 Treatment of Stress Fracture of the Lower Extremity

Activity Progression

1. Non-weight bearing, non-impact activities like swimming or biking.

2. Weight bearing, non-impacting activities like a stair machine or a cross country machine.

3. Weight bearing, impacting activities like walking.

Chart 2 Treatment of Stress Fracture of the Lower Extremity

Intensity Progression

1. Low intensity, short duration.

2. Low intensity, increased duration.

3. Higher intensity, short duration.

4. Higher intensity, increased duration.

5. Advance to next activity level.

Stress Fractures in Female Athletes

Stress fractures have two primary causes. They result from excessive bone strain resulting in micro damage to the bone coupled with an inability to keep up with appropriate repair of the bone, or a depressed response to normal strain at the cellular and molecular levels where bone remodeling occurs. The former occurs most often in otherwise healthy female athletes and military recruits, while the latter is likely to occur with other physical problems, such as osteoporosis.

There were 2.4 million high school girls competing in sports in 1997, an 800% increase over 1971. And stress fractures occur more often in female athletes than male athletes. The risk of stress fractures in female recruits in the U.S. military is up to 10 times higher than men undergoing the same training program.

There are many contributing factors to the greater frequency of stress fractures in women. Male athletes may have greater muscle mass, which absorbs shock better. In a study of female athletes, decreased calf girth was a predictor of stress fractures of the tibia. The larger width of male bones may also absorb shock better.

Bone mass and bone mineral density can vary widely in females due to several factors, including hormonal influences and menstrual irregularities. Low calcium intake and eating disorders may contribute to the development of stress fractures. Conversely, oral contraceptive pills appear to help prevent stress fractures in female athletes.

For both men and women, a rigid, high-arched foot absorbs less stress and transmits greater force to the leg bones, which may increase stress fracture risk. And studies of female athletes have shown that having one leg slightly longer than the other can increase the risk of stress fractures.

Other risk factors for stress fractures, in general, include training regimen, footwear, and training surface. For example, higher weekly running mileage has been shown to correlate with increased incidence of stress fractures. In another study, ballet dancers who trained more than five hours a day had a significantly higher risk of stress fractures than those who trained less than five hours per day. A sudden change in frequency, duration, or intensity of training also affects the risk of stress fractures.

In addition, research has shown that training in athletic shoes older than six months increased the risk for stress fractures. Shoe age, rather than shoe cost, was a better indicator of shock absorbing ability. In theory, training on uneven surfaces, or hard surfaces like cement, could also increase stress fracture risk.

Female Athlete Triad

Stress fractures may be the first sign of a more serious underlying condition, such as the "female athlete triad." This is an interrelated problem consisting of amenorrhea (no menstruation), disordered eating, and osteoporosis, a potentially lethal combination. Female athletes, particularly those participating in individual sports, may feel significant pressure to excel where leanness and a low body weight are seen as advantageous.

Abnormal eating patterns include food restriction or fasting, bingeing and purging, or the use of laxatives and diet pills. In combination with decreased body weight and excessive training, this can lead to menstrual disturbance, and in turn, low estrogen levels. Women with disordered eating, estrogen deficiency, and menstrual dysfunction are predisposed to osteoporosis. Female athlete triad sufferers are at a significant risk for stress fractures.

Several studies have shown that stress fractures occur more commonly in women who have stopped menstruating or have irregular periods than those who have a regular menstrual cycle. Athletes with menstrual disturbances have lower estrogen levels and this may lead to lower bone mineral densities. Estrogen deprivation may affect the bone's ability to adapt to stress.

There is some evidence that beginning to menstruate at a later age may be a factor in stress fractures. Another issue for young female athletes is abnormally low levels of estrogen and poor nutrition during adolescence. This can lead to lower bone mass, which may be irreversible after a certain age.

Diagnosis and Treatment

A very specific and accurate diagnosis is the key to proper treatment. Pain from a stress fracture of the neck of the femur (thigh bone), for example, may cause pain in the groin, hip, front of the thigh or the knee. Often standard x-rays do not disclose stress fractures. A bone scan, CT (computerized tomography) scan, or magnetic resonance imaging (MRI) may be more effective, depending on the site of the suspected fracture. The pelvis, sacrum (in the lower back), and the femur are areas where females tend to have a higher occurrence of stress fractures. The patella (knee cap), tibia (shin bone), and bones on the outside of the foot are other common areas of stress fractures, the tibia being the most common of all.

The type of stress fracture and its location generally determine treatment. In most cases, rest is the cure for stress fractures. Nonweight bearing exercise, such as swimming, may be prescribed so that the athlete can maintain aerobic fitness. However, some stress fractures require surgery to fix the bone in place so that it can heal properly.

Additional Reading

"Stress Injury to the Bone among Women Athletes" in *Physical Medicine and Rehabilitation Clinics of North America,* November 2000.

Additional Information

The American Orthopaedic Society for Sports Medicine
6300 N. River Road, Suite 200
Rosemont, IL 60018
Tel: 847-292-4900
Fax: 847-292-4905
Website: www.sportsmed.org

Chapter 12

Sprains and Strains

This chapter contains general information about sprains and strains, which are both very common injuries. Individual sections describe what sprains and strains are, where they usually occur, what their signs and symptoms are, how they are treated, and how they can be prevented. At the end is a list of key words to help you understand the terms used in the chapter. If you have further questions, you may wish to discuss them with your doctor.

What Is the Difference between a Sprain and a Strain?

A sprain is an injury to a ligament—a stretching or a tearing. One or more ligaments can be injured during a sprain. The severity of the injury will depend on the extent of injury to a single ligament (whether the tear is partial or complete) and the number of ligaments involved.

A strain is an injury to either a muscle or a tendon. Depending on the severity of the injury, a strain may be a simple overstretch of the muscle or tendon, or it can result in a partial or complete tear.

What Causes a Sprain?

A sprain can result from a fall, a sudden twist, or a blow to the body that forces a joint out of its normal position. This results in an

"Questions and Answers about Sprains and Strains," National Institute of Arthritis and Musculoskeletal and Skin Diseases (NIAMS), December 1999.

115

overstretch or tear of the ligament supporting that joint. Typically, sprains occur when people fall and land on an outstretched arm, slide into base, land on the side of their foot, or twist a knee with the foot planted firmly on the ground.

Where Do Sprains Usually Occur?

Although sprains can occur in both the upper and lower parts of the body, the most common site is the ankle. Ankle sprains are the most common injury in the United States and often occur during sports or recreational activities. Approximately 1 million ankle injuries occur each year, and 85 percent of them are sprains.

The talus bone and the ends of two of the lower leg bones (tibia and fibula) form the ankle joint. This joint is supported by several lateral (outside) ligaments and medial (inside) ligaments. Most ankle sprains happen when the foot turns inward as a person runs, turns, falls, or lands on the ankle after a jump. This type of sprain is called

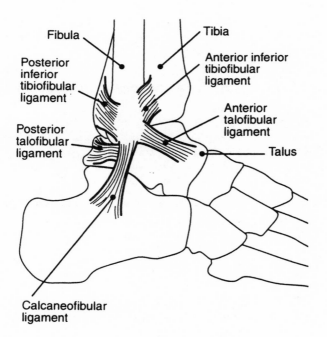

Figure 12.1. *Lateral View of the Ankle*

an inversion injury. One or more of the lateral ligaments are injured, usually the anterior talofibular ligament. The calcaneofibular ligament is the second most frequently torn ligament.

The knee is another common site for a sprain. A blow to the knee or a fall is often the cause; sudden twisting can also result in a sprain.

Sprains frequently occur at the wrist, typically when people fall and land on an outstretched hand.

What Are the Signs and Symptoms of a Sprain?

The usual signs and symptoms include pain, swelling, bruising, and loss of the ability to move and use the joint (called functional ability). However, these signs and symptoms can vary in intensity, depending on the severity of the sprain. Sometimes people feel a pop or tear when the injury happens.

Doctors use many criteria to diagnose the severity of a sprain. In general, **a grade I or mild sprain** causes overstretching or slight

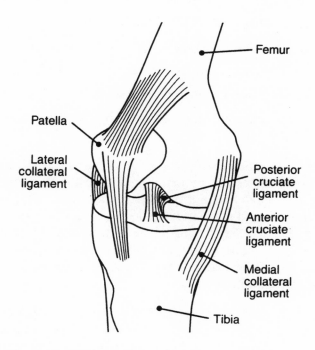

Figure 12.2. Lateral View of the Knee

tearing of the ligaments with no joint instability. A person with a mild sprain usually experiences minimal pain, swelling, and little or no loss of functional ability. Bruising is absent or slight, and the person is usually able to put weight on the affected joint. People with mild sprains usually do not need an x-ray, but one is sometimes performed if the diagnosis is unclear.

When to See a Doctor for a Sprain

- You have severe pain and cannot put any weight on the injured joint.

- The area over the injured joint or next to it is very tender when you touch it.

- The injured area looks crooked or has lumps and bumps (other than swelling) that you do not see on the uninjured joint.

- You cannot move the injured joint.

- You cannot walk more than four steps without significant pain.

- Your limb buckles or gives way when you try to use the joint.

- You have numbness in any part of the injured area.

- You see redness or red streaks spreading out from the injury.

- You injure an area that has been injured several times before.

- You have pain, swelling, or redness over a bony part of your foot.

- You are in doubt about the seriousness of the injury or how to care for it.

A grade II or moderate sprain causes partial tearing of the ligament and is characterized by bruising, moderate pain, and swelling. A person with a moderate sprain usually has some difficulty putting weight on the affected joint and experiences some loss of function. An x-ray may be needed to help the doctor determine if a fracture is causing the pain and swelling. Magnetic resonance imaging is occasionally used to help differentiate between a significant partial injury and a complete tear in a ligament.

People who sustain a grade III or severe sprain completely tear or rupture a ligament. Pain, swelling, and bruising are usually severe, and the patient is unable to put weight on the joint. An x-ray is usually taken to rule out a broken bone.

When diagnosing any sprain, the doctor will ask the patient to explain how the injury happened. The doctor will examine the affected joint and check its stability and its ability to move and bear weight.

What Causes a Strain?

A strain is caused by twisting or pulling a muscle or tendon. Strains can be acute or chronic. An acute strain is caused by trauma or an injury such as a blow to the body; it can also be caused by improperly lifting heavy objects or overstressing the muscles. Chronic strains are usually the result of overuse—prolonged, repetitive movement of the muscles and tendons.

Where Do Strains Usually Occur?

Two common sites for a strain are the back and the hamstring muscle (located in the back of the thigh). Contact sports such as soccer, football, hockey, boxing, and wrestling put people at risk for strains. Gymnastics, tennis, rowing, golf, and other sports that require extensive gripping can increase the risk of hand and forearm strains. Elbow strains sometimes occur in people who participate in racquet sports, throwing, and contact sports.

What Are the Signs and Symptoms of a Strain?

Typically, people with a strain experience pain, muscle spasm, and muscle weakness. They can also have localized swelling, cramping, or inflammation, and with a minor or moderate strain, usually some loss of muscle function. Patients typically have pain in the injured area and general weakness of the muscle when they attempt to move it. Severe strains that partially or completely tear the muscle or tendon are often very painful and disabling.

How Are Sprains and Strains Treated?

Reduce Swelling and Pain

Treatment for sprains and strains is similar and can be thought of as having two stages. The goal during the first stage is to reduce swelling and pain. At this stage, doctors usually advise patients to follow a formula of rest, ice, compression, and elevation (RICE) for the first 24 to 48 hours after the injury. The doctor may also recommend an over-the-counter or prescription nonsteroidal anti-inflammatory drug, such as aspirin or ibuprofen, to help decrease pain and inflammation.

For people with a moderate or severe sprain, particularly of the ankle, a hard cast may be applied. Severe sprains and strains may require surgery to repair the torn ligaments, muscle, or tendons. Surgery is usually performed by an orthopaedic surgeon.

It is important that moderate and severe sprains and strains be evaluated by a doctor to allow prompt, appropriate treatment to begin. A person who has any concerns about the seriousness of a sprain or strain should always contact a doctor for advice.

RICE Therapy

Rest: Reduce regular exercise or activities of daily living as needed. Your doctor may advise you to put no weight on an injured area for 48 hours. If you cannot put weight on an ankle or knee, crutches may help. If you use a cane or one crutch for an ankle injury, use it on the uninjured side to help you lean away and relieve weight on the injured ankle.

Ice: Apply an ice pack to the injured area for 20 minutes at a time, 4 to 8 times a day. A cold pack, ice bag, or plastic bag filled with crushed ice and wrapped in a towel can be used. To avoid cold injury and frostbite, do not apply the ice for more than 20 minutes.

Compression: Compression of an injured ankle, knee, or wrist may help reduce swelling. Examples of compression bandages are elastic wraps, special boots, air casts, and splints. Ask your doctor for advice on which one to use.

Elevation: If possible, keep the injured ankle, knee, elbow, or wrist elevated on a pillow, above the level of the heart, to help decrease swelling.

Begin Rehabilitation

The second stage of treating a sprain or strain is rehabilitation. The overall goal is to improve the condition of the injured part and restore its function. The health care provider will prescribe an exercise program designed to prevent stiffness, improve range of motion, and restore the joint's normal flexibility and strength. Some patients may need physical therapy during this stage.

When the acute pain and swelling have diminished, the health care provider or physical therapist will instruct the patient to do a series of exercises several times a day. These are very important because they help reduce swelling, prevent stiffness, and restore normal, pain-free range of motion. The health care provider can recommend many different types of exercises, depending on the injury. For example, people with an ankle sprain may be told to rest their heel on the floor and write the alphabet in the air with their big toe. A patient with an injured knee or foot will work on weight bearing and balancing exercises. The duration of the program depends on the extent of the injury, but the regimen commonly lasts for several weeks.

Another goal of rehabilitation is to increase strength and regain flexibility. Depending on the patient's rate of recovery, this process begins about the second week after the injury. The health care provider or physical therapist will instruct the patient to do a series of exercises designed to meet these goals. During this phase of rehabilitation, patients progress to more demanding exercises as pain decreases and function improves.

The final goal is the return to full daily activities, including sports when appropriate. Patients must work closely with their health care provider or physical therapist to determine their readiness to return to full activity. Sometimes people are tempted to resume full activity or play sports despite pain or muscle soreness. Returning to full activity before regaining normal range of motion, flexibility, and strength increases the chance of reinjury and may lead to a chronic problem.

The amount of rehabilitation and the time needed for full recovery after a sprain or strain depend on the severity of the injury and individual rates of healing. For example, a moderate ankle sprain may require 3 to 6 weeks of rehabilitation before a person can return to full activity. With a severe sprain, it can take 8 to 12 months before the ligament is fully healed. Extra care should be taken to avoid reinjury.

Can Sprains and Strains Be Prevented?

There are many things people can do to help lower their risk of sprains and strains:

- Maintain a healthy, well-balanced diet to keep muscles strong.
- Maintain a healthy weight.

- Practice safety measures to help prevent falls (for example, keep stairways, walkways, yards, and driveways free of clutter, and salt or sand icy patches in the winter).

- Wear shoes that fit properly.

- Replace athletic shoes as soon as the tread wears out or the heel wears down on one side. Do stretching exercises daily.

- Be in proper physical condition to play a sport.

- Warm up and stretch before participating in any sports or exercise.

- Wear protective equipment when playing.

- Avoid exercising or playing sports when tired or in pain.

- Run on even surfaces.

Additional Information

National Institute of Arthritis and Musculoskeletal and Skin Diseases Information Clearinghouse
NIAMS/National Institutes of Health
1 AMS Circle
Bethesda, MD 20892-3675
Toll-Free: 877-22-NIAMS
Tel: 301-495-4484
TTY: 301-565-2966
Fax: 301-718-6366
Website: www.nih.gov/niams
E-mail: niamsinfo@mail.nih.gov

American Academy of Orthopaedic Surgeons
6300 North River Road
Rosemont, IL 60018-4262
Toll-Free: 800-346-2267
Tel: 847-823-7186
Fax: 847-823-8125
Fax on Demand: 800-999-2939
Website: www.aaos.org
E-mail: custserv@aaos.org

This professional association of orthopaedic surgeons publishes a variety of patient education brochures on common orthopaedic problems.

Key Words

Acute: An illness or injury that lasts for a short time and may be intense.

Chronic: An illness or injury that lasts for a long time.

Femur: The upper leg or thigh bone, which extends into the hip socket at its upper end and down to the knee at its lower end.

Fibula: The thin, outer bone of the leg that forms part of the ankle joint at its lower end.

Inflammation: A characteristic reaction of tissues to disease or injury; it is marked by four signs: swelling, redness, heat, and pain.

Joint: A junction where two bones meet.

Ligament: A band of tough, fibrous tissue that connects two or more bones at a joint and prevents excessive movement of the joint.

Muscle: Tissue composed of bundles of specialized cells that contract and produce movement when stimulated by nerve impulses.

Range of motion: The arc of movement of a joint from one extreme position to the other; range-of-motion exercises help increase or maintain flexibility and movement in muscles, tendons, ligaments, and joints.

Tendons: Tough, fibrous cords of tissue that connect muscle to bone.

Tibia: The thick, long bone of the lower leg (also called the shin) that forms part of the knee joint at its upper end and the ankle joint at its lower end.

Acknowledgments

The NIAMS gratefully acknowledges the assistance of James S. Panagis, M.D., M.P.H., of NIAMS; Jo A. Hannafin, M.D., Ph.D., of the Hospital for Special Surgery, New York, NY; and Harold B. Kitaoka, M.D., of the Mayo Clinic, Rochester, MN, in the preparation and review of this document.

123

Chapter 13

Knee Injuries

Knee problems commonly occur in young people and adults. This chapter contains general information about several knee problems. It includes descriptions and a diagram of the different parts of the knee. Individual sections describe the symptoms, diagnosis, and treatment of specific types of knee injuries and conditions. Information on how to prevent these problems is also provided.

What Do the Knees Do? How Do They Work?

The knees provide stable support for the body and allow the legs to bend and straighten. Both flexibility and stability are needed for standing and for motions like walking, running, crouching, jumping, and turning.

Several kinds of supporting and moving parts, including bones, cartilage, muscles, ligaments, and tendons, help the knees do their job. Any of these parts can be involved in pain or dysfunction.

"Questions and Answers about Knee Problems," National Institute of Arthritis and Musculoskeletal and Skin Diseases (NIAMS), NIH Publication No. 01-4912, May 2001, updated in October 2001 by Dr. David A. Cooke, MD, Diplomate, American Board of Internal Medicine; and text reprinted from Malone, T., Finke, C., and Mangine, R., "Taking Care of Your Knees," in the Public Information area of the American Physical Therapy Association Website © 1999 American Physical Therapy Association available at <www.apta.org/Consumer/ptandyourbody/knee> with permission of the American Physical Therapy Association.

What Causes Knee Problems?

There are two general kinds of knee problems: mechanical and inflammatory.

Mechanical Knee Problems

Some knee problems result from injury, such as a direct blow or sudden movements that strain the knee beyond its normal range of movement. Other problems, such as osteoarthritis in the knee, result from wear and tear on its parts.

Inflammatory Knee Problems

Inflammation that occurs in certain rheumatic diseases, such as rheumatoid arthritis and systemic lupus erythematosus, can damage the knee.

Joint Basics

The point at which two or more bones are connected is called a joint. In all joints, the bones are kept from grinding against each other by padding called cartilage. Bones are joined to bones by strong, elastic bands of tissue called ligaments. Tendons are tough cords of tissue that connect muscle to bone. Muscles work in opposing pairs to bend and straighten joints. While muscles are not technically part of a joint, they're important because strong muscles help support and protect joints.

What Are the Parts of the Knee?

Like any joint, the knee is composed of bones and cartilage, ligaments, tendons, and muscles.

Bones and Cartilage

The knee joint is the junction of three bones: the femur (thigh bone or upper leg bone), the tibia (shin bone or larger bone of the lower leg), and the patella (knee cap). The patella is 2 to 3 inches wide and 3 to 4 inches long. It sits over the other bones at the front of the knee joint and slides when the leg moves. It protects the knee and gives leverage to muscles.

The ends of the three bones in the knee joint are covered with articular cartilage, a tough, elastic material that helps absorb shock and allows the knee joint to move smoothly. Separating the bones of the knee are pads of connective tissue. One pad is called a meniscus (muh-NISS-kus). The plural is menisci (muh-NISS-sky). The menisci are divided into two crescent-shaped discs positioned between the tibia and femur on the outer and inner sides of each knee. The two menisci in each knee act as shock absorbers, cushioning the lower part of the leg from the weight of the rest of the body as well as enhancing stability.

Muscles

There are two groups of muscles at the knee. The quadriceps muscle comprises four muscles on the front of the thigh that work to straighten the leg from a bent position. The hamstring muscles, which

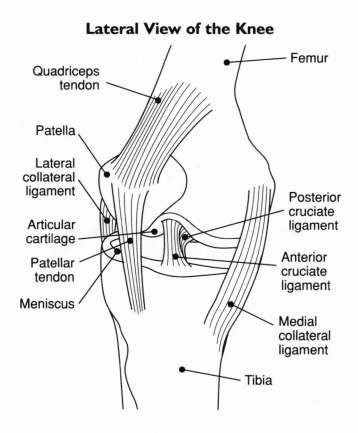

Figure 13.1. Lateral View of the Knee

bend the leg at the knee, run along the back of the thigh from the hip to just below the knee. Keeping these muscles strong with exercises such as walking up stairs or riding a stationary bicycle helps support and protect the knee.

Tendons and Ligaments

The quadriceps tendon connects the quadriceps muscle to the patella and provides the power to extend the leg. Four ligaments connect the femur and tibia and give the joint strength and stability:

- The medial collateral ligament (MCL) provides stability to the inner (medial) part of the knee.

- The lateral collateral ligament (LCL) provides stability to the outer (lateral) part of the knee.

- The anterior cruciate ligament (ACL), in the center of the knee, limits rotation and the forward movement of the tibia.

- The posterior cruciate ligament (PCL), also in the center of the knee, limits backward movement of the tibia.

Other ligaments are part of the knee capsule, which is a protective, fiber-like structure that wraps around the knee joint. Inside the capsule, the joint is lined with a thin, soft tissue called synovium.

How Are Knee Problems Diagnosed?

Doctors use several methods to diagnose knee problems.

Medical history—The patient tells the doctor details about symptoms and about any injury, condition, or general health problem that might be causing the pain.

Physical examination—The doctor bends, straightens, rotates (turns), or presses on the knee to feel for injury and discover the limits of movement and the location of pain. The patient may be asked to stand, walk, or squat to help the doctor assess the knee's function.

Diagnostic tests—The doctor uses one or more tests to determine the nature of a knee problem.

- **X-ray** (radiography)—An x-ray beam is passed through the knee to produce a two-dimensional picture of the bones.

- **Computerized axial tomography** (CAT) scan—X-rays lasting a fraction of a second are passed through the knee at different angles, detected by a scanner, and analyzed by a computer. This produces a series of clear cross-sectional images (slices) of the knee tissues on a computer screen. CAT scan images show soft tissues such as ligaments or muscles more clearly than conventional x-rays. The computer can combine individual images to give a three-dimensional view of the knee.

- **Bone scan** (radionuclide scanning)—A very small amount of radioactive material is injected into the patient's bloodstream and detected by a scanner. This test detects blood flow to the bone and cell activity within the bone and can show abnormalities in these processes that may aid diagnosis.

- **Magnetic resonance imaging** (MRI)—Energy from a powerful magnet (rather than x-rays) stimulates knee tissue to produce signals that are detected by a scanner and analyzed by a computer. This creates a series of cross-sectional images of a specific part of the knee. An MRI is particularly useful for detecting soft tissue damage or disease. Like a CAT scan, a computer is used to produce three-dimensional views of the knee during MRI.

- **Arthroscopy**—The doctor manipulates a small, lighted optic tube (arthroscope) that has been inserted into the joint through a small incision in the knee. Images of the inside of the knee joint are projected onto a television screen. While the arthroscope is inside the knee joint, removal of loose pieces of bone or cartilage or the repair of torn ligaments and menisci is also possible.

- **Biopsy**—The doctor removes tissue to examine under a microscope.

Knee Injuries and Problems

Arthritis

Arthritis of the knee is most often osteoarthritis. In this disease, the cartilage in the joint gradually wears away. In rheumatoid arthritis, which can also affect the knees, the joint becomes inflamed and cartilage may be destroyed. Arthritis not only affects joints; it can also affect supporting structures such as muscles, tendons, and ligaments.

Osteoarthritis may be caused by excess stress on the joint from deformity, repeated injury, or excess weight. It most often affects middle-aged and older people. A young person who develops osteoarthritis may have an inherited form of the disease or may have experienced continuous irritation from an unrepaired torn meniscus or other injury. Rheumatoid arthritis often affects people at an earlier age than osteoarthritis.

Signs and Diagnosis

Someone who has arthritis of the knee may experience pain, swelling, and a decrease in knee motion. A common symptom is morning stiffness that lessens as the person moves around. Sometimes the joint locks or clicks when the knee is bent and straightened, but these signs may occur in other knee disorders as well. The doctor may confirm the diagnosis by performing a physical examination and examining x-rays, which typically show a loss of joint space. Blood tests may be helpful for diagnosing rheumatoid arthritis, but other tests may be needed too. Analyzing fluid from the knee joint may be helpful in diagnosing some kinds of arthritis. The doctor may use arthroscopy to directly see damage to cartilage, tendons, and ligaments and to confirm a diagnosis, but arthroscopy is usually done only if a repair procedure is to be performed.

Treatment

Most often osteoarthritis of the knee is treated with pain-reducing medicines, such as aspirin or acetaminophen (Tylenol); nonsteroidal anti-inflammatory drugs (NSAIDs), such as ibuprofen (Motrin, Nuprin, Advil); and exercises to restore joint movement and strengthen the knee. Glucosamine, a dietary supplement, has been shown in multiple studies to reduce pain and improve joint quality. However, it may take one to two months to work. Losing excess weight can also help people with osteoarthritis.

Rheumatoid arthritis of the knee may require physical therapy and more powerful medications. In people with arthritis of the knee, a seriously damaged joint may need to be replaced with an artificial one. (A new procedure designed to stimulate the growth of cartilage by using a patient's own cartilage cells is being used experimentally to repair cartilage injuries at the end of the femur at the knee. It is not, however, a treatment for arthritis.)

Cartilage Injuries and Disorders

Chondromalacia (KON-dro-mah-LAY-she-ah), also called chondromalaciapatellae, refers to softening of the articular cartilage of the knee cap. This disorder occurs most often in young adults and can be caused by injury, overuse, parts out of alignment, or muscle weakness. Instead of gliding smoothly across the lower end of the thigh bone, the knee cap rubs against it, thereby roughening the cartilage underneath the knee cap. The damage may range from a slightly abnormal surface of the cartilage to a surface that has been worn away to the bone. Chondromalacia related to injury occurs when a blow to the knee cap tears off either a small piece of cartilage or a large fragment containing a piece of bone (osteochondral fracture).

Symptoms and Diagnosis

The most frequent symptom is a dull pain around or under the knee cap that worsens when walking down stairs or hills. A person may also feel pain when climbing stairs or when the knee bears weight as it straightens. The disorder is common in runners and is also seen in skiers, cyclists, and soccer players. A patient's description of symptoms and a follow-up x-ray usually help the doctor make a diagnosis. Although arthroscopy can confirm the diagnosis, it's not performed unless the condition requires extensive treatment.

Treatment

Many doctors recommend that patients with chondromalacia perform low-impact exercises that strengthen muscles, particularly the inner part of the quadriceps, without injuring joints. Swimming, riding a stationary bicycle, and using a cross-country ski machine are acceptable as long as the knee doesn't bend more than 90 degrees. Electrical stimulation may also be used to strengthen the muscles. If these treatments don't improve the condition, the doctor may perform arthroscopic surgery to smooth the surface of the cartilage and "wash out" the cartilage fragments that cause the joint to catch during bending and straightening. In more severe cases, surgery may be necessary to correct the angle of the knee cap and relieve friction with the cartilage or to reposition parts that are out of alignment.

Injuries to the Meniscus

The meniscus is easily injured by the force of rotating the knee while bearing weight. A partial or total tear may occur when a person quickly twists or rotates the upper leg while the foot stays still (for example, when dribbling a basketball around an opponent or turning to hit a tennis ball). If the tear is tiny, the meniscus stays connected to the front and back of the knee; if the tear is large, the meniscus may be left hanging by a thread of cartilage. The seriousness of a tear depends on its location and extent.

Symptoms

Generally, when people injure a meniscus, they feel some pain, particularly when the knee is straightened. If the pain is mild, the person may continue moving. Severe pain may occur if a fragment of the meniscus catches between the femur and the tibia. Swelling may occur soon after injury if blood vessels are disrupted, or swelling may occur several hours later if the joint fills with fluid produced by the joint lining (synovium) as a result of inflammation. If the synovium is injured, it may become inflamed and produce fluid to protect itself. This makes the knee swell. Sometimes, an injury that occurred in the past but was not treated becomes painful months or years later, particularly if the knee is injured a second time. After any injury, the knee may click, lock, or feel weak. Although symptoms of meniscal injury may disappear on their own, they frequently persist or return and require treatment.

Diagnosis

In addition to listening to the patient's description of the onset of pain and swelling, the doctor may perform a physical examination and take x-rays of the knee. The examination may include a test in which the doctor bends the leg, then rotates the leg outward and inward while extending it. Pain or an audible click suggests a meniscal tear. An MRI may be recommended to confirm the diagnosis. Occasionally, the doctor may use arthroscopy to help diagnose and treat a meniscal tear.

Treatment

If the tear is minor and the pain and other symptoms go away, the doctor may recommend a muscle strengthening program. Exercises for meniscal problems are best started with guidance from a doctor and physical therapist or exercise therapist. The therapist will make sure that the patient does the exercises properly and without risking new or repeat injury. The following exercises after injury to the meniscus are designed to build up the quadriceps and hamstring muscles and increase flexibility and strength.

- Warming up the joint by riding a stationary bicycle, then straightening and raising the leg (but not straightening it too much).

- Extending the leg while sitting (a weight may be worn on the ankle for this exercise).

- Raising the leg while lying on the stomach.

- Exercising in a pool (walking as fast as possible in chest-deep water, performing small flutter kicks while holding onto the side of the pool, and raising each leg to 90 degrees in chest-deep water while pressing the back against the side of the pool).

If the tear is more extensive, the doctor may perform arthroscopic or open surgery to see the extent of injury and to repair the tear. The doctor can sew the meniscus back in place if the patient is relatively young, if the injury is in an area with a good blood supply, and if the ligaments are intact. Most young athletes are able to return to active sports after meniscus repair.

If the patient is elderly or the tear is in an area with a poor blood supply, the doctor may cut off a small portion of the meniscus to even the surface. In some cases, the doctor removes the entire meniscus. However, osteoarthritis is more likely to develop in the knee if the meniscus is removed. Medical researchers are investigating a procedure called an allograft, in which the surgeon replaces the meniscus with one from a cadaver. A grafted meniscus is fragile and will shrink and tear easily. Researchers have also attempted to replace a meniscus with an artificial one, but this procedure is even less successful than an allograft.

Recovery after surgical repair takes several weeks, and postoperative activity is slightly more restricted than when the meniscus is removed. Nevertheless, putting weight on the joint actually fosters recovery. Regardless of the form of surgery, rehabilitation usually includes walking, bending the legs, and doing exercises that stretch and build up leg muscles. The best results of treatment for meniscal injury are obtained in people who do not show articular cartilage changes and who have an intact ACL.

Ligament Injuries

What Are the Causes of Anterior and Posterior Cruciate Ligament Injuries?

Injury to the cruciate ligaments is sometimes referred to as a sprain. The ACL is most often stretched or torn (or both) by a sudden twisting motion (for example, when the feet are planted one way and

133

the knees are turned another). The PCL is most often injured by a direct impact, such as in an automobile accident or football tackle.

Symptoms and Diagnosis

Injury to a cruciate ligament may not cause pain. Rather, the person may hear a popping sound, and the leg may buckle when he or she tries to stand on it. The doctor may perform several tests to see whether the parts of the knee stay in proper position when pressure is applied in different directions. A thorough examination is essential. A MRI is very accurate in detecting a complete tear, but arthroscopy may be the only reliable means of detecting a partial one.

Treatment

For an incomplete tear, the doctor may recommend that the patient begin an exercise program to strengthen surrounding muscles. The doctor may also prescribe a brace to protect the knee during activity. For a completely torn ACL in an active athlete and motivated person, the doctor is likely to recommend surgery. The surgeon may reattach the torn ends of the ligament or reconstruct the torn ligament by using a piece (graft) of healthy ligament from the patient (autograft) or from a cadaver (allograft). Although synthetic ligaments have been tried in experiments, the results have not been as good as with human tissue. One of the most important elements in a patient's successful recovery after cruciate ligament surgery is a 4-6 month exercise and rehabilitation program that may involve using special exercise equipment at a rehabilitation or sports center. Successful surgery and rehabilitation will allow the patient to return to a normal lifestyle.

What Is the Most Common Cause of Medial and Lateral Collateral Ligament Injuries?

The MCL is more easily injured than the LCL. The cause is most often a blow to the outer side of the knee that stretches and tears the ligament on the inner side of the knee. Such blows frequently occur in contact sports like football or hockey.

Symptoms and Diagnosis

When injury to the MCL occurs, a person may feel a pop and the knee may buckle sideways. Pain and swelling are common. A thorough examination is needed to determine the kind and extent of the injury. To diagnose a collateral ligament injury, the doctor exerts pressure on the side of the knee to determine the degree of pain and the looseness of the joint. A MRI is helpful in diagnosing injuries to these ligaments.

Treatment

Most sprains of the collateral ligaments will heal if the patient follows a prescribed exercise program. In addition to exercise, the doctor may recommend ice packs to reduce pain and swelling and a small sleeve-type brace to protect and stabilize the knee. A sprain may take 2 to 4 weeks to heal. A severely sprained or torn collateral ligament may be accompanied by a torn ACL, which usually requires surgical repair.

Tendon Injuries and Disorders

What Causes Tendinitis and Ruptured Tendons?

Knee tendon injuries range from tendinitis (inflammation of a tendon) to a ruptured (torn) tendon. If a person overuses a tendon during certain activities such as dancing, cycling, or running, the tendon stretches like a worn-out rubber band and becomes inflamed. Also, trying to break a fall may cause the quadriceps muscles to contract and tear the quadriceps tendon above the patella or the patellar tendon below the patella. This type of injury is most likely to happen in older people whose tendons tend to be weaker. Tendinitis of the patellar tendon is sometimes called jumper's knee because in sports that require jumping, such as basketball, the muscle contraction and force of hitting the ground after a jump strain the tendon. After repeated stress, the tendon may become inflamed or tear.

Symptoms and Diagnosis

People with tendinitis often have tenderness at the point where the patellar tendon meets the bone. In addition, they may feel pain during running, hurried walking, or jumping. A complete rupture of the quadriceps or patellar tendon is not only painful, but also makes it difficult for a person to bend, extend, or lift the leg against gravity. If there is not much swelling, the doctor will be able to feel a defect in the tendon near the tear during a physical examination. An x-ray will show that the patella is lower than normal in a quadriceps tendon

135

tear and higher than normal in a patellar tendon tear. The doctor may use a MRI to confirm a partial or total tear.

Treatment

Initially, the doctor may ask a patient with tendinitis to rest, elevate, and apply ice to the knee and to take medicines such as aspirin or ibuprofen to relieve pain and decrease inflammation and swelling. If the quadriceps or patellar tendon is completely ruptured, a surgeon will reattach the ends. After surgery, the patient will wear a cast for 3 to 6 weeks and use crutches. For a partial tear, the doctor might apply a cast without performing surgery.

Rehabilitating a partial or complete tear of a tendon requires an exercise program that is similar to but less vigorous than that prescribed for ligament injuries. The goals of exercise are to restore the ability to bend and straighten the knee and to strengthen the leg to prevent repeat injury. A rehabilitation program may last 6 months, although the patient can return to many activities before then.

What Causes Osgood-Schlatter Disease?

Osgood-Schlatter disease is caused by repetitive stress or tension on part of the growth area of the upper tibia (the apophysis). It is characterized by inflammation of the patellar tendon and surrounding soft tissues at the point where the tendon attaches to the tibia. The disease may also be associated with an injury in which the tendon is stretched so much that it tears away from the tibia and takes a fragment of bone with it. The disease most commonly affects active young people, particularly boys between the ages of 10 and 15, who play games or sports that include frequent running and jumping.

Symptoms and Diagnosis

People with this disease experience pain just below the knee joint that usually worsens with activity and is relieved by rest. A bony bump that is particularly painful when pressed may appear on the upper edge of the tibia (below the knee cap). Usually, the motion of the knee is not affected. Pain may last a few months and may recur until the child's growth is completed.

Osgood-Schlatter disease is most often diagnosed by the symptoms. An x-ray may be normal, or show an injury, or, more typically, show that the growth area is in fragments.

Treatment

Usually, the disease resolves without treatment. Applying ice to the knee when pain begins helps relieve inflammation and is sometimes used along with stretching and strengthening exercises. The doctor may advise the patient to limit participation in vigorous sports. Children who wish to continue moderate or less stressful sports activities may need to wear knee pads for protection and apply ice to the knee after activity. If there is a great deal of pain, sports activities may be limited until discomfort becomes tolerable.

What Causes Iliotibial Band Syndrome?

This is an overuse condition in which inflammation results when a band of a tendon rubs over the outer bone (lateral condyle) of the knee. Although iliotibial band syndrome may be caused by direct injury to the knee, it is most often caused by the stress of long-term overuse, such as sometimes occurs in sports training.

Symptoms and Diagnosis

A person with this syndrome feels an ache or burning sensation at the side of the knee during activity. Pain may be localized at the side of the knee or radiate up the side of the thigh. A person may also feel a snap when the knee is bent and then straightened. Swelling is usually absent and knee motion is normal. The diagnosis of this disorder is typically based on the symptoms, such as pain at the outer bone, and exclusion of other conditions with similar symptoms.

Treatment

Usually, iliotibial band syndrome disappears if the person reduces activity and performs stretching exercises followed by muscle-strengthening exercises. In rare cases when the syndrome doesn't disappear, surgery may be necessary to split the tendon so it isn't stretched too tightly over the bone.

Other Knee Injuries

What Is Osteochondritis Dissecans?

Osteochondritis dissecans results from a loss of the blood supply to an area of bone underneath a joint surface and usually involves the knee. The affected bone and its covering of cartilage gradually

137

loosen and cause pain. This problem usually arises spontaneously in an active adolescent or young adult. It may be due to a slight blockage of a small artery or to an unrecognized injury or tiny fracture that damages the overlying cartilage. A person with this condition may eventually develop osteoarthritis.

Lack of a blood supply can cause bone to break down (avascular necrosis). The involvement of several joints or the appearance of osteochondritis dissecans in several family members may indicate that the disorder is inherited.

Symptoms and Diagnosis

If normal healing doesn't occur, cartilage separates from the diseased bone and a fragment breaks loose into the knee joint, causing weakness, sharp pain, and locking of the joint. An x-ray, MRI, or arthroscopy can determine the condition of the cartilage and can be used to diagnose osteochondritis dissecans.

Treatment

If cartilage fragments have not broken loose, a surgeon may fix them in place with pins or screws that are sunk into the cartilage to stimulate a new blood supply.

If fragments are loose, the surgeon may scrape down the cavity to reach fresh bone and add a bone graft and fix the fragments in position. Fragments that cannot be mended are removed, and the cavity is drilled or scraped to stimulate new cartilage growth. Research is being done to assess the use of cartilage cell and other tissue transplants to treat this disorder.

What Is Plica Syndrome?

Plica (PLI-kah) syndrome occurs when plicae (bands of synovial tissue) are irritated by overuse or injury. Synovial plicae are the remains of tissue pouches found in the early stages of fetal development.

As the fetus develops, these pouches normally combine to form one large synovial cavity. If this process is incomplete, plicae remain as four folds or bands of synovial tissue within the knee. Injury, chronic overuse, or inflammatory conditions are associated with this syndrome.

Symptoms and Diagnosis

People with this syndrome are likely to experience pain and swelling, a clicking sensation, and locking and weakness of the knee. Because the symptoms are similar to those of some other knee problems, plica syndrome is often misdiagnosed. Diagnosis usually depends on excluding other conditions that cause similar symptoms.

Treatment

The goal of treatment is to reduce inflammation of the synovium and thickening of the plicae. The doctor usually prescribes medicine such as ibuprofen to reduce inflammation. The patient is also advised to reduce activity, apply ice and an elastic bandage to the knee, and do strengthening exercises. A cortisone injection into the plica folds helps about half of those treated. If treatment fails to relieve symptoms within 3 months, the doctor may recommend arthroscopic or open surgery to remove the plicae.

What Kinds of Doctors Treat Knee Problems?

Extensive injuries and diseases of the knees are usually treated by an orthopaedic surgeon, a doctor who has been trained in the non-surgical and surgical treatment of bones, joints, and soft tissues such as ligaments, tendons, and muscles. Patients seeking nonsurgical treatment of arthritis of the knee may also consult a rheumatologist (a doctor specializing in the diagnosis and treatment of arthritis and related disorders).

Taking Care of Your Knees—A Physical Therapist's Perspective

When the mother of the hero Achilles dipped him in the River Styx, she held him by the heel, leaving that spot unprotected. For most of us mortals, however, that most vulnerable spot is two joints higher.

The knee is a relatively simple joint that is required to do a complicated job—to provide flexible mobility while bearing considerable weight. While walking down the street, our knees bear three to five times our body weight. When climbing stairs, that force can multiply to seven times our body weight.

That force is borne by compact structures of bone and cartilage, supported by muscles and ligaments. When the knee is overstressed in sports or in everyday activities, those structures can break down— and knee injury occurs.

This section will discuss knee injury and how your licensed physical therapist can help you recover function. Also discussed are ways you can prevent future injury and reduce your risk of knee injury in the first place.

The Knee Joint

The knee joint is really two joints: the patello-femoral joint, where the large bone of the upper leg connects with the knee cap; and the tibio-femoral joint, where the upper leg bone hinges with the large bone of the lower leg. These bones are held in place by a system of passive restraints, the fibrous ligaments that hold the joint in place. The joint is further supported by muscle tissue, a system of dynamic restraints. When conditioned and strengthened, these muscles apply forces that help hold the joint together. The menisci are pads of cartilage that further stabilize the bones, and provide shock absorbency.

Anatomy of a Bad Knee

Injuries to the knee can be grouped into two categories: acute macro-traumatic, or injuries that result from a single event; and micro-traumatic, repetitive injuries that occur over time.

Acute Macro-Traumatic Injury. An example of this type of injury is a rupture or tear of a ligament, part of the passive restraint system of the knee. Perhaps most common among these injuries is rupture of the anterior cruciate ligament, a condition usually caused by over-rotation of the joint. This type of injury can occur in both sports and occupations where there is excessive twisting.

Micro-Traumatic Injury. Micro-trauma due to overstress of normal tissue. Instead of damage from one event, the knee suffers many repetitive injuries over a period of time. Another name for this condition is overuse syndrome. Micro-trauma often occurs with a sudden increase in exercise level, such as when a runner increases distance or a tennis player plays extra sets.

Treatment of Knee Injuries

There is, unfortunately, no quick cure for a knee injury. Physical therapy plays a key role in treating and rehabilitating the knee, but you and your attitude toward recovery are the biggest factor in achieving a successful outcome.

Physical Therapy

Your licensed physical therapist will design a phased treatment plan with two main components:

1.   Maximum protection, a series of exercises designed to help motion. Activities in this phase might include water walking, swimming, leg presses, and mini-squats; and

2.   Return to function and maintenance, an exercise sequence to restore strength. These activities are a functional progression, that is, a gradual return to normal activities using exercises that simulate the knee stresses of your normal activities.

Surgery

Advances in surgical approaches to the knee joint have made repair to these structures practical in many cases. Arthroscopic surgery employs small incisions to access the joint. The surgeon views the damaged area through an arthroscope, hence the name. These procedures are quick, involve a minimum of discomfort, and enjoy an excellent success rate. Such surgery is indicated when:

• Repair is needed for ruptured ligaments or torn menisci, or

• Some level of disability accompanies injury.

Preventing Your Knee Injury

Your knee's tolerance for stressful activities will decrease with age and loss of conditioning. So, stresses that would not have caused injury last year could hurt your knee today. A decrease in your level of activity over a period of time will also contribute to the vulnerability of your knees.

But there are things you can do to help prevent injury so you can continue to enjoy sports and exercise. Pursuing an exercise program designed by your physical therapist, and applying some good common sense, can be your best protection from injury.

The first step in designing your exercise program is an evaluation by your physical therapist. He or she can identify your predisposing factors, those body traits that may make you more or less vulnerable to a knee injury. Based on this assessment, your physical therapist can design a program that will help you gain your optimum levels of strength and conditioning.

How Physical Therapy Can Help Your Knee Problems

One way to think about your physical therapist's role is as a coach—a caregiver and mentor to lead you through a course of action toward achieving your goals for your comfort and lifestyle.

It's important to recognize that you, the patient, are the most important participant in the healing and prevention process. They are, after all, your knees. Whatever treatment you receive from others, the treatment you give them, day in and day out, is just as important.

Whether you're currently suffering from a knee injury, or trying to avoid one, your physical therapist has the skills to help. It all starts with a careful evaluation.

Evaluation. Physical therapy places great emphasis on this process. Your therapist will take the time to talk with you and perform a thorough physical evaluation to identify your knee condition or predisposing factors.

Therapy. Your physical therapist will plan a treatment regimen suited to your individual condition, and begin working to restore motion and muscular performance.

Teaching. You don't need to become an expert to avoid or overcome injury, but you may need to learn some new habits. Your physical therapist will help you continue therapy on your own, with a home program of exercises designed to fit your needs.

Aftercare. The goal of physical therapy is to return you to normal life as soon as possible, with the skills you need to prevent reinjury. You probably won't need to visit your therapist again unless you have another injury or pain.

As respected members of the professional health care community, licensed physical therapists work in private practice, hospitals, rehabilitation centers, industrial and sports settings, home care, and public schools.

Additional Information

National Institute of Arthritis and Musculoskeletal and Skin Diseases Information Clearinghouse
National Institutes of Health
1 AMS Circle
Bethesda, MD 20892-3675

Toll-Free: 877-22-NIAMS (226-4267)
Tel: 301-495-4484
TTY: 301-565-2966
Fax: 301-718-6366
Website: www.niams.nih.gov
E-mail: niamsinfo@mail.nih.gov

The clearinghouse provides information about various forms of arthritis and rheumatic disease and bone, muscle, and skin diseases. It distributes patient and professional education materials and refers people to other sources of information. Additional information and updates can also be found on the NIAMS website.

American Academy of Orthopaedic Surgeons

6300 North River road
Rosemont, IL 60018-4262
Toll-Free: 800-346-AAOS
Tel: 847-823-7186
Fax: 847-823-8125
Website: www.aaos.org
E-mail: custserv@aaos.org

The academy publishes several brochures on the knee. Single copies of a brochure are available free of charge by sending a self-addressed, stamped (business-size) envelope to (name of brochure) at the address above.

American College of Rheumatology

1800 Century Place, Suite 250
Atlanta, GA 30345
Tel: 404-633-3777
Fax: 404-633-1870
Website: www.rheumatology.org
E-mail: acr@rheumatology.org

This national professional organization can provide referrals to rheumatologists and allied health professionals, such as physical therapists. One-page fact sheets are available on various forms of arthritis. Lists of specialists by geographic area and fact sheets are also available on this website.

American Physical Therapy Association

1111 N. Fairfax Street
Alexandria, VA 22314-1488

American Physical Therapy Association (continued)
Toll-Free: 800-999-APTA (2782)
Tel: 703-684-2782
Fax: 703-683-6743
TDD: 703-683-6748
Website: www.apta.org

The association publishes a free brochure titled "Taking Care of the Knees."

Arthritis Foundation
1330 West Peachtree Street
Atlanta, GA 30309
Toll-Free: 800-283-7800
Tel: 404-872-7100 or call your local chapter (listed in the local telephone directory)
Website: www.arthritis.org

The foundation has several free brochures about coping with arthritis, taking nonsteroid and steroid medicines, and exercise. A free brochure on protecting your joints is titled "Using Your Joints Wisely." The foundation also can provide addresses and phone numbers for local chapters and physician and clinic referrals.

Chapter 14

Shoulder Injuries

This chapter first answers general questions about the shoulder and shoulder problems. It then answers questions about specific shoulder problems (dislocation, separation, tendinitis, bursitis, impingement syndrome, torn rotator cuff, frozen shoulder, and fracture) as well as shoulder pain caused by arthritis of the shoulder.

How Common Are Shoulder Problems?

According to the American Academy of Orthopaedic Surgeons, about 4 million people in the United States seek medical care each year for shoulder sprain, strain, dislocation, or other problems. Each year, shoulder problems account for about 1.5 million visits to orthopaedic surgeons—doctors who treat disorders of the bones, muscles, and related structures.

What Are the Structures of the Shoulder and How Does the Shoulder Function?

The shoulder joint is composed of three bones: the clavicle (collarbone), the scapula (shoulder blade), and the humerus (upper arm bone). Two joints facilitate shoulder movement. The acromioclavicular (AC) joint is located between the acromion (part of the scapula that

"Questions and Answers about Shoulder Problems," National Institute of Arthritis and Musculoskeletal and Skin Diseases (NIAMS), NIH Publication No. 01-4865, May 2001.

forms the highest point of the shoulder) and the clavicle. The gleno-humeral joint, commonly called the shoulder joint, is a ball-and-socket type joint that helps move the shoulder forward and backward and allows the arm to rotate in a circular fashion or hinge out and up away from the body. (The ball is the top, rounded portion of the upper arm bone or humerus; the socket, or glenoid, is a dish-shaped part of the outer edge of the scapula into which the ball fits.) The capsule is a soft tissue envelope that encircles the glenohumeral joint. It is lined by a thin, smooth synovial membrane.

The bones of the shoulder are held in place by muscles, tendons, and ligaments. Tendons are tough cords of tissue that attach the shoulder muscles to bone and assist the muscles in moving the shoulder.

Structure of the Shoulder

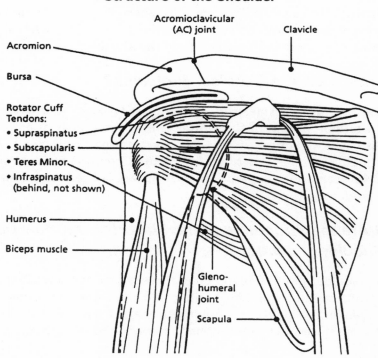

Figure 14.1. Structure of the Shoulder

Ligaments attach shoulder bones to each other, providing stability. For example, the front of the joint capsule is anchored by three gleno-humeral ligaments.

The rotator cuff is a structure composed of tendons that, with associated muscles, holds the ball at the top of the humerus in the glenoid socket and provides mobility and strength to the shoulder joint.

Two filmy sac-like structures called bursae permit smooth gliding between bone, muscle, and tendon. They cushion and protect the rotator cuff from the bony arch of the acromion.

What Are the Origin and Causes of Shoulder Problems?

The shoulder is the most movable joint in the body. However, it is an unstable joint because of the range of motion allowed. It is easily subject to injury because the ball of the upper arm is larger than the shoulder socket that holds it. To remain stable, the shoulder must be anchored by its muscles, tendons, and ligaments. Some shoulder problems arise from the disruption of these soft tissues as a result of injury or from overuse or underuse of the shoulder. Other problems arise from a degenerative process in which tissues break down and no longer function well.

Shoulder pain may be localized or may be referred to areas around the shoulder or down the arm. Disease within the body (such as gallbladder, liver, or heart disease, or disease of the cervical spine of the neck) also may generate pain that travels along nerves to the shoulder.

How Are Shoulder Problems Diagnosed?

Following are some of the ways doctors diagnose shoulder problems:

- **Medical history** (the patient tells the doctor about an injury or other condition that might be causing the pain).

- **Physical examination** to feel for injury and discover the limits of movement, location of pain, and extent of joint instability.

- **Tests** to confirm the diagnosis of certain conditions. Some of these tests include:
  - x-ray
  - arthrogram—Diagnostic record that can be seen on an x-ray after injection of a contrast fluid into the shoulder joint to outline structures such as the rotator cuff. In disease or injury, this contrast fluid may either leak into an

147

area where it does not belong, indicating a tear or opening, or be blocked from entering an area where there normally is an opening.

- MRI (magnetic resonance imaging)—A non-invasive procedure in which a machine produces a series of cross-sectional images of the shoulder.

- Other diagnostic tests, such as injection of an anesthetic into and around the shoulder joint, are discussed in specific sections of this chapter.

Dislocation

What Is a Shoulder Dislocation?

The shoulder joint is the most frequently dislocated major joint of the body. In a typical case of a dislocated shoulder, a strong force that pulls the shoulder outward (abduction) or extreme rotation of the joint pops the ball of the humerus out of the shoulder socket. Dislocation commonly occurs when there is a backward pull on the arm that either catches the muscles unprepared to resist or overwhelms the muscles. When a shoulder dislocates frequently, the condition is referred to as shoulder instability. A partial dislocation where the upper arm bone is partially in and partially out of the socket is called a subluxation.

What Are the Signs of a Dislocation and How Is It Diagnosed?

The shoulder can dislocate either forward, backward, or downward. Not only does the arm appear out of position when the shoulder dislocates, but the dislocation also produces pain. Muscle spasms may increase the intensity of pain. Swelling, numbness, weakness, and bruising are likely to develop. Problems seen with a dislocated shoulder are tearing of the ligaments or tendons reinforcing the joint capsule and, less commonly, nerve damage. Doctors usually diagnose a dislocation by a physical examination, and x-rays may be taken to confirm the diagnosis and to rule out a related fracture.

How Is a Dislocated Shoulder Treated?

Doctors treat a dislocation by putting the ball of the humerus back into the joint socket—a procedure called a reduction. The arm is then immobilized in a sling or a device called a shoulder immobilizer for several weeks. Usually the doctor recommends resting the shoulder and applying ice three or four times a day. After pain and swelling have been controlled, the patient enters a rehabilitation program that includes exercises to restore the range of motion of the shoulder and strengthen the muscles to prevent future dislocations. These exercises may progress from simple motion to the use of weights.

After treatment and recovery, a previously dislocated shoulder may remain more susceptible to reinjury, especially in young, active individuals. Ligaments may have been stretched or torn, and the shoulder may tend to dislocate again. A shoulder that dislocates severely or often, injuring surrounding tissues or nerves, usually requires surgical repair to tighten stretched ligaments or reattach torn ones.

Sometimes the doctor performs surgery through a tiny incision into which a small scope (arthroscope) is inserted to observe the inside of the joint. After this procedure, called arthroscopic surgery, the shoulder is generally immobilized for about 6 weeks and full recovery takes several months. Arthroscopic techniques involving the shoulder are relatively new and many surgeons prefer to repair a recurrent dislocating shoulder by the time-tested open surgery under direct vision. There are usually fewer repeat dislocations and improved movement following open surgery, but it may take a little longer to regain motion.

Separation

What Is a Shoulder Separation?

A shoulder separation occurs where the collarbone (clavicle) meets the shoulder blade (scapula). When ligaments that hold the joint together are partially or completely torn, the outer end of the clavicle may slip out of place, preventing it from properly meeting the scapula. Most often the injury is caused by a blow to the shoulder or by falling on an outstretched hand.

What Are the Signs of a Shoulder Separation and How Is It Diagnosed?

Shoulder pain or tenderness and, occasionally, a bump in the middle of the top of the shoulder (over the AC joint) are signs that a separation may have occurred. Sometimes the severity of a separation can be detected by taking x-rays while the patient holds a light weight that pulls on the muscles, making a separation more pronounced.

How Is a Shoulder Separation Treated?

A shoulder separation is usually treated conservatively by rest and wearing a sling. Soon after injury, an ice bag may be applied to relieve pain and swelling. After a period of rest, a therapist helps the patient perform exercises that put the shoulder through its range of motion. Most shoulder separations heal within 2 or 3 months without further intervention. However, if ligaments are severely torn, surgical repair may be required to hold the clavicle in place. A doctor may wait to see if conservative treatment works before deciding whether surgery is required.

Tendinitis, Bursitis, and Impingement Syndrome

What Are Tendinitis, Bursitis, and Impingement Syndrome of the Shoulder?

These conditions are closely related and may occur alone or in combination. If the rotator cuff and bursa are irritated, inflamed, and swollen, they may become squeezed between the head of the humerus and the acromion. Repeated motion involving the arms, or the aging process involving shoulder motion over many years, may also irritate and wear down the tendons, muscles, and surrounding structures. Tendinitis is inflammation (redness, soreness, and swelling) of a tendon. In tendinitis of the shoulder, the rotator cuff and/or biceps tendon become inflamed, usually as a result of being pinched by surrounding structures. The injury may vary from mild inflammation to involvement of most of the rotator cuff. When the rotator cuff tendon becomes inflamed and thickened, it may get trapped under the acromion. Squeezing of the rotator cuff is called impingement syndrome.

Tendinitis and impingement syndrome are often accompanied by inflammation of the bursa sacs that protect the shoulder. An inflamed bursa is called bursitis. Inflammation caused by a disease such as rheumatoid arthritis may cause rotator cuff tendinitis and bursitis. Sports involving overuse of the shoulder and occupations requiring frequent overhead reaching are other potential causes of irritation to the rotator cuff or bursa and may lead to inflammation and impingement.

What Are the Signs of Tendinitis and Bursitis?

Signs of these conditions include the slow onset of discomfort and pain in the upper shoulder or upper third of the arm and/or difficulty sleeping on the shoulder. Tendinitis and bursitis also cause pain when the arm is lifted away from the body or overhead. If tendinitis involves the biceps tendon (the tendon located in front of the shoulder that helps bend the elbow and turn the forearm), pain will occur in the front or side of the shoulder and may travel down to the elbow and forearm. Pain may also occur when the arm is forcefully pushed upward overhead.

How Are These Conditions Diagnosed?

Diagnosis of tendinitis and bursitis begins with a medical history and physical examination. X-rays do not show tendons or the bursae but may be helpful in ruling out bony abnormalities or arthritis. The doctor may remove and test fluid from the inflamed area to rule out infection. Impingement syndrome may be confirmed when injection of a small amount of anesthetic (lidocaine hydrochloride) into the space under the acromion relieves pain.

How Are Tendinitis, Bursitis, and Impingement Syndrome Treated?

The first step in treating these conditions is to reduce pain and inflammation with rest, ice, and anti-inflammatory medicines such as aspirin, naproxen (Naprosyn), ibuprofen (Advil, Motrin, or Nuprin), or cox-2 inhibitors (Celebrex, Vioxx, or Mobic). In some cases the doctor or therapist will use ultrasound (gentle sound wave vibrations) to warm deep tissues and improve blood flow. Gentle stretching and strengthening exercises are added gradually. These may be preceded or followed by use of an ice pack. If there is no improvement, the doctor may inject a corticosteroid medicine into the space under the acromion. While steroid injections are a common treatment, they must be used with caution because they may lead to tendon rupture. If there is still no improvement after 6 to 12 months, the doctor may perform either arthroscopic or open surgery to repair damage and relieve pressure on the tendons and bursae.

Torn Rotator Cuff

What Is a Torn Rotator Cuff?

One or more rotator cuff tendons may become inflamed from overuse, aging, a fall on an outstretched hand, or a collision. Sports requiring repeated overhead arm motion or occupations requiring heavy lifting also place a strain on rotator cuff tendons and muscles. Normally, tendons are strong, but a longstanding wearing down process may lead to a tear.

151

What Are the Signs of a Torn Rotator Cuff?

Typically, a person with a rotator cuff injury feels pain over the deltoid muscle at the top and outer side of the shoulder, especially when the arm is raised or extended out from the side of the body. Motions like those involved in getting dressed can be painful. The shoulder may feel weak, especially when trying to lift the arm into a horizontal position. A person may also feel or hear a click or pop when the shoulder is moved.

How Is a Torn Rotator Cuff Diagnosed?

Pain or weakness on outward or inward rotation of the arm may indicate a tear in a rotator cuff tendon. The patient also feels pain when lowering the arm to the side after the shoulder is moved backward and the arm is raised. A doctor may detect weakness but may not be able to determine from a physical examination where the tear is located. X-rays, if taken, may appear normal. A MRI can help detect a full tendon tear, but does not detect partial tears. If the pain disappears after the doctor injects a small amount of anesthetic into the area, impingement is likely to be present. If there is no response to treatment, the doctor may use an arthrogram, rather than a MRI, to inspect the injured area and confirm the diagnosis.

How Is a Torn Rotator Cuff Treated?

Doctors usually recommend that patients with a rotator cuff injury rest the shoulder, apply heat or cold to the sore area, and take medicine to relieve pain and inflammation. Other treatments might be added, such as electrical stimulation of muscles and nerves, ultrasound, or a cortisone injection near the inflamed area of the rotator cuff. The patient may need to wear a sling for a few days. If surgery is not an immediate consideration, exercises are added to the treatment program to build flexibility and strength and restore the shoulder's function. If there is no improvement with these conservative treatments and functional impairment persists, the doctor may perform arthroscopic or open surgical repair of the torn rotator cuff.

Frozen Shoulder (Adhesive Capsulitis)

What Is a Frozen Shoulder?

As the name implies, movement of the shoulder is severely restricted in people with a frozen shoulder. This condition, which doctors call adhesive capsulitis, is frequently caused by injury that leads to lack of use due to pain. Rheumatic disease progression and recent shoulder surgery can also cause frozen shoulder. Intermittent periods of use may cause inflammation. Adhesions (abnormal bands of tissue) grow between the joint surfaces, restricting motion. There is also a lack of synovial fluid, which normally lubricates the gap between the arm bone and socket to help the shoulder joint move. It is this restricted space between the capsule and ball of the humerus that distinguishes adhesive capsulitis from a less complicated painful, stiff shoulder. People with diabetes, stroke, lung disease, rheumatoid arthritis, and heart disease, or who have been in an accident, are at a higher risk for frozen shoulder. The condition rarely appears in people under 40 years old.

What Are the Signs of a Frozen Shoulder and How Is It Diagnosed?

With a frozen shoulder, the joint becomes so tight and stiff that it is nearly impossible to carry out simple movements, such as raising the arm. People complain that the stiffness and discomfort worsen at night. A doctor may suspect the patient has a frozen shoulder if a physical examination reveals limited shoulder movement. An arthrogram may confirm the diagnosis.

How Is a Frozen Shoulder Treated?

Treatment of this disorder focuses on restoring joint movement and reducing shoulder pain. Usually, treatment begins with nonsteroidal anti-inflammatory drugs and the application of heat, followed by gentle stretching exercises. These stretching exercises, which may be performed in the home with the help of a therapist, are the treatment of choice. In some cases, transcutaneous electrical nerve stimulation (TENS) with a small battery-operated unit may be used to reduce pain by blocking nerve impulses. If these measures are unsuccessful, the doctor may recommend manipulation of the shoulder under general anesthesia. Surgery to cut the adhesions is only necessary in some cases.

Fracture

What Happens When the Shoulder Is Fractured?

A fracture involves a partial or total crack through a bone. The break in a bone usually occurs as a result of an impact injury, such as a fall or blow to the shoulder. A fracture usually involves the clavicle or the neck (area below the ball) of the humerus.

What Are the Signs of a Shoulder Fracture and How Is It Diagnosed?

A shoulder fracture that occurs after a major injury is usually accompanied by severe pain. Within a short time, there may be redness and bruising around the area. Sometimes a fracture is obvious because the bones appear out of position. Both diagnosis and severity can be confirmed by x-rays.

How Is a Shoulder Fracture Treated?

When a fracture occurs, the doctor tries to bring the bones into a position that will promote healing and restore arm movement. If the clavicle is fractured, the patient must at first wear a strap and sling around the chest to keep the clavicle in place. After removing the strap and sling, the doctor will prescribe exercises to strengthen the shoulder and restore movement. Surgery is occasionally needed for certain clavicle fractures. Fracture of the neck of the humerus is usually treated with a sling or shoulder immobilizer. If the bones are out of position, surgery may be necessary to reset them. Exercises are also part of restoring shoulder strength and motion.

Arthritis of the Shoulder

What Is Arthritis of the Shoulder?

Arthritis is a degenerative disease caused by either wear and tear of the cartilage (osteoarthritis) or an inflammation (rheumatoid arthritis) of one or more joints. Arthritis not only affects joints; it may also affect supporting structures such as muscles, tendons, and ligaments.

What Are the Signs of Shoulder Arthritis and How Is It Diagnosed?

The usual signs of arthritis of the shoulder are pain, particularly over the AC joint, and a decrease in shoulder motion. A doctor may suspect the patient has arthritis when there is both pain and swelling in the joint. The diagnosis may be confirmed by a physical examination and x-rays. Blood tests may be helpful for diagnosing rheumatoid arthritis, but other tests may be needed as well. Analysis of synovial fluid from the shoulder joint may be helpful in diagnosing some kinds of arthritis. Although arthroscopy permits direct visualization of damage to cartilage, tendons, and ligaments, and may confirm a diagnosis, it is usually done only if a repair procedure is to be performed.

How Is Arthritis of the Shoulder Treated?

Most often osteoarthritis of the shoulder is treated with nonsteroidal anti-inflammatory drugs, such as aspirin, ibuprofen, or cox-2 inhibitors. (Rheumatoid arthritis of the shoulder may require physical therapy and additional medicine, such as corticosteroids.) When non-operative treatment of arthritis of the shoulder fails to relieve pain or improve function, or when there is severe wear and tear of the joint causing parts to loosen and move out of place, shoulder joint replacement (arthroplasty) may provide better results. In this operation, a surgeon replaces the shoulder joint with an artificial ball for the top of the humerus and a cap (glenoid) for the scapula. Passive shoulder exercises (where someone else moves the arm to rotate the shoulder joint) are started soon after surgery. Patients begin exercising on their own about 3 to 6 weeks after surgery. Eventually, stretching and strengthening exercises become a major part of the rehabilitation program. The success of the operation often depends on the condition of rotator cuff muscles prior to surgery and the degree to which the patient follows the exercise program.

If you receive a shoulder injury, here's what you can do:

RICE = Rest, Ice, Compression, and Elevation

- **Rest**—Reduce or stop using the injured area for 48 hours.

- **Ice**—Put an ice pack on the injured area for 20 minutes at a time, 4 to 8 times per day. Use a cold pack, ice bag, or a plastic bag filled with crushed ice that has been wrapped in a towel.

- **Compression**—Compression may help reduce the swelling. Compress the area with bandages, such as an elastic wrap, to help stabilize the shoulder.

- **Elevation**—Keep the injured area elevated above the level of the heart. Use a pillow to help elevate the injury.

If pain and stiffness persist, see a doctor.

Additional Information

National Institute of Arthritis and Musculoskeletal and Skin Diseases Information Clearinghouse
National Institutes of Health
1 AMS Circle
Bethesda, MD 20892-3675

National Institute of Arthritis and Musculoskeletal and Skin Diseases Information Clearinghouse (continued)
Toll-Free: 877-22-NIAMS (226-4267)
Tel: 301-495-4484
TTY: 301-565-2966
Fax: 301-718-6366
Website: www.niams.nih.gov
E-mail: NIAMSinfo@mail.nih.gov

The clearinghouse provides information about various forms of arthritis and rheumatic disease and bone, muscle, and skin diseases. It distributes patient and professional education materials and refers people to other sources of information.

American Academy of Orthopaedic Surgeons
6300 North River Road
Rosemont, IL 60018-4262
Toll-Free: 800-346-AAOS (2267)
Tel: 847-823-7186
Fax: 847-823-8125
Website: www.aaos.org
E-mail: custserv@aaos.org

The academy publishes brochures on total joint replacement, arthritis, arthroscopy, and other subjects. Single copies of a brochure are available free of charge by sending a self-addressed, stamped (business-size) envelope to (name of brochure) at their address.

American College of Rheumatology
1800 Century Place
Suite 250
Atlanta, GA 30345
Tel: 404-633-3777
Fax: 404-633-1870
Website: www.rheumatology.org
E-mail: acr@rheumatology.org

This national professional organization can provide referrals to rheumatologists and allied health specialists, such as physical therapists. One-page fact sheets are also available on various forms of arthritis. Lists of specialists by geographic area and fact sheets are also available on their website.

American Physical Therapy Association
1111 North Fairfax Street
Alexandria, VA 22314-1488
Toll-Free: 800-999-2782, ext. 3395
Tel: 703-684-2782
Fax: 703-683-6743
TDD: 703-683-6748
Website: www.apta.org

This national professional organization represents physical thera-pists, allied personnel, and students. Its objectives are to improve re-search, public understanding, and education in the physical therapies. A free brochure titled "Taking Care of Your Shoulder: A Physical Therapist's Perspective" is available on the association's website or by sending a business-size, stamped, self-addressed envelope to their address.

Arthritis Foundation
1330 West Peachtree Street
Atlanta, GA 30309
Toll-Free: 800-283-7800
Tel: 404-872-7100 or call your local chapter (listed in the telephone directory)
Website: www.arthritis.org

This is the major voluntary organization devoted to arthritis. The foundation publishes pamphlets on arthritis, such as "Arthritis An-swers," that may be obtained by calling the toll-free telephone num-ber. The foundation also can provide physician and clinic referrals. Local chapters also provide information and organize exercise pro-grams for people who have arthritis.

Acknowledgments

The NIAMS gratefully acknowledges the assistance of James Panagis, M.D., M.P.H., of the NIAMS; Frank A. Pettrone, M.D., of Ar-lington, Virginia; and Thomas J. Neviaser, M.D., of Fairfax, Virginia, in the preparation and review of this information.

Chapter 15

Growth Plate Injuries

This chapter contains general information about growth plate injuries. It describes what the growth plate is, how injuries occur, and how they are treated. At the end is a list of additional resources. If you have further questions after reading this chapter, you may wish to discuss them with your doctor.

What Is the Growth Plate?

The growth plate, also known as the physis, is the area of developing tissue near the end of the long bones in children and adolescents. Each long bone has at least two growth plates: one at each end. The growth plate determines the future length and shape of the mature bone. When growth is complete—sometime during adolescence— the growth plates are replaced by solid bone.

Who Gets Growth Plate Injuries?

These injuries occur in children and adolescents. The growth plate is the weakest area of the growing skeleton, weaker than the nearby ligaments and tendons that connect bones to other bones and muscles. In a growing child, a serious injury to a joint is more likely to damage a growth plate than the ligaments that stabilize the joint. An injury that would cause a sprain in an adult can be a potentially serious growth plate injury in a young child.

"Questions and Answers about Growth Plate Injuries," National Institute of Arthritis and Musculoskeletal and Skin Diseases (NIAMS), March 1999.

Most injuries to the growth plate are fractures. Growth plate fractures comprise 15 to 30 percent of all childhood fractures. They occur twice as often in boys as in girls, with the greatest incidence among 14 year-old boys and 11-12 year-old girls. Older girls experience these fractures less often because their bodies mature at an earlier age than boys. As a result, their bones finish growing sooner, and growth plates are replaced by stronger, solid bone.

Growth plate fractures occur most often in the long bones of the fingers (phalanges), followed by the outer bone of the forearm (radius) at the wrist. These injuries also occur frequently in the lower bones of the leg: the tibia and fibula. They can also occur in the upper leg bone (femur) or in the ankle, foot, or hip bone.

What Causes Growth Plate Injuries?

While growth plate injuries can be caused by an acute event, such as a fall or a blow to the body, they can also result from overuse. For example, a gymnast who practices for hours on the uneven bars, a long-distance runner, or a baseball pitcher perfecting his curve ball can all have growth plate injuries.

In one large study of growth plate injuries in children, the majority resulted from a fall, usually while running or playing on furniture or playground equipment. Competitive sports, such as football, basketball, softball, track and field, and gymnastics, accounted for one-third of all injuries. Recreational activities, such as biking, sledding, skiing, and skateboarding, accounted for one-fifth of all growth plate fractures, while car, motorcycle, and all-terrain-vehicle accidents accounted for only a small percentage of fractures.

Whether an injury is acute or due to overuse, a child who has pain that persists or affects athletic performance or the ability to move or put pressure on a limb should be examined by a doctor. A child should never be allowed or expected to "work through the pain."

Children who participate in athletic activity often experience some discomfort as their bones and muscles grow and they practice new movements. Some aches and pains can be expected, but a child's complaints always deserve careful attention. Some injuries, if left untreated, can cause permanent damage and interfere with proper physical growth.

Although many growth plate injuries are caused by accidents that occur during play or athletic activity, growth plates are also susceptible to other types of injury, infection, and diseases that can alter their normal growth and development.

Additional Reasons for Growth Plate Injuries

- Child abuse can result in skeletal injuries. These more often occur in very young children, who still have years of bone growth ahead of them. One study reported that half of all fractures due to child abuse were found in children younger than age 1, whereas only 2 percent of accidental fractures occurred in this age group.

- Injury from cold or frostbite can also damage the growth plate in children and result in short, stubby fingers or premature degenerative arthritis.

- Radiation, which is used to treat certain cancers in children, can damage the growth plate. Moreover, a recent study has suggested that chemotherapy given for childhood cancers may also negatively affect bone growth.

- Children with certain neurological disorders that result in sensory deficit, muscular imbalance, or looseness in the ligaments are prone to growth plate fractures, especially at the ankle and knee. Similar types of injury are seen in children who are born with insensitivity to pain.

- The growth plates are the site of many inherited disorders that affect the musculoskeletal system. Scientists are just beginning to understand the genes involved in skeletal formation, growth, and development. This new information is raising hopes for improving treatment of children who are born with poorly formed or improperly functioning growth plates.

How Are Growth Plate Fractures Diagnosed?

After learning how the injury occurred and examining the child, the doctor will probably use x-rays to determine the type of fracture and decide on a treatment plan. Because growth plates have not yet hardened into solid bone, they don't show on x-rays. Instead, they appear as gaps between the shaft of a long bone, called the metaphysis, and the end of the bone, called the epiphysis. Because injuries to the growth plate may be hard to see on x-ray, an x-ray of the noninjured side of the body may be taken so the two sides can be compared. In some cases, other diagnostic tests, such as magnetic resonance imaging (MRI), computed tomography (CT), or ultrasound, will be used.

Since the 1960s, the Salter-Harris classification, which divides most growth plate fractures into five categories based on the type of damage, has been the standard. The categories are as follows:

Type I

The epiphysis is completely separated from the end of the bone, or the metaphysis. The vital portions of the growth plate remain attached to the epiphysis. Only rarely will the doctor have to put the fracture back into place, but all type I injuries generally require a cast to keep the fracture in place as it heals. Unless there is damage to the blood supply, the likelihood that the bone will grow normally is excellent.

Type II

This is the most common type of growth plate fracture. The epiphysis, together with the growth plate, is partially separated from the metaphysis, which is cracked. Unlike type I fractures, type II fractures typically have to be put back into place and immobilized for normal growth to continue. Because these fractures usually return to their normal shape during growth, sometimes the doctor does not have to manipulate this fracture back into position.

Type III

This fracture occurs only rarely, usually at the lower end of the tibia, one of the long bones of the lower leg. It happens when a fracture runs completely through the epiphysis and separates part of the epiphysis and growth plate from the metaphysis. Surgery is sometimes necessary to restore the joint surface to normal. The outlook or prognosis for growth is good if the blood supply to the separated portion of the epiphysis is still intact, if the fracture is not displaced, and if a bridge of new bone has not formed at the site of the fracture.

Type IV

This fracture runs through the epiphysis, across the growth plate, and into the metaphysis. Surgery is needed to restore the joint surface to normal and to perfectly align the growth plate. Unless perfect alignment is achieved and maintained during healing, prognosis for growth is poor. This injury occurs most commonly at the end of the humerus (the upper arm bone) near the elbow.

Type V

This uncommon injury occurs when the end of the bone is crushed and the growth plate is compressed. It is most likely to occur at the knee or ankle. Prognosis is poor, since premature stunting of growth is almost inevitable.

A newer classification, called the Peterson classification, adds a type VI fracture, in which a portion of the epiphysis, growth plate, and metaphysis is missing. This usually occurs with an open wound or compound fracture, often involving lawnmowers, farm machinery, snowmobiles, or gunshot wounds. All type VI fractures require surgery, and most will require later reconstructive or corrective surgery. Bone growth is almost always stunted.

What Kind of Doctor Treats Growth Plate Injuries?

For all but the simplest injuries, the doctor may recommend that the injury be treated by an orthopaedic surgeon, a doctor who specializes in bone and joint problems in children and adults. Some problems may require the services of a pediatric orthopaedic surgeon, who specializes in injuries and musculoskeletal disorders in children.

How Are Growth Plate Injuries Treated?

As indicated in the previous section, treatment depends on the type of fracture. Treatment, which should be started as soon as possible after injury, generally involves a mix of the following:

Immobilization

The affected limb is often put in a cast or splint, and the child is told to limit any activity that puts pressure on the injured area. The doctor may also suggest that ice be applied to the area.

Manipulation or Surgery

In about 1 out of 10 cases, the doctor will have to put the bones or joints back in their correct positions, either by using his or her hands (called manipulation) or by performing surgery. After the procedure, the bone will be set in place so it can heal without moving. This is usually done with a cast that encloses the injured growth plate and the joints on both sides of it. The cast is left in place until the injury heals, which can take anywhere from a few weeks to several months for serious injuries. The need for manipulation or surgery depends on the location and extent of the injury, its effect on nearby nerves and blood vessels, and the child's age.

Strengthening and Range-of-Motion Exercises

These treatments may also be recommended after the fracture is healed.

Long-Term Follow-Up

Long-term follow-up is usually necessary to monitor the child's recuperation and growth. Evaluation may include x-rays of matching limbs at 3- to 6-month intervals for at least 2 years. Some fractures require periodic evaluations until the child's bones have finished growing. Sometimes a growth arrest line may appear as a marker of the injury. Continued bone growth away from that line may mean that there will not be a long-term problem, and the doctor may decide to stop following the patient.

What Is the Prognosis for a Child with a Growth Plate Injury?

Most growth plate fractures heal without any lasting harm. Whether long-term damage occurs depends on the following factors, in descending order of importance:

- **Severity of the injury**. If the injury causes the blood supply to the epiphysis to be cut off, growth can be stunted. If the growth plate is shifted, shattered, or crushed, a bony bridge is more likely to form and the risk of growth retardation is higher. An open injury in which the skin is broken carries the risk of infection, which could destroy the growth plate.

- **Age of the child.** In a younger child, the bones have a great deal of growing to do; therefore, growth arrest can be more serious, and closer surveillance is needed.

- **Which growth plate is injured.** Some growth plates are more responsible for extensive bone growth than others.

- **Type of growth plate fracture.** The five fracture types are described in the section, "How Are Growth Plate Fractures Diagnosed?"

The treatment depends on the listed factors and also bears on the prognosis.

The most frequent complication of a growth plate fracture is premature arrest of bone growth. The affected bone grows less than it would have without the injury, and the resulting limb could be shorter than the opposite, uninjured limb. If only part of the growth plate is injured, growth may be lopsided and the limb may be crooked.

Growth plate injuries at the knee are at greatest risk of complications. Nerve and blood vessel damage occurs most frequently there. Injuries to the knee have a much higher incidence of premature growth arrest and crooked growth.

What Are Researchers Trying to Learn about Growth Plate Injuries?

Researchers continue to develop methods to optimize the diagnosis and treatment of growth plate injuries and to improve patient outcomes. Examples of such work include:

- Removal of a growth-blocking bridge or bar of bone that can form across a growth plate following a fracture. After the bridge is removed, fat, cartilage, or other materials are inserted in its place to prevent the bridge from forming again.

- Use of distraction osteogenesis, a procedure in which a bone that is prematurely shortened is surgically cut and gradually lengthened.

- Development of methods to regenerate musculoskeletal tissue by using principles of tissue engineering.

Additional Information

American Academy of Orthopaedic Surgeons
6300 North River Road
Rosemont, IL 60018-4262
Toll-Free: 800-346-AAOS
Tel: 847-823-7186
Fax: 847-823-8125
Fax on Demand: 800-999-2939
Website: www.aaos.org
E-mail: custserv@aaos.org

American Academy of Orthopaedic Surgeons (continued)

The academy provides education and practice management services for orthopaedic surgeons and allied health professionals. It also serves as an advocate for improved patient care and informs the public about the science of orthopaedics. The orthopaedist's scope of practice includes disorders of the body's bones, joints, ligaments, muscles, and tendons.

American Academy of Pediatrics

141 Northwest Point Boulevard
Elk Grove Village, IL 60007-1098
Tel: 847-434-4000
Fax: 847-434-8000
Website: www.aap.org
E-mail: kidsdocs@aap.org

The American Academy of Pediatrics (AAP) and its member pediatricians dedicate their efforts and resources to the health, safety, and well-being of infants, children, adolescents, and young adults. Activities of the AAP include advocacy for children and youth, public education, research, professional education, and membership service and advocacy for pediatricians.

American Orthopaedic Society for Sports Medicine

6300 N. River Road, Suite 200
Rosemont, IL 60018
Tel: 847-292-4900
Fax: 847-292-4905
Website: www.sportsmed.org

The society is an organization of orthopaedic surgeons and allied health professionals dedicated to educating health care professionals and the general public about sports medicine. It promotes and supports educational and research programs in sports medicine, including those concerned with fitness, as well as programs designed to advance our knowledge of the recognition, treatment, rehabilitation, and prevention of athletic injuries.

National Institute of Arthritis and Musculoskeletal and Skin Diseases Information Clearinghouse (NAMSIC)

National Institutes of Health
1 AMS Circle
Bethesda, MD 20892-3675

Toll-Free: 877-22-NIAMS
Tel: 301-495-4484
Fax: 301-718-6366
TTY: 301-565-2966
Website: www.nih.gov/niams
E-mail: niamsinfo@mail.nih.gov

This clearinghouse, a public service sponsored by the NIAMS, provides information on arthritis and musculoskeletal and skin diseases. The clearinghouse distributes patient and professional education materials and also refers people to other sources of information.

Chapter 16

Emotional Abuse in Youth Sports Activities

Desirable Outcomes of Participation

Ideally, well organized youth sports programs provide a safe, wholesome environment where children can enjoy their spare time and sports experience. Desirable outcomes of this experience include having fun, the development of sound character, self-esteem, confidence, friendships, trust, and the accomplishment of goals. Unfortunately, not all children have a positive experience in youth sports programs. Certain behaviors and philosophies have been found to create a destructive environment causing some children to be scarred for life.

Emotional Abuse

Emotions, defined by Richard Lazarous, Professor Emeritus at Cal-Berkeley are as follows: "Negative emotions include: anger, anxiety, fright, sadness, guild, shame, envy, jealousy, and disgust. Positive emotions we would like developed include: relief, hope, happiness/joy, pride, love, gratitude, and compassion."

Emotional abuse occurs when an individual treats a child in a negative manner which impairs the child's concept of self. This may include a parent/guardian/caregiver, coach, teacher, brother, sister, or a

"Emotional Injuries," Fact Sheet, © 2001 NYSSF. This material is reprinted with permission of the National Youth Sports Safety Foundation, One Beacon Street, Suite 3333, Boston, Massachusetts 02108. All Rights Reserved.

friend. Emotional abuse is, perhaps, the most difficult abuse to identify and the most common form of maltreatment in youth sports. Examples include: rejecting; ignoring; isolating; terrorizing; name calling; making fun of someone; putting someone down, saying things that hurt feelings; and/or yelling.

Additional examples of emotional abuse:

- Forcing a child to participate in sports

- Not speaking to a child after he/she plays poorly in a youth sports game or practice

- Asking your child why he/she played poorly when it meant so much to you

- Hitting a child when his/her play disappoints you

- Yelling at a child for not playing well or for losing

- Punishing a child for not playing well or for losing

- Criticizing and/or ridiculing a child for his/her sports performance

Statements such as: "You're stupid, you're an embarrassment, you're not worth the uniform you play in," are damaging and hurt a young athlete's self-esteem and their value as a human being. If said long enough or strong enough these statement or other negative statements may become beliefs of the athlete and may carry forth into their adult life.

Philosophical Abuse

Healthy philosophies foster emotionally healthy children. They are based on sound objectives and nurture the concept that the well being of a child is more important than his/her performance or winning. The American Sport Education Program suggests, "Athletes First, Winning Second."

Examples of destructive philosophies:

- Win at all cost philosophy—"winning is the only thing"

- Making a child believe his/her self worth relies on wins and losses. The following illustration demonstrates how this belief is established: the first thing you ask a child when he/she comes home is, "Did you win—what was the score?"

Parental Misconduct at Youth Sports Events

It has been widely reported and well documented that parental rage in youth sports is becoming a commonplace occurrence. Examples of parental misconduct:

- Booing or taunting

- Using profane language or gestures

- Physically hitting another parent, official, or player

- Yelling at or arguing with game officials, parents, or players

How Common Is Abuse in Youth Sports?

The Minnesota Amateur Sports Commission conducted a survey in 1993 and found the following incidences of abuse in sports in Minnesota:

- 45.3% of males and females surveyed said they have been called names, yelled at or insulted while participating in sports.

- 17.5% of people surveyed said they have been hit, kicked, or slapped while participating in sports.

- 21% said they have been pressured to play with an injury.

- 8.2% said they have been pressured into sex or sexual touching.

- 8% of all surveyed said they have been called names with sexual connotations while participating in sports.

What Are the Effects of Abuse or Witnessing Parental Misconduct?

- Children who have strong reactions to viewing violence or aggression could develop post traumatic stress disorder.

- The trauma associated with witnessing violence can adversely affect a child's ability to learn.

- Childhood abuse increases the likelihood that the youth will engage in health risk behaviors including suicidal behavior, and delinquent and aggressive behaviors in adolescence.

- Abuse in childhood has been linked to a variety of adverse health outcomes in adulthood. These include mood and anxiety disorders and diseases.

- Violence is a learned behavior; our children are often learning violence from places where they should be learning positive life skills.

- Abuse will "turn the child off" to exercise and sports participation and prevent the development of healthy lifestyles that will promote wellness through their life.

Barriers to Prevention

- People may not be clear what behaviors constitute maltreatment or abuse.

- Young athletes may not recognize that what is happening to them is abusive.

Resources

Lazarus, RS. (2000), How emotions influence performance in competitive sports. *The Sport Psychologist*, 14, 229-252.

Additional Information

National Youth Sports Safety Foundation
One Beacon Street, Suite 3333
Boston, MA 02108
Tel: 617-277-1771
Fax: 617-722-9999
Website: www.nyssf.org
E-mail: NYSSF@aol.com

Arizona Sports Summit Accord
Josephson Institute
4640 Admiralty Way, #1001
Marina del Rey, CA 90292
Tel: 310-306-1868
Fax: 310-306-2140
Website: www.charactercounts.org/sports/accord.htm

American Sport Education Program (ASEP)
Box 5076
Champaign, IL 61825-5076
Toll-free: 800-747-3698

Minnesota Amateur Sports Commission
1700 105th Ave. NE
Blaline, MN 55449
Tel: 763-785-5630
Fax: 763-785-5699
Website: www.masc.state.mn.us/resources/index.html

National Institute of Child Centered Coaching
3160 Pinebrook Road
Park City, UT 84060
Toll-Free: 801-649-5822

National Alliance for Youth Sports
2050 Vista Parkway
West Palm Beach, FL 33411
Toll-Free: 800-729-2057
Tel: 561-684-1141
Fax: 561-684-2546
Website: www.nays.org
E-mail: nays@nays.org

Positive Coaching Alliance
c/o Stanford Athletic Department
Stanford, CA 94305
Tel: 650-725-0024
Fax: 650-725-7242
Website: www.positivecoach.org
E-mail: pca@positivecoach.org

Part Three

Injuries Frequently Associated with Specific Sports

Chapter 17

Basketball Injuries in Young Adults

Each year, more than 200,000 young people under age 15 are treated for basketball-related injuries in hospital emergency departments. Many of these injuries can be prevented if players condition and train properly and follow the rules of the game. A safe playing environment also lowers the risk of injury.

Who Is Affected?

Basketball is a popular sport, especially among children and young adults. But the sport carries a risk for injury, whether played in an organized league or with friends on a local park court. More than 200,000 young people under age 15 are treated in hospital emergency departments each year for basketball-related injuries. This makes basketball the fourth leading cause of injury in both unorganized settings and organized community team sports.

Injuries to basketball players are usually minor, mostly sprains and strains. The ankle and knee are the most common sites of injury, followed by the lower back, hand, and wrist. Eye injuries also occur frequently, as a result of being hit with fingers or elbows.

At the high school and recreational levels, injuries occur more frequently during practice; college players are injured more often during games. Girls and women appear to have a higher rate of injury than boys and men. And many of the injuries female players sustain are more serious than those of their male counterparts (e.g., knee injuries).

"Basketball Safety," SafeUSA™, updated February 27, 2001.

Preventing Basketball Injuries

To help your child avoid sports injuries, follow these safety tips from the American Academy of Orthopaedic Surgeons, the National SAFE KIDS Campaign, and other sports and health organizations. (Note: These tips apply to adults, too.)

- Before your child starts a training program or plays competitive basketball, take him or her to the doctor for a physical exam. The doctor can help assess any special injury risks your child may have.

- Make sure your child wears all the required safety gear every time he or she plays and practices. Knee and elbow pads protect against scrapes and bruises, and mouth guards prevent serious dental injuries. Eye protection is recommended (eye injuries account for about 2 percent of injuries, according to the National Collegiate Athletic Association). If your child wears glasses, talk to the eye doctor about sports eyewear.

- If your child is under age seven, encourage the league to use smaller, mini-foam or rubber balls. These balls are lighter weight and easier for young players to handle.

- Insist that your child warm up and stretch before playing.

- Teach your child not to play through pain. If your child gets injured, see your doctor. Follow all the doctor's orders for recovery, and get the doctor's approval before your child returns to play.

- Make sure first aid is available at all games and practices.

- Talk to and watch your child's coach. Coaches should enforce all the rules of the game, encourage safe play, and understand the special injury risks that young players face. They should never allow players to hold, block, push, trip, or charge opponents.

- Inspect the court for safety. Baskets and boundary lines should not be close to walls, fences, bleachers, or water fountains. The goals and the walls behind them should be padded. If your child plays outside, make sure the court is free of holes and debris.

- Above all, keep basketball fun. Putting too much focus on winning can make your child push too hard and risk injury.

Safety Resources

American Academy of Ophthalmology
P.O. Box 7424
San Francisco, CA 94120
Tel: 415-561-8500
Fax: 415-561-8533
Website: www.aao.org
E-mail: customer_service@aao.org

American Academy of Orthopaedic Surgeons
6300 North River Road
Rosemont, IL 60018-4262
Toll-Free: 800-346-2267
Tel: 847-823-7186
Fax: 847-823-8125
AAOS Fax on Demand: 800-999-2939
Website: www.aaos.org
E-mail: custserv@aaos.org

National Athletic Trainers Association
2952 Stemmons Freeway
Dallas, TX 75247-6916
Toll-Free: 800-879-6282
Tel: 214-637-6282
Fax: 214-637-2206
Website: www.nata.org
E-mail: natanews@nata.org

National SAFE KIDS Campaign
1301 Pennsylvania Ave NW, Suite 1000
Washington, DC 20003
Tel: 202-662-0600
Fax: 202-393-2072
Website: www.safekids.org
E-mail: info@safekids.org

National Youth Sports Safety Foundation
One Beacon Street, Suite 3333
Boston, MA 02108
Tel: 617-277-1171
Fax: 617-722-9999

179

National Youth Sports Safety Foundation (continued)
Website: www.nyssf.org
E-mail: nyssf@aol.com

References

The data and safety tips in this fact sheet were obtained from the following sources:

American Academy of Orthopaedic Surgeons. Basketball. Available at http://www.aaos.org/wordhtml/pat_educ/basketba.htm. Accessed July 7, 1999.

American Academy of Pediatrics. Sports Medicine: Health care for young athletes. Elk Grove Village, IL: *The Academy*, 1991:152,169.

Caine D, Caine C, Lindner K, editors. Epidemiology of Sports Injuries. Champaign, IL: *Human Kinetics*, 1996:86-97.

Chapter 18

High School and College Football Injuries

In 1931 the American Football Coaches Association initiated the
First Annual Survey of Football Fatalities. The original survey committee was chaired by Marvin A. Stevens, M.D., of Yale University,
who served from 1931-1942. Floyd R. Eastwood, Ph.D., Purdue University, succeeded Dr. Stevens in 1942 and served through 1964. Carl
S. Blyth, Ph.D., University of North Carolina at Chapel Hill, was
appointed in 1965 and served through the 1979 football season. In
January 1980, Frederick O. Mueller, Ph.D., University of North Carolina at Chapel Hill, was appointed by the American Football Coaches
Association and the National Collegiate Athletic Association to continue this research under the new title, *Annual Survey of Football
Injury Research.*

The primary purpose of the *Annual Survey of Football Injury Research* is to make the game of football a safer, and therefore, a more
enjoyable sports activity. Because of these surveys the game of football has realized many benefits in regard to rule changes, improvement of equipment, improved medical care, and improved coaching
techniques. The 1976 rule change that made it illegal to make initial

contact with the head while blocking and tackling was the direct result of this research.

The 1990 report was historic in that it was the first year since the beginning of the research, 1931, that there was not a direct fatality in football at any level of play. This clearly illustrates that data collection and analysis is important and plays a major role in injury prevention.

Data Collection

Throughout the year, upon notification of a suspected football fatality, immediate contact is made with the appropriate officials (coaches, administrators, physicians, trainers). Pertinent information is collected through questionnaires and personal contact.

Football fatalities are classified for this report as direct and indirect. The criteria used to classify football fatalities are as follows:

- Direct—Those fatalities which resulted directly from participation in the fundamental skills of football.

- Indirect—Those fatalities which are caused by systemic failure as a result of exertion while participating in football activity or by a complication which was secondary to a non-fatal injury.

In several instances of reported football fatalities, the respondent stated the fatality should not be attributed to football. Reasons for these statements are that the fatality was attributed to physical defects that were unrelated to football injuries.

Participation numbers were updated in the 1989 report. The National Federation of State High School Associations has estimated that there are approximately 1,500,000 high school, junior high school, and non-federation school football participants in the United States. The college figure of 75,000 participants includes the National Collegiate Athletic Association, the National Association of Intercollegiate Athletics, the National Junior College Athletic Association, and an estimate of schools not associated with any national organization. Sandlot and professional football have been estimated at 225,000 participants. These figures give an estimate of 1,800,000 total football participants in the United States for the 2000 football season.

Dr. Mueller compiled and prepared the survey report on college, professional, and sandlot levels, and Mr. Jerry Diehl of the National Federation of State High School Associations assumed responsibility for collecting and preparing the senior and junior high school phase of the study. Sandlot is defined as non-school football, but organized and using full protective equipment.

At the conclusion of the football season, both reports are compiled into this Annual Survey of Football Injury Research. This report is sponsored by the American Football Coaches Association, the National Collegiate Athletic Association, and The National Federation of State High School Associations.

Medical data for the 2000 report were compiled by Dr. Robert C. Cantu, Chairman, Department of Surgery and Chief, Neurosurgery Service, Emerson Hospital, in Concord, MA. Dr. Cantu is a Past-President of the American College of Sports Medicine and is the Medical Director for the National Center for Catastrophic Sports Injury Research at the University of North Carolina at Chapel Hill.

Summary

1. There were eight fatalities directly related to football during the 2001 football season. Seven were associated with high school football and one Pop Warner recreational play.

2. The rate of direct fatal injuries is very low on a 100,000 player exposure basis. For the approximately 1,800,000 participants in 2001, the rate of direct fatalities was 0.44 per 100,000 participants.

3. The rate of direct fatalities in high school and junior high school football was 0.44 per 100,000 participants. The rate of direct fatalities in college was 0.00 per 100,000 participants.

4. Most direct fatalities usually occur during regularly scheduled games. In 2001 all eight of the direct fatalities happened in games.

5. The 2001 survey shows that one fatality happened in August, two in September, four in October, and one in November.

6. The major activities in football would naturally account for the greatest number of fatalities. In 2001 one fatality occurred while tackling, two being tackled, one being blocked on a kick-off, two tackled on a kick-off, one falling on the ball, and one in other football activity.

7. In 2001 six of the direct fatalities resulted from an injury to the brain, one from a fractured neck, and one from a ruptured spleen.

8. In many cases football cannot be directly responsible for fatal injuries (heat stroke, heart related and so forth). In 2001 there were 15 indirect fatalities. Ten were associated with high school football, three were associated with college football, and two were associated with professional football. Six of the high school indirect deaths were heart related, one was heat related, and the cause of three were unknown at this time. One of the college indirect fatalities was heat related, one heart related, and one to an asthma attack. The professional indirect fatalities included a heat stroke death and the cause of one was unknown. The heat related deaths are a major concern since they are preventable with the proper precautions.

Discussions and Recommendations

After a slight rise in the number of football fatalities during the 1986 season, the 1990 data revealed the elimination of direct football fatalities. That was the first time in the past 59 years that there have been no direct football fatalities. The 2001 data continues the trend of single digit direct fatalities that started in the 1978 football season, but there was an increase from three in 2000 to eight in 2001. The data illustrates the importance of data collection and the analysis of this data in making changes in the game of football that help reduce the incidence of serious injuries. This effort must be continued in order to keep these numbers low and to strive for the elimination of football fatalities.

Head and Neck Injuries

Past efforts that were successful in reducing fatalities to the levels indicated from 1990 through 2001, and the elimination of direct fatalities in 1990 should again be emphasized. Rule changes for the 1976 football season which eliminated the head as a primary and initial contact area for blocking and tackling are of utmost importance. *Coaches who are teaching helmet or face to the numbers tackling and blocking are not only breaking the football rules, but are placing their players at risk for permanent paralysis or death.* This type of tackling and blocking technique was the direct cause of 36 football fatalities and 30 permanent paralysis injuries in 1968. In addition, if a catastrophic football injury case goes to a court of law, there is no defense for using this type of tackling or blocking technique. Since

1960 most of the direct fatalities have been caused by head and neck injuries. We must continue to reduce head and neck injuries.

Several suggestions for reducing head and neck injuries are as follows:

1. Athletes must be given proper conditioning exercises which will strengthen their necks so that participants will be able to hold their heads firmly erect when making contact.

2. Coaches should drill the athletes in the proper execution of the fundamental football skills, particularly blocking and tackling. Contact should always be made with the head up and never with the top of the head/helmet. Initial contact should never be made with the head/helmet or face mask.

3. Coaches and officials should discourage the players from using their heads as battering rams when blocking and tackling. The rules prohibiting spearing should be enforced in practice and in games. The players should be taught to respect the helmet as a protective device and that the helmet should not be used as a weapon.

4. All coaches, physicians, and trainers should take special care to see that the player's equipment is properly fitted, particularly the helmet.

5. When a player has experienced or shown signs of head trauma (loss of consciousness, visual disturbances, headache, inability to walk correctly, obvious disorientation, memory loss), he should receive immediate medical attention and should not be allowed to return to practice or game without permission from the proper medical authorities.

6. A number of the players associated with brain trauma complained of headaches or had a previous concussion prior to their deaths. Players should be made aware of these signs by the team physician, athletic trainer, or coach. Players should also be encouraged to inform the team physician, athletic trainer, or coach if they are experiencing any of the mentioned signs of brain trauma.

7. Coaches should never make the decision whether a player returns to a game or active participation in a practice if that player experiences brain trauma.

Another important effort has been and continues to be the improvement of football protective equipment. It is imperative that old and worn equipment be properly renovated or discarded and continued emphasis is placed on developing the best equipment possible. Manufacturers, coaches, trainers, and physicians should continue their joint and individual efforts toward this end.

The authors of this research are convinced that the current rules which eliminate the head in blocking and tackling, coaches teaching the proper fundamentals of blocking and tackling, the helmet research conducted by NOCSAE, excellent physical conditioning, proper medical supervision, and a good data collection system have played the major role in reducing fatalities and serious head and neck injuries in football. This is best illustrated by Table 18.1 which shows the increase in both head and cervical spine fatalities during the decade from 1965-1974. This time period was associated with blocking and tackling techniques that involved the head as the initial point of contact. The reduction in head and cervical spine injuries is shown in the decade from 1975-1984. This decade was associated with the 1976 rule change that eliminated the head as the initial contact point in blocking and tackling. There is no doubt that the 1976 rule change has made a difference and that a continued effort should be made to keep the head out of the fundamental skills of football. Data from the decade 1985-1994 continues to illustrate the reduction in head and neck fatalities.

Heat Stroke

A continuous effort should be made to eliminate heat stroke deaths associated with football. Since the beginning of the survey through 1959 there were five cases of heat stroke death reported. From 1960 through 2001 there have been 100 heat stroke cases which resulted in death (Table 18.2). *The 2001 data show three cases of heat stroke death. There is no excuse for any number of heat stroke deaths since they are all preventable with the proper precautions. In the past seven years 20 young football players have died from heat stroke.* Every effort should be made to continuously educate coaches concerning the proper procedures and precautions when practicing or playing in the heat. Since 1974 there has been a dramatic reduction in heat stroke deaths with the exception of 1978, 1995, 1998, and 2000 when there were four each year. There were no heat stroke deaths in 1993 and 1994. All coaches, trainers, and physicians should place special emphasis on eliminating football fatalities which result from physical activity in hot weather.

Heat stroke and heat exhaustion are prevented by careful control of various factors in the conditioning program of the athlete. When football activity is carried on in hot weather, the following suggestions and precautions should be taken:

1. Each athlete should have a complete physical examination with medical history and an annual health history update. History of previous heat illness and type of training activities before organized practice begins should be included.

2. Acclimatize athletes to heat gradually by providing graduated practice sessions for the first seven to ten days and other abnormally hot or humid days.

3. Know both the temperature and the humidity since it is more difficult for the body to cool itself in high humidity. Use of a sling psychrometer is recommended to measure the relative humidity and anytime the wet-bulb temperature is over 78 degrees practice should be altered.

4. Adjust activity level and provide frequent rest periods. Rest in cool, shaded areas with some air movement and remove helmets and loosen or remove jerseys. Rest periods of 15-30 minutes should be provided during workouts of one hour.

5. Provide adequate cold water replacement during practice. Water should always be available and in unlimited quantities to the athletes. *Give Water Regularly*.

Table 18.1. Head and Cervical Spine Fatalities

Year	Head Frequency	Head Percent	Cervical Spine Frequency	Cervical Spine Percent
1945-1954	87	17.4	32	27.3
1955-1964	115	23.0	23	19.7
1965-1974	162	32.4	42	35.9
1975-1984	69	13.8	14	12.0
1985-1994	33	6.6	5	4.3
1995-2001	34	6.8	1	0.8

6. Salt should be replaced daily and liberal salting of the athletes' food will accomplish this purpose. Coaches should not provide salt tablets to athletes. Attention must be directed to water replacement.

Table 18.2. Heat Stroke Fatalities 1931-2001

Year	Total	Year	Total
1931–1954*	0	1979	2
1955	1	1980	1
1956–1958	0	1981	2
1959	4	1982	2
1960	3	1983	1
1961	3	1984	3
1962	5	1985	0
1963	0	1986	0
1964	4	1987	1
1965	6	1988	2
1966	1	1989	1
1967	2	1990	1
1968	5	1991	0
1969	5	1992	1
1970	8	1993	0
1971	4	1994	0
1972	7	1995	4
1973	3	1996	2
1974	1	1997	1
1975	0	1998	4
1976	1	1999	2
1977	1	2000	4
1978	4	2001	3

*No study was conducted in 1942.

7. Athletes should weigh each day before and after practice and weight charts checked in order to treat the athlete who loses excessive weight each day. Generally, a three percent body weight loss through sweating is safe, and a five percent loss is in the danger zone.

8. Clothing is important and a player should avoid use of long sleeves, long stockings, and any excess clothing. Never use rubberized clothing or sweatsuits.

9. Some athletes are more susceptible to heat injury. These individuals are not accustomed to work in the heat, may be overweight, and may be the eager athlete who constantly competes at his capacity. Athletes with previous heat problems should be watched closely.

10. It is important to observe for signs of heat illness. Some trouble signs are nausea, incoherence, fatigue, weakness, vomiting, cramps, weak rapid pulse, flushed appearance, visual disturbances, and unsteadiness. Heat stroke victims, contrary to popular belief, may sweat profusely. If heat illness is suspected, seek a physician's immediate service. Recommended emergency procedures are vital.

11. An increasing number of medical personnel are using treatment for heat illnesses that involves applying either alcohol or cool water to the victim's skin and is followed by vigorous fanning. The fanning causes evaporation and cooling. (Source: *The First Aider,* September 1987)

Recommendations

Specific recommendations resulting from the 2001 survey data are as follows:

1. Mandatory medical examinations and medical history should be taken before allowing an athlete to participate in football. The NCAA recommends a thorough medical examination when the athlete first enters the college athletic program and an annual health history update with use of referral exams when warranted. If the physician or coach has any questions about the athlete's readiness to participate, the athlete should not be allowed to play. High school coaches should follow the recommendations set by their State High School Athletic Associations.

2. All personnel concerned with training football athletes should emphasize proper, gradual, and complete physical conditioning. Particular emphasis should be placed on neck strengthening exercises.

3. A physician should be present at all games and practice sessions. If it is impossible for a physician to be present at all practice sessions, emergency measures must be provided.

4. All personnel associated with football participation should be cognizant of the problems and safety measures related to physical activity in hot weather.

5. Each institution should strive to have a team trainer who is a regular member of the faculty and is adequately prepared and qualified.

6. Cooperative liaison should be maintained by all groups interested in the field of Athletic Medicine (coaches, trainers, physicians, manufacturers, administrators, and so forth).

7. There should be strict enforcement of game rules, and administrative regulations should be enforced to protect the health of the athlete. Coaches and school officials must support the game officials in their conduct of the athletic contests.

8. There should be a renewed emphasis on employing well-trained athletic personnel, providing excellent facilities, and securing the safest and best equipment possible.

9. There should be continued research concerning the safety factor in football (rules, facilities, equipment, and so forth).

10. Coaches should continue to teach and emphasize the proper fundamentals of blocking and tackling to help reduce head and neck fatalities. *Keep the head out of football!*

11. Strict enforcement of the rules of the game by both coaches and officials will help reduce serious injuries.

12. When a player has experienced or shown signs of head trauma (loss of consciousness, visual disturbances, headache, inability to walk correctly, obvious disorientation, or memory loss), he should receive immediate medical attention and should not be allowed to return to practice or game without permission from the proper medical authorities.

Case Studies Direct Fatalities

High School

A 17-year-old high school football player suffered a severe brain injury while trying to break the wedge on a kick-off. The accident took place in a game on September 28, 2001. The player had a previous concussion on September 15, 2001. Cause of death was second impact syndrome brain injury.

A 16-year-old high school running back was injured on November 15, 2001, while being tackled in a game. Cause of death was a fractured cervical vertebra.

A 17-year-old high school running back was injured on August 30, 2001, while being tackled returning a kick-off. He received a severe brain injury and died on August 31, 2001.

A 17-year-old high school quarterback was injured in the first quarter of a game on October 13, 2001. After contact he fell on the ball and had a ruptured spleen. He died the same day from the ruptured spleen.

A 17-year-old defensive end was injured in a game on October 20, 2001. Cause of death was a subdural hematoma

A 15-year-old high school running back was injured in a game on October 30, 2001, while being tackled. He received a severe brain injury and cause of death was a subdural hematoma.

An 18-year-old high school football player was injured in a game on September 7, 2001. He was a linebacker making a tackle and the knee of the running back hit him in the top of the head. Cause of death was a subdural hematoma. He died on September 15, 2001.

Sandlot

An 11-year-old Pop Warner football player was tackled in a game while running back the kick-off. After being tackled his head struck the ground. The injury took place on October 3, 2001. Cause of death was a brain injury.

Case Studies Indirect Fatalities

High School

A 14-year-old high school football player collapsed and died at practice on June 20, 2001. Cause of death was heart-related.

A 13-year-old middle school football player collapsed at practice on August 15, 2001. He died later at the hospital. Cause of death was a defective coronary artery.

A 14-year-old high school football player collapsed at practice on August 19, 2001. He later died of hypertrophic cardiomyopathy.

A 17-year-old high school football player collapsed at practice on November 12, 2001. He died later that day. The player had failed a physical exam earlier in year but was later cleared to play by a cardiologist. Cause of death was heart-related.

A middle school football player collapsed while running laps and later died. The accident happened on September 24, 2001. Cause of death was heart-related.

A 16-year-old high school football player died of unknown causes on May 17, 2001. He collapsed at practice.

A 17-year-old high school football player died of heatstroke on August 1, 2001. The player was six feet tall and weighed 220 pounds. The accident happened on the second day of practice during a non-contact workout. The temperature was in the 90s with high humidity.

A 15-year-old high school football player died after returning home from a morning practice on August 19, 2001. Cause of death was heart-related.

A 16-year-old high school football player collapsed during a game on October 12, 2001. He had made a tackle three plays before collapsing. Cause of death was unknown.

A 14-year-old high school football player collapsed before practice on September 12, 2001. Cause of death was unknown.

College

A 22-year-old college football player collapsed during summer conditioning drills on August 3, 2001. He was six feet tall and weighed 212 pounds. Cause of death was exercise induced asthma.

An 18-year-old college football player died during summer conditioning drills on July 25, 2001. Cause of death was heatstroke. The player was six feet two inches tall and weighed 255 pounds.

An 18-year-old college football player died after a morning workout on February 26, 2001. Possible cause of death was listed as sickle cell trait.

Professional

A 35-year-old semi-professional football player collapsed and died in the locker room after a game. The player had no physical examination and there was no medical help available at the game. Cause of death was unknown.

A 27-year-old professional football player died of heatstroke on July 31, 2001. The accident took place at 11:30 AM in 99 degree weather. The player also weighed over 300 pounds and was affected by the heat the day before.

Annual Survey of Catastrophic Football Injuries 1977– 2000

In 1977 the National Collegiate Athletic Association initiated funding for the First Annual Survey of Catastrophic Football Injuries. Frederick O. Mueller, Ph.D., and Carl S. Blyth, Ph.D., both professors in the Department of Physical Education at the University of North Carolina at Chapel Hill were selected to conduct the research. The research is now being conducted as part of the National Center for Catastrophic Sports Injury Research, University of North Carolina at Chapel Hill, Frederick O. Mueller, Director and Robert C. Cantu, Medical Director.

The *Annual Survey of Catastrophic Football Injuries* was part of a concerted effort put forth by many individuals and research organizations to reduce the steady increase of football head and neck injuries taking place during the 1960s and 1970s. The primary purpose of the research was and is to make the game of football a safer sport.

Data Collection

Since 1977 and the initiation of this research, catastrophic injuries were defined as football injuries which resulted in brain or spinal cord injury or skull or spine fracture. It should be noted that all cases involved some disability at the time of the injury. Neurological recovery is either complete or incomplete (quadriplegia or quadriparesis). Yearly follow-up is not done, thus neurological status (complete or incomplete recovery) refers to when the athlete is entered into the registry which is usually two to three months after injury. Injuries which result in death are not included in this report.

Data were complied with the assistance of high school and college coaches, athletic directors, school administrators, physicians, athletic trainers, executive officers of state and national athletic organizations, sporting goods dealers and manufacturers' representatives, a national newspaper clipping service, and professional associates of the researchers. Data collection would have been impossible without the help of the National Federation of State High School Associations and the National Collegiate Athletic Association. The research was funded by a grant provided by the National Collegiate Athletic Association.

Upon receiving information concerning a possible catastrophic football injury, contact by telephone, personal letter, and questionnaire is made with the injured player's coach, physician, and athletic director. The questionnaire provides background data on the athlete (age, height, weight, experience, previous injury, etc.), accident information, immediate and post-accident treatment, and equipment data.

In 1987, a joint endeavor was initiated with the section on Sports Medicine of the American Association of Neurological Surgeons. The purpose of this collaboration was to enhance the collection of medical data. Dr. Robert C. Cantu, Chairman, Department of Surgery and Chief, Neurosurgery Service, Emerson Hospital, in Concord, MA, and the Medical Director of the National Center for Catastrophic Sports Injury Research has been responsible for collecting the medical data.

Background

An early investigation into serious head and neck football injuries was conducted by Schneider.[1] He reported 30 permanent cervical spinal cord injuries in high school and college football during the period from 1959–1963. A later study by Torg indicated a total of 99 permanent cervical spinal cord injuries in high school and college football from 1971–1975.[3] Torg has discontinued his research, but his data show a decline in permanent cervical cord injuries in high school and college from 34 cases in 1976 to 5 cases in 1984. A study published in 1976 reported the incidence of neck injuries based on roentgenographic evidence was as high as 32% in a sample of 104 high school students and 75 college freshmen in Iowa.[2]

In order to help alleviate this problem the National Collegiate Athletic Association and the National Federation of State High School Associations implemented rule changes in 1976 to prohibit using the head as the initial contact point when blocking and tackling. Furthermore, the American Football Coaches Association Ethics Committee went on record opposing this type of blocking and tackling. Emphasis on complete physical examinations and improved physical conditioning programs have also been recommended to mitigate the injury issue.

Discussion

For the past 24 years there have been a total of 217 football players with incomplete neurological recovery from cervical cord injuries.

One hundred and seventy-seven of these injuries have been to high school players, twenty-nine to college players, four to sandlot players, and seven to professionals. This data indicates a reduction in the number of cervical cord injuries with incomplete neurological recovery when compared to data published in the early 1970s. While the 1995, 1996, and 1997 data suggested a gradual increase in these types of injuries, the 1998 data showed a reduction. The 1999 and 2000 data show an increase to nine and eight respectively. The numbers remain in single digits, but the increase to nine and eight is a concern. The six cerebral injuries with incomplete recovery is a slight increase from the four in 1999. Since 1984 there were 77 cerebral injuries with incomplete recovery. These numbers also are a concern, and if the cervical cord injuries and the cerebral injuries with incomplete recovery are combined, the number of incomplete recovery injuries is 294. That is an average of 12 for the past 24 years. Coaches, players, trainers, physicians, and administrators must continue the emphasis on eliminating paralyzing injuries to football players.

The latest participation figures show 1,500,000 players participating in junior and senior high school football and 75,000 in college football. The incidence rate per 100,000 participants is less than one per 100,000 at the high school level and 2.66 at the college level. In looking at the incidence rates for the past 24 years, the high school incidence is 0.53 per 100,000 participants and the college incidence is 1.61 per 100,000 participants.

As indicated in past reports a majority of the permanent cervical cord injuries are taking place in games. In 2000 seven of the injuries took place in games and one in practice.

When comparing cervical cord injuries to offensive and defensive players, it is safer playing offensive football. During the 24 year period from 1977–2000, 153 (70.5%) of the 217 players with cervical cord injuries were playing defense. A majority of the defensive players were tackling when injured. In 2000, five of the eight injured players were tackling. Coaches have indicated that their players have been taught to tackle with the head up, but for some reason many of the players are lowering their heads before making contact. Fifty-three or 24.4% of the injured players were tackling with the head in a down position (chin to chest and contact with the top or crown of the helmet). These are the only players we are sure had their heads down, but it is possible that there were others tackling with the head down. In addition to tackling with the head down, ball carriers are being injured with their heads in a down position while being tackled. It is important for coaches to emphasize head up tackling, but it is also important to emphasize head up blocking and head up ball carrying when being tackled. Many coaches teach their ball carriers to lower the head before being tackled and to run over the tackler, but this can be a dangerous activity and can cause cervical spine and cerebral injuries with incomplete recovery.

Past reports have revealed that defensive backs were injured at a higher rate than other positions. In 2000 four of the injured players were defensive backs, two were ball carriers, one was a quarterback, and one was a tight end.

In 2000 there were five subdural hematoma injuries with incomplete neurological recovery. Four of the injuries were at the high school level and one at the college level. There was also one fractured skull with incomplete neurological recovery at the high school. In addition to the injuries with incomplete recovery, there were 12 injuries with complete recovery. The high school injuries included three brain injuries, four cervical spine fractures, and three cervical spine contusions. College injuries with complete recovery included one brain injury and one cervical spine contusion.

Recommendations

As stated in earlier reports, there has been a reduction of permanent cervical cord injuries when compared to data from the early 1970s. The 1995, 1996, and 1997 data indicated an increase, but were fewer than the early 1970s. The 1991 and 1994 data show a dramatic reduction to one permanent cervical cord injury in high school football. That was a great accomplishment and every effort should be made to continue that trend. For the past ten years, including 2000, there has been an average of 6.8 cervical cord injuries with incomplete neurological recovery, and 4.9 cerebral injuries with incomplete recovery in football. The eight cerebral injuries in 1997 were the highest number since we started to collect this data in 1984.

The initial reduction of permanent disability injuries was the result of efforts put forth by the total athletic community concerned with safety of football participants. Major areas of emphasis that once again should receive attention are the 1976 rule change that eliminated the head as the initial point of contact during blocking and tackling, improved medical care both at the game site and in medical facilities, improved coaching techniques in teaching the fundamentals of tackling and blocking, and the increased concern and awareness of football coaches.

A concerted effort must be made to continue the reduction of cervical spine and cerebral injuries and to aim for the elimination of these injuries. Following are several suggestions for reducing these catastrophic injuries:

1. Rule changes initiated for the 1976 football season which eliminated the head as a primary and initial contact area for blocking and tackling are of utmost importance. Coaches should drill the players in the proper execution of the fundamentals of football—particularly blocking and tackling. *Shoulder block and tackle with the head up—Keep the head out of football.*

2. Athletes must be given proper conditioning exercises which will strengthen their necks in order to be able to hold their heads firmly erect while making contact during a tackle or block. Strengthening of the neck muscles may also protect the neck from injury.

3. Coaches and officials should discourage the players from using their heads as battering rams when blocking, tackling, and ball carrying. The rules prohibiting spearing should be enforced in practice and games. The players should be taught to respect the helmet as a protective device and that the helmet should not be used as a weapon. Ball carriers should also be taught not to lower their heads when making contact with the tackler.

4. Football officials can play a major role in reducing catastrophic football injuries. The use of the helmet-face mask in making initial contact while blocking and tackling is illegal and should be called for a penalty. Officials should concentrate on helmet-face mask contact and call the penalty. If more of these penalties are called there is no doubt that both players and coaches will get the message and discontinue this type of play. A reduction in helmet-face mask contact will result in a reduction of catastrophic football injuries.

5. All coaches, physicians, and trainers should take special care to see that the players' equipment is properly fitted, particularly the helmet.

6. It is important, whenever possible, for a physician to be on the field of play during game and practice. When this is not possible, arrangements must be made in advance to obtain a physician's immediate services when emergencies arise. Each

institution should have a team trainer who is a regular member of the institution's staff and who is qualified in the emergency care of both treating and preventing injuries.

7. Coaches must be prepared for a possible catastrophic head or neck injury. Everyone involved must know what to do. Being prepared and knowing what to do may be the difference that prevents permanent disability. Have a written emergency plan and give copies to all personnel. Areas that should be covered are, 1) an evacuation plan, 2) available transportation, 3) portable and open communication, and 4) game/practice schedule awareness in local hospital emergency department.

8. When a player has experienced or shown signs of head trauma (loss of consciousness, visual disturbances, headache, inability to walk correctly, obvious disorientation, or memory loss), he should receive immediate medical attention and should not be allowed to return to practice or game without permission from the proper medical authorities.

9. Both past and present data show that the football helmet does not cause cervical spine injuries but that poorly executed tackling and blocking technique is the major problem.

Football catastrophic injuries may never be totally eliminated, but continued research has resulted in rule changes, equipment standards, improved medical care both on and off the playing field, and changes in teaching the fundamental techniques of the game. These changes were the result of a united effort by coaches, administrators, researchers, equipment manufacturers, physicians, trainers, and players.

Research based on reliable data is essential if progress is to be made. Research provides data that indicate the problems and reveal the adequacy of preventive measures.

References

1. Schneider, R.C.: *Head and Neck Injuries in Football*. Baltimore, William and Wilkins Co., 1973.

2. Albright, J.P., Moses, J.M., Feldick, H.G., et al.: Nonfatal Cervical Spine Injuries in Interscholastic Football. *JAMA* 236: 1243 - 1245, 1976.

3. Torg, J.S., Trues, R., Quedenfeld, T.C., et al.: The National Football Head and Neck Injury Registry. *JAMA* 241: 1477 - 1479, 1979.

4. Mueller, F.O., Schindler, R.D.: *Annual Survey of Football Injury Research 1931 - 1996.* National Collegiate Athletic Association, National Federation of State High School Associations and the American Football Coaches Association, 1997.

Catastrophic Injury Case Studies

High School

A high school football player was injured while being tackled in a game in September 2000. His fourth cervical vertebra was fractured and the athlete is quadriplegic.

A 17-year-old high school football player was injured making a headfirst tackle during a game on September 8, 2000. He had a four-hour surgery to fuse the fourth and fifth vertebrae. The athlete is quadriplegic.

A 16-year-old high school football player was injured during a game on September 22, 2000. He was playing quarterback and was injured after an awkward fall. The athlete is quadriplegic.

A 16-year-old high school football player was injured in a game on September 13, 2000. He was playing tight end and was injured while being tackled. The athlete is quadriplegic.

A 17-year-old high school football player was injured in a practice on November 8, 2000. He fractured a cervical vertebra while making a tackle. The athlete is quadriplegic.

An 18-year-old high school football player was injured in a game on December 9, 2000. He was a defensive back and was injured when colliding with an opposing player. The opposing player's helmet struck the athlete in the shoulder. He suffered complete avulsion of three nerve roots to his arm and has lost the use of his right arm.

A 17-year-old high school football player was injured during a game on September 15, 2000. He collapsed during the game from a head injury. The injury was a subdural hematoma and the athlete has short-term memory losses and weakness on the right side of his body.

A 17-year-old high school football player was injured during a game on October 6, 2000 while being tackled. The athlete suffered a brain injury, had surgery, was in critical condition, and recovery is incomplete.

A 15-year-old junior high school football player was injured in a game on September 28, 2000. He came to the sideline complaining of a headache, collapsed, and lost consciousness. He suffered brain trauma and recovery was incomplete.

A 16-year-old high school football player suffered a subdural hematoma during a game on September 8, 2000. He was making a tackle and a second tackler hit him head to head. The athlete had a concussion one-week prior to the injury. Recovery was incomplete.

A 16-year-old high school football player was injured in a summer passing league when he ran into another player and suffered a fractured skull. The players were not wearing helmets. He was in a coma for nine days. Recovery is incomplete.

A 16-year-old high school football player was injured during a tackling drill in practice in September 2000. He suffered an aneurysm, had surgery, and had a full recovery. He also suffered a concussion during the previous spring football practice. He will not play anymore football.

A 17-year-old running back was injured in a game while being tackled. He had surgery for a blood clot. Recovery was complete but he will not play anymore football.

A high school football player was injured after being hit by an opposing player. He complained of a headache the next day and was taken to a physician. He had surgery for a fractured cervical vertebra and had full recovery.

A 17-year-old high school football player fractured his 4th and 5th cervical vertebrae while making a tackle in a game on November 24, 2000. He had surgery and a full recovery.

A 16-year-old high school football player was injured in a game while making a tackle. He made the initial hit and other defensive players joined in the tackle. He fractured three cervical vertebrae, had surgery, and recovery was complete.

A high school football player was injured in a game on August 8, 2000 after being tackled by two defenders. He fractured a cervical vertebra and recovery was complete.

A 14-year-old high school football player was hit on the helmet by a tackler after catching a pass. He had transient paralysis for several days before a full recovery.

A high school football player suffered transient paralysis and returned to play three weeks later. No other information was available.

A high school football player was injured in a game and suffered bruises to his neck and spine. He experienced initial paralysis but had a full recovery.

An 18-year-old high school running back was tackled in a game on September 8, 2000. He suffered a torn peroneal nerve and has ankle and foot paralysis.

A high school football player suffered a fractured cervical vertebra while tackling with his head down in a game. The game was played in September of 1997. Recovery was complete.

A high school football player was tackling with his head down during a game in 1998. He fractured a cervical vertebra and recovery was complete.

A 17-year-old high school football player was injured in a game on September 3, 1998. He fractured the 6th cervical vertebra and recovery was complete.

An eighth grade football player suffered a broken blood vessel in his brain during an eighth grade game. He was in a coma for two weeks and recovery was incomplete. The game was played in September of 1999.

A 16-year-old high school football player was injured in a game on September 3, 1999. He was being tackled and bruised his spinal cord. He has recovered but will not play anymore football.

A 15-year-old high school football player was injured while being blocked head to head on a punt return. He was unconscious for approximately four minutes. He was injured on September 9, 1999 and has fully recovered.

College

A 22-year-old college football player was injured in a game on October 28, 2000, while tackling in a game. He suffered damage to cervical vertebrae 1 and 2 and is quadriplegic.

A 20-year-old college football player collapsed during the first spring football practice. He had emergency surgery to repair a blood clot on the brain and two collapsed lungs. Recovery was incomplete.

An 18-year-old college football player was injured while making a tackle in a game on September 23, 2000. He suffered a fractured cervical vertebra and recovery was incomplete.

A 21-year-old college defensive back was injured while making a tackle in a game on October 7, 2000. He suffered a brain hemorrhage and had surgery. Recovery was complete and he was cleared to play again, but most likely will not play.

A college football player suffered a spinal contusion in a game on September 20, 2000. Recover was complete. No other information was available.

A 20-year-old college football player suffered an open fracture of the tibia and fibula in a game on October 14, 2000. He had a severe infection of the leg and had to have his right lower leg amputated.

Chapter 19

Soccer Injuries Hit Below the Belt

Soccer is the most participated sport in the world and one of the most popular sports in this country. The World Cup tournament in France only increases the interest in the sport. Participation in soccer is great fun and excellent exercise. Unfortunately, injuries do occur, and they most commonly occur below the belt line.

Hip injuries usually involve muscles and tendons because the hip flexors generate kicking power. Muscle and tendon strains occur from over-contraction and over-stretching of the hip flexors. Treatment involves rest, ice, anti-inflammatory medication, and possibly a rehabilitation program. Before returning to action, a compression wrap or compression shorts are also helpful.

Knee injuries are common in soccer. Most soccer injuries are non-contact, involving twisting stress to the knee. A moderately significant twist can tear the meniscus, commonly referred to as "cartilage." Meniscus tears cause a small or moderate amount of swelling, possibly locking or catching of the joint, and a sharp pain on the side of the knee. Treatment of significant meniscus tears usually requires arthroscopy. Arthroscopy involves looking inside the joint with a small

---

"Soccer Injuries Hit Below the Belt," by Donald Zoltan, M.D., Orthopedic Surgeon, © Sports Medicine Performance Center of St. Francis Hospital, Milwaukee, Wisconsin, reprinted with permission; and "Injuries during Competitive Youth Soccer—Abstract," by Selim Suner, *Academic Emergency Medicine* Volume 8, Number 5, p.457, © 2001 Society for Academic Emergency Medicine, reprinted with permission.

telescope about half the diameter of a pen. Through small incisions, the meniscus tear can be repaired or partially removed.

A more severe twisting injury to the knee can cause a tear of the anterior cruciate ligament (ACL). The ACL is the most important stabilizing ligament in the knee. If this ligament is torn, the knee usually blows up like a balloon. Left untreated, ACL tears will likely cause significant problems with instability of the knee.

Athletes that wish to return to soccer and other twisting sports should strongly consider surgical reconstruction of the ligament. The procedure requires a significant investment of time and rehabilitation, but has a high success rate in returning the athlete to action.

Finally, ankle injuries, usually sprains also occur. As with most musculoskeletal injuries, the initial treatment involves rest, ice, compression, and elevation (R.I.C.E.). A rehabilitation program is also very important. Stretching, strengthening, and balance retraining are critical to reducing the risk of re-injury.

Participating in soccer provides great exercise and coordination. It is an excellent way to experience the fun of teamwork and competition. However, injuries can occur and when they do, they usually hit below the belt.

Injuries during Competitive Youth Soccer

Objectives: To implement an injury tracking system, and to identify and describe injury patterns in competitive youth soccer.

Methods: A prospective observational study was conducted in 2 consecutive youth (ages 11-19) soccer tournaments in July 1999 and 2000 with 8,000 athletes competing in 846 games. All visits to the medical facility (MF) were recorded on standardized forms including detailed description of injury. Treatment was provided by members of a team comprised of EMTs, nurses, resident and attending emergency physicians in an on-site field MF. All patients with injury and illness were initially taken to the MF.

Results: A total of 251 patients, 54% female, were treated. Of these, 213 (85%), with a mean age of 15.9 +/- 2.8 years, were athletes from games in progress. Rate of injury was 26 per 1,000 athletes and 0.25 per game. 23 patients (11%) required transportation to hospitals, of whom 4 (2%) were admitted. Concussion (13%), fractures (28, 13%), sprains (59, 28%), soft-tissue injury (80, 38%), and heat illness (27, 13%) accounted for most visits. Three patients (1%) had significant abdominal trauma (splenic laceration, pancreatic injury, and duodenal hematoma), all from a kick by the opponent. Seventy-eight (43%) of the injuries were caused by the opponent, 27 (15%) by falls, 13 (7%) by the ball, and 64 (35%) were self-induced (tripping, twisting, turning, etc.). Fourteen (7%) of the injuries were incurred while jumping for a header. Contact with the opponent (CWO) was associated with injury to the abdomen, head, and lower extremity (Fisher's exact p=0.027, p=0.02, p=0.01, respectively). Falls were associated with injury to the upper extremity and contact with the ball with head injury (Fisher's exact p=0.038 and p<0.0001, respectively). Recurrent injury was present in 17% of patients.

Conclusions: Rate of injury is high among youth athletes during competitive soccer tournaments. Contact with the opponent and headers accounted for most of the significant injuries and should be considered as targets for injury prevention initiatives.

Chapter 20

Bicycle Injuries

In 1996, more than half a million people were treated in emergency departments for bicycle-related injuries. Seventy-three percent were children and teens under age 21. In 1997, 813 bicyclists—31% of them under age 16—were killed in crashes with motor vehicles, an increase of 7% over the previous year. Only 3% of those killed were wearing helmets.

The Scope of the Problem

- About 67 million Americans ride bicycles; half of them are children or teenagers.

- Children account for one-third of the nation's hours spent riding, one-third of bicycle-related deaths, and two-thirds of bicycle-related injuries. Bicycles are associated with more childhood injuries than any other consumer product except motor vehicles.

- A review of hospital discharge data in Washington State found that nonfatal bicycle injuries among children age 14 and under cost more than $113 million each year.

- Among children age 14 and under, more than 80% of bicycle-related deaths are associated with the bicyclist's behavior—for example, riding into a street without stopping, swerving into

"Bicycle-Related Injuries," *Fact Book for the Year 2000*, National Center for Injury Prevention and Control, 2000.

traffic that is coming from behind, running a stop sign, or riding against the flow of traffic.

- An estimated 127,000 children and teens (under age 21) and 29,200 adults are treated each year in emergency departments for injuries to the brain, face, eye, or ear sustained while bicycling. Of these, about 33,000 are traumatic brain injuries such as concussions and hemorrhages—almost 80% are sustained by children.

- Head injuries are the leading cause of death in crashes with motor vehicles and the most important determinant of permanent disability. A helmet is the single most effective safety device available to reduce injury to the brain and upper face from bicycle crashes, but relatively few riders wear them.

- Only 25% of children ages 5 to 14 wear a helmet when riding. The most common complaints from young riders are that helmets are not fashionable or cool, that their friends don't wear them, and that helmets are uncomfortable (usually too hot).

- The Healthy People 2010 goal is to have 50% of ninth- through twelfth-graders wear bicycle helmets when they ride. The current percentage is close to zero.

Working Toward a Solution

- CDC-funded extramural research has demonstrated that wearing a bicycle helmet reduces the risk of head injury by 85% and the risk of traumatic brain injury by 88%.

- Researchers found that if every rider wore a helmet, 500 deaths and 151,000 nonfatal head injuries could be prevented each year. That's more than one death per day and one nonfatal head injury every 4 minutes.

- Some evidence suggests that legislative efforts related to helmet use are more effective than school or community programs alone. By early 1999, 15 states and more than 65 local governments had enacted some form of bicycle-helmet legislation; most pertain to children and adolescents. These laws help increase helmet use among all income groups, but especially among high-income families.

- Measures should be developed to prevent crashes between bicycles and motor vehicles. Strategies include traffic and road engineering (e.g., building speed bumps and creating bike lanes or paths) and educating drivers and riders on the rules of sharing the road safely.

- NCIPC funds bicycle safety programs in 15 communities throughout California, Colorado, Florida, Oklahoma, and Rhode Island. The multifaceted programs coordinate education, helmet giveaways, and other efforts to promote bicycle safety and increased helmet use, especially among children ages 5 to 12. Evaluation conducted halfway through the three-year projects has shown promising results.

- In some communities, helmet use doubled.

- Helmet use among all communities was 51%, double the national average and exceeding the Healthy People 2010 objective.

- Collectively, these programs have provided helmets to more than 36,000 children, supported helmet legislation and ordinances, educated more than 30,000 children at school or in the community, and mounted bicycle safety awareness campaigns that have reached more than 200,000 households.

- In Florida, where a statewide helmet-use law is in effect, some school policies mandate helmet use. Preliminary data from a 1999 survey by the Florida Bicycle Safety Program found that children in that state are 8 times more likely to wear a helmet while riding to or from school if they live in a county that mandates helmet use.

These bicycle safety programs have demonstrated the following: a multifaceted approach is more effective than a single intervention; state or local laws increase helmet use; helmet give-aways are most effective when accompanied by safety education and instruction on proper helmet fit; and helmet use is increased by such programs across a wide range of socioeconomic groups, although the programs require several years to reach their maximum potential.

- NCIPC and the National Highway Traffic Safety Administration, U.S. Department of Transportation, co-chair the National Bicycle Safety Network (NBSN), a group of about 20 federal, nonprofit, and advocacy agencies and organizations that support efforts to promote bicycle safety and increase the number of riders to promote physical activity. To share information more effectively among member organizations and the people they serve, NBSN created a web site called the Bike Hub (www.cdc.gov/ncipc/bike). The site provides information on safety programs, legislation, research, and technical aspects of bicycle helmets. In May 1999, NBSN sponsored a national, grassroots youth safety campaign during Bicycle Safety Month. The program culminated in a bike rodeo in front of the U.S. Capitol, with several members of Congress in attendance.

- A project at the University of Washington will develop and evaluate a bicycle helmet promotion intervention in King County, Washington, targeting young adolescents ages 12 to 14. The program will use community-based coalitions to increase bicycle helmet use and reduce bicycle-related head injuries among this group.

- To find clues to the nature and severity of head impacts, small business researchers are using computerized tomography scanning to image the internal structure of a damaged helmet. The outcome of this research will be the development of a common method for assessing helmet damage, which should greatly enhance the ability to define head protection standards for head gear.

- A study at the University of Alabama to determine perceptions of caregivers of children that relate to bicycle safety and their provision of proper safety gear for their children found that caregivers perceive the dangers associated with bicycling but are not aware of available programs and methods that prevent risk. This study resulted in recommendations to improve comprehensive education on bicycle safety for caregivers and also urged health professionals to educate caregivers of children about bicycle safety in routine health care visits.

- Researchers from the University of North Carolina will evaluate a law in British Columbia that requires all cyclists regardless of age to wear helmets. Data from an observational survey of helmet use before the law will be compared with survey data after the law was implemented to determine changes in correct and incorrect helmet use as well as changes in the amount of bicycling.

Additional Information

National Center for Injury Prevention and Control
Mailstop K65
4770 Buford Highway NE
Atlanta, GA 30341-3724

Tel: 770-488-1506
Fax: 770-488-1667
Website: www.cdc.gov/ncipc
E-mail: OHCINFO@cdc.gov

National Bike Safety Network
Website: *The Bike Hub* at www.cdc.gov/ncipc/bike

Chapter 21

Running and Jogging Injuries

Aerobic exercise has become one of the most popular forms of endurance training today. In the United States, the most popular forms of aerobic exercise are running and jogging (jogging is a slow, rhythmic form of running). In fact, it is estimated that 15% of Americans run, jog, or walk regularly.

The aim of aerobic conditioning is to improve the function and efficiency of the cardiovascular system. To be effective, exercise must be at a pace great enough to reach 75-80% of the maximum heart rate and continued for least 25 minutes. It is not necessary to exercise everyday to obtain the maximum aerobic effect. Three to four times per week is sufficient.

Some of the benefits of jogging or distance running include:

- Prevention or postponement of coronary disease
- Personal gratification and enjoyment
- Low cost sport that both sexes can enjoy and participate

An unfortunate by-product of this broad interest in running has been the growing incidence of injury. The primary causes seem to be lack of adherence to proper training techniques, wearing improper footwear, and initial poor conditioning, which then leads to overuse injuries.

"Preventing Running and Jogging Injuries," Matthew Matava, MD, consultant, revised 2001, © American Orthopaedic Society for Sports Medicine, reprinted with permission.

Causes of Running Injuries

Most running injuries tend to be caused by a few recurring factors including shoe problems, training errors, environmental factors, or anatomic abnormalities that can predispose an athlete to certain injuries. As a result, runners can directly prevent the majority (60-70%) of running and jogging injuries.

Shoes

An appropriate running shoe is very important in training and may help prevent running injuries. Shoes should provide shock absorption, motion control, and stability for the runner. When selecting a running shoe, the athlete should look for a style that will provide all of the above benefits as well as fit comfortably. Fortunately, all of the major shoe brands make a shoe appropriate for the vast majority of runners.

Laboratory studies that analyzed an athlete's gait (pattern of walking or running) have determined that during running on level surfaces, the forces exerted on the lower extremities are two to three times body weight. Under this heavy pounding, shoes will lose approximately 60% or more of their shock absorption capability after 250-500 miles of use. A runner who puts in 10 miles per week, therefore, should consider buying new shoes after nine to 12 months. When a shoe's mileage exceeds 500-600 miles, it should be discarded for running purposes. Resoling will not revitalize the dead shoe. Sole wear should also be checked regularly because it can be an indicator of other problems.

Training Errors

The rule of too's: Too much, too fast, too soon, and too little rest appear to be the hallmarks of training errors. Every runner has a physiologic limit and trying to exceed that limit can lead to injury. The mileage one runs should be gradually increased, on an individual basis. A good rule of thumb is 10% per week. Overall, injuries are most likely to occur in one or more of the following situations:

- Over distancing without adequate stretching

- Rapid changes in mileage

- An increase in hill training

- Interval training (going from slow speeds over long distances to fast speeds covering less ground)

- Insufficient rest between training sessions

Anatomic Abnormalities

Preexisting structural or biomechanical problems such as a high foot arch, a limb length discrepancy, scoliosis (curvature of the spine), or excessive muscle tightness, may increase a runner's susceptibility to injury during intense training. The athlete can compensate for these abnormalities by following special training guidelines, incorporating a stretching regimen into the conditioning program, and the use of semi-rigid orthotics (shoe inserts). Following are some common physical abnormalities that can lead to running injuries.

Ankle laxity (joint instability) can lead to frequent ankle sprains and pain. Beneficial treatment includes muscle strengthening to increase stability, shoe modification to alter gait, and change of a running surface.

Knee joint and kneecap (patellofemoral) injuries are common sites of overuse injuries. A twenty-minute ice massage to the involved area, stretching of the hamstring and quadriceps muscles, a program of strengthening exercises, and a short course of an over-the-counter anti-inflammatory medication may also be added.

Foot problems in runners are related to foot types. Non-operative treatment such as orthotics and shoe modifications should be used if necessary.

Hip and back injuries account for a smaller but growing number of running injuries and should be treated on an individual basis.

Environmental Factors

Running is a flexible exercise that can be done anywhere and anytime. However, the runner is often faced with a variety of environmental factors—such as terrain, altitude, temperature variations, and air quality—that can adversely affect performance and physical health.

The same runner will recognize potential environmental problems and make adjustment in training routines, terrain, clothing, and fluid intake to reduce the risk of injury.

In choosing a place to run, keep in mind that the ideal surface on which to run is flat, smooth, resilient, and reasonably soft.

Avoid concrete or rough road surfaces. If possible, use community trails that have been developed specifically for jogging and running; they usually have the appropriate surface and are isolated from vehicular traffic and poor air quality.

Hills should be avoided at first because of the increased stress placed on joints and muscles. The ankle and foot are stressed most by running uphill, while downhill running stresses the knee and lower leg. For the competitive runner, hills often cannot be avoided, so care should be taken when running on such terrain.

Temperature variation, air quality, and altitude are significant environmental factors affecting the runner. During warmer, humid weather, take care to increase fluid intake, in cool weather, dress appropriately. It is often helpful to weigh yourself before and after running on a hot, humid day. One pint of water should be consumed for every pound of weight lost. Avoid running during temperature extremes—both hot and cold—or when the air pollution levels are high. The entire body is stressed by exercising in these conditions and the risk of injury is increased. When running at higher altitudes, the runner should gradually acclimate to the lower oxygen levels by slow, steady increases in speed and distance.

Common Running and Jogging Injuries

Foot

Plantar Fasciitis—Inflammation of the fibrous connective tissue of the sole of the foot. It is a common cause of low-grade, insidious heel pain. Treatment consists of activity modification, nonsteroidal anti-inflammatory medications, stretching exercises to the heel and foot, ice massage, and use of a soft heel pad.

Metatarsalgia—Pain in the region of the five long bones (metatarsals) of the foot (ball of the foot). Its causes may be excessive pressure on the ball of the foot, abnormality in foot type or metatarsal phalangeal joint, and stress fractures. Treatment includes use of orthotics if necessary, activity modification, and change to a softer running surface.

Stress fracture—A complete or incomplete hairline break in a foot bone resulting from abnormal stress to normal bone. It usually occurs in the heel and forefoot/midfoot bones and results from fatigue or stress produced by frequent, repeated physical activity (overuse). It constitutes 10% or more of all running injures. Treatment consists of rest or immobilization. Running should be resumed gradually after four to six weeks.

Posterior tibial tendinitis—Inflammation of the tendon behind the inner heel. Treatment consists of activity modification, ice massage, aspirin, and, occasionally, shoe appliance.

Leg

Stress fracture—A complete or incomplete hairline break in the fibula or tibia. It results in localized pain over the affected bone. Treatment includes activity modification, use of an orthotic with a stirrup or possible immobilization with a cast or brace. Gradual return to running or jogging, after four to six weeks, will allow the fracture to heal.

Exertional compartment syndromes—Caused by overuse of leg muscles resulting in decreased blood supply to a particular group (compartment) of muscles. Treatment consists of rest or, in severe cases, surgery to relieve the pressure constricting the leg muscles.

Achilles tendinitis—Inflammation of the heel tendon producing pain and tightness in the calf of the leg is caused by repetitive overuse of the Achilles tendon typically from running up hills. The condition may become incapacitating particularly to the competitive athlete. Treatment includes rest until acute inflammation subsides, Achilles stretching, ice massage, anti-inflammatory medication, and shoe appliance such as heel lifts to relieve tension on the tendon.

Medial tibial stress syndrome (shin splints)—Pain in the lower leg due to inflammation of the lining surrounding the shin bone. This is usually caused by an imbalance in calf muscle strength. Treatment consists of discontinuing exercise until the athlete is able to resume without pain, icing of the affected area, stretching, and occasionally taping of the leg to relieve tension on the lining of the bone.

Knee

Patellofemoral joint pain—As one of the most common injuries that affect runners, it centers on the kneecap (patella). Its onset is usually insidious and related to increased mileage, a change in terrain, or a change in running shoe. Treatment consists of anti-inflammatory medication, alteration in running terrain (avoidance of hills), and strengthening exercises for the quadriceps muscles (the four divisions of muscles at the front of the thigh).

Internal derangements—Tearing of internal structures such as the meniscus (cartilage) will cause pain, swelling, joint locking, and giving way. It is a rare injury in runners.

Tendinitis—Inflammation resulting in pain and tenderness in one of the tendons surrounding the knee. Tendinitis is usually caused by overuse. Treatment includes rest until the acute symptoms subside, icing, stretching, and anti-inflammatory medication. The conditions can become chronic if not treated.

Thigh and Pelvis

Bursitis—Inflammation of a bursa (fluid-filled sac between a tendon or muscle and a bony prominence) of the side of the hip. Bursitis occurs when a bursa becomes inflamed as result of chronic, repetitive use. Treatment includes rest until acute symptoms subside, icing, and anti-inflammatory medication.

Hamstring strains and Tendinitis—Pain, tenderness, and swelling in the hamstring muscle in the back of the thigh. Treatment consists of rest, ice massage, and non-steroidal anti-inflammatory medication.

Back

Sciatica—Sharp, burning pain and numbness that radiates down the sciatic nerve into the buttock and down the back of the leg. It may indicate a ruptured disc and should be evaluated and treated promptly by a physician.

Lumbosacral strain—Abnormal strain of the lower back muscles. This condition produces pain, spasms, and tenderness in the lower back. It can be relieved by rest, stretching, and ice massage.

Spinal stenosis—Gradual narrowing of the spinal canal in the lower back causing back and hip pain particularly in the older runner. Lying down usually relieves the symptoms within minutes. It can be treated by activity modification and stretching. Occasionally, cortisone injections or surgery are required for the condition.

Guidelines for Managing Running Injuries

General Guidelines

The basic principle of treatment for running injuries includes rest or modification of activity to allow healing and reduction of inflammation. A gradual return to running (10% increase in mileage per week) can be allowed after flexibility, strength, and endurance have returned.

Mild Injuries

Minimal pain occurs at onset or during running and decreases as running progresses. There is no limitation of motion. Stretching, reducing mileage, and icing can manage this type of injury.

Moderate Injuries

Moderate pain is present throughout the running session or occurs just after running starts. This type of injury can often be managed by activity modification and use of anti-inflammatory medication.

Severe Injuries

Severe pain, swelling, loss of motion and/or alterations in running form are representative of more significant injuries. Immediate medical treatment is advised.

Rehabilitation

Following an injury, there are no definite guidelines for determining when an athlete may resume activity. However, runners should remember that there are four periods of time when they are most likely to break down:

- During the initial four to six months of running
- Upon returning to running after an injury
- When the quantity of running is increased (distance)
- When the quality of running is increased (speed or terrain)

219

The goal of rehabilitation of injuries suffered by runners and joggers is to return safely to the desired level of running. Remember, training errors constitute the most common cause of injuries. A well-planned program prevents injury while benefiting the athlete.

This is general information. It does not purport to encompass all risks associated with running and jogging, nor is it a substitute for your own good judgment.

Chapter 22

Mountain Biking Injuries

During the past 20 years, off-road bicycling, or mountain biking, has grown from its origins on a California hillside to a worldwide sport with a multibillion dollar market. Mountain bikes account for more than half of U.S. bicycle sales and are owned by at least 25 million Americans.[1] This tremendous growth has fueled the bicycle industry, and technical innovations and new designs flood the market each year. Competition within the sport has also increased, and over 85,000 Americans now participate in organized races annually.[2] Rising international participation led to the first Olympic mountain bike race at the 1996 summer games in Atlanta.

With the increased popularity of the sport has come an increased number of injuries. Research regarding these injuries has begun to reveal injury patterns in the sport. Awareness of these patterns as well as the unique character and demands of the sport can help healthcare professionals manage the traumatic and overuse injuries that mountain bikers may sustain.

The Shape of the Sport

Although the physiologic characteristics of elite mountain bikers are similar to those of elite road cyclists,[3] the differences in equipment, terrain, and competition make the two activities distinct. The mountain

"Mountain Biking Injuries: Fitting Treatment to the Causes," by Robert L. Kronisch, MD, *The Physician and Sportsmedicine*, Vol. 26, No.3, March 1998, © The McGraw-Hill Companies, reprinted with permission.

bicycle has evolved far from the road bicycle, and many models are now constructed of exotic materials shaped in new geometries that have departed considerably from the standard double-triangle steel bike design. Wide knobby tires with lower inflation pressures, advanced braking systems, and shock-absorbing suspensions make the mountain bike suitable for off-road riding.

The cross-country race is the most popular form of competition and typically involves a large number of riders that must maneuver an uphill and downhill course for 2 to 3 hours. Other types of competition include the downhill race, an individual, 5- to 10-minute time trial in which speeds may exceed 50 miles per hour. The dual slalom event has an elimination format and takes place on a pair of short downhill courses featuring multiple gates and small jumps.

Whether off-road cyclists are competitors or recreational riders, the rough, varied terrain they negotiate places a premium on bike handling skills and makes them vulnerable to acute and chronic injuries. Although these injuries may resemble road-biking injuries, the contributing factors are often quite distinct.

Traumatic Injuries

Unfortunately, crashes appear to be inherent in off-road bicycling. More than 80% of 650 mountain bikers who participated in surveys[4-7] were injured in off-road crashes during a 1-year period. However, many of those injuries were minor and self-treated. In one study,[7] 20% reported a traumatic injury in the preceding year that was severe enough to require medical attention and limit their ability to ride.

Types and incidence. Most crashes result in only minor injuries such as abrasions, contusions, and lacerations. These superficial wounds accounted for 60% to 70% of injuries in most studies.[7-11] Fractures and concussions are less common (20% to 30% and 3% to 12% of injuries requiring medical attention, respectively) but have been consistently reported.[7-11] The majority of fractures occur to the upper extremity and most commonly involve the fingers, metacarpals, wrist, and radial head.

The shoulder is particularly vulnerable to injury. Clavicle fractures and acromioclavicular separations commonly occur when a cyclist falls and lands on the shoulder. Shoulder dislocations can occur if the cyclist's arm is raised during a forward fall.

Serious injuries have been reported, including pelvic fractures,[12] intra-abdominal injuries,[13] facial fractures,[14] and severe brain injuries.[11,15]

One death from a head injury in an unhelmeted off-road cyclist has been reported.[11]

Fortunately, helmets are used by 80% to 90% of off-road cyclists.[4,7,11] One study[11] found that mountain bikers were more than four times as likely as other cyclists to wear helmets, which probably accounts for the low rate of head injuries in the sport.

Contributing factors. A number of factors contribute to acute injuries. A retrospective survey[4] of recreational mountain bikers found that off-road crashes were commonly associated with excessive speed, unfamiliar terrain, inattentiveness, and riding beyond one's ability. A similar survey[7] of recreational and competitive off-road cyclists identified loss of control, high-speed descent, and competition as factors related to acute injuries; competitors were four times more likely than noncompetitors to be acutely injured.

Many studies[4-10] indicate that the majority of injuries take place on downhill rides. Flat tires and other mechanical problems are more commonly associated with accidents that occur during downhill than during cross-country races.[9,10] Other causes of accidents are multifactorial and include hitting a bump or rock during a high-speed descent, losing traction while turning, or losing control of the bike while riding too fast.[8]

Whatever the cause, injuries tend to be more severe when a rider is thrown forward over the handlebars than when he or she falls off the bike to the side.[9,10] In one study, female cross-country racers were more likely to be thrown forward off their bikes and injured than their male counterparts.[10]

Prevention strategies. To prevent injuries, the importance of bicycle maintenance, bike-handling skills, and common sense cannot be overemphasized. Helmet use is clearly effective in decreasing head injuries and should remain a key preventive measure.[11,16] However, since most bicycle helmets provide little protection to the lower face,[15,17] some helmets have been redesigned to offer improved facial protection, and these are especially popular among downhill cyclists. Significant facial injuries have still occurred despite the use of these newer helmets (author's unpublished data, July 1997), and the optimally protective mountain bike helmet is probably yet to be developed.

Other protective gear, such as chest, shoulder, and extremity padding, is also used by many downhill cyclists. These devices probably help decrease superficial injuries to the bicyclist, but their ability to prevent serious injury has not been demonstrated.[9]

Overuse Injuries

Like other cyclists, mountain bikers can suffer overuse injuries. Such injuries have been studied little in mountain bikers, but studies in road cyclists indicate that overuse injuries of the knee are common.[18] Other overuse syndromes have also been reported, including problems in other parts of the lower extremity,[19] the spine,[20] upper extremity,[21] and saddle region.[22] In one study[7] involving 265 off-road cyclists, 30% had recently experienced knee pain associated with mountain biking, and 37% reported low-back pain while riding; wrist pain and hand numbness were each reported by 19%.

Contributing factors. Overuse injuries in off-road cyclists are related to interactions between the cyclist's body, the bicycle, and the terrain on which they ride. The effects of anatomic variations and small errors in bike fit are magnified by long hours spent riding and by highly repetitive lower-extremity motions. A combination of these factors is usually responsible for overuse injuries of the lower extremity. In contrast, upper body overuse syndromes are more often related to weight bearing on the handlebars and vibrations transmitted from rough riding surfaces to the cyclist via the bicycle.

Training errors frequently contribute to overuse injuries. The abundance of hills available for off-road riding can easily tempt a rider to push beyond his or her established level of conditioning, especially early in the season. Common training errors include inadequate preseason conditioning, riding in too high a gear by overrelying on the large chainring, and suddenly increasing mileage, hill climbing, or riding intensity.

Evaluation, treatment, and prevention. The office evaluation of a cycling overuse injury should include a training history to detect common training errors. Riders should be encouraged to establish a basic level of conditioning at the beginning of the season before increasing their mileage, hill climbing, or intensity. Injured cyclists may require temporary modifications of their riding habits until symptoms decrease. Rather than taking a complete break from cycling, the injured off-road cyclist can often benefit from relative rest, i.e., temporarily decreasing mileage and hill climbing and emphasizing low-resistance easy pedaling with avoidance of the large chainring. As symptoms subside, the cyclist can gradually increase the amount and level of riding.

The physical examination should include a search for anatomic variations that could negatively interact with the mechanical restraints of the bicycle. When present, these malalignments can usually be compensated for with adjustments to the bicycle, as described in Table 22.1.[19] The cyclist's position on the bicycle should be checked whenever possible by following the guidelines that accompany this article. The riding position thus obtained is considered a neutral position and is a good starting point for most riders. Sometimes an overuse injury can be treated simply by putting the cyclist in a neutral riding position. If this treatment does not resolve the symptoms or if a cyclist with an overuse injury already rides in a neutral position, specific adjustments to the bicycle may be indicated.[18-22] Adjustments to consider for a number of common problems are summarized in Table 22.2.

For lower-extremity problems such as tendinitis and patellofemoral pain, the key to successful treatment is usually in detecting anatomic malalignments or errors in bike fit and correcting the rider's position on the bicycle with adjustments to the saddle and pedals.

Table 22.1. Lower-Extremity Malalignments, Associated Overuse Injuries, and Suggested Adjustments to the Mountain Bike and Equipment (continued on next page)

Malalignment	Associated Injuries	Suggested Equipment Adjustments
Valgus alignment (evaluated while standing)	Hamstring tendinitis, Medial synovial plica irritation, Patellar tendinitis, Patellofemoral pain, Pes anserine bursitis, Quadriceps tendinitis	Use rigid orthoses* in cycling shoes or medial wedge between shoe and cleat
Varus alignment (evaluated while standing)	Hamstring tendinitis, Iliotibial band friction syndrome, Quadriceps tendinitis	Add threaded spacer between crankarm and pedal
Internal tibial torsion (evaluated while seated)	Iliotibial band friction syndrome, Medial synovial plica irritation, Patellar tendinitis	Adjust cleats to reflect alignment (toes pointing inward)
External tibial torsion (evaluated while seated)	Pes anserine bursitis	Adjust cleats to reflect alignment (toes pointing outward)

Upper body syndromes such as ulnar nerve compression and neck soreness often respond to unloading of the upper extremities by raising the handlebars and/or decreasing the cyclist's reach. Adding or adjusting a front suspension system and allowing the elbows to flex during rough riding may also be helpful in relieving upper body symptoms. Low-back pain is often related to inflexibility and inadequate conditioning and tends to decrease as the season progresses. Raising the handlebars early in the season and gradually lowering them to

Table 22.1. Lower-Extremity Malalignments, Associated Overuse Injuries, and Suggested Adjustments to the Mountain Bike and Equipment (continued from previous page)

Malalignment	Associated Injuries	Suggested Equipment Adjustments
Overpronation (evaluated while pedaling; usually with associated pes planus and internal tibial rotation)	Achilles tendinitis, Iliotibial band friction syndrome, Medial synovial plica irritation, Patellar tendinitis, Patellofemoral pain, Pes anserine bursitis, Tibialis posterior tendinitis	Use rigid orthoses* in cycling shoes or medial wedge between shoe and cleat
Leg-length discrepancy	Achilles tendinitis, Hamstring tendinitis, Pes anserine bursitis	First correct overpronation, if present; then fit bike to long leg and correct short leg with orthosis or shim between shoe and cleat (the thickness of the shim should be less than the measured discrepancy)
Patellofemoral malalignment (at rest or with pedaling)	Patellar tendinitis, Patellofemoral pain	Ensure optimal saddle and cleat adjustment; correct for other associated malalignments (eg, overpronation or valgus alignment)

*Cycling orthoses are rigid and extend to the metatarsal heads in order to provide foot control; running orthoses will not work for cycling.

the desired position as flexibility and conditioning improve may be helpful to some cyclists with low-back pain.

Other treatment options for overuse injuries in off-road cyclists include all of the same approaches used with other athletes, such as physical therapy, ice, and anti-inflammatory medication. However, without attention to the bicycle as well as the bicyclist, overuse injuries are likely to persist.

Table 22.2. Common Mountain Biking Overuse Injuries, Bicycle-Related Causes, and Suggested Adjustments (continued on next page)

Injury or Symptom	Possible Cause	Suggested Adjustments
Achilles tendinitis	Foot too far back on pedal	Move foot forward on pedal (move cleat backward on shoe)
Hamstring tendinitis	Cleats incorrectly placed	Adjust cleats to reflect lower-extremity alignment (see Table 22.1)
	Saddle too far back	Move saddle forward
	Saddle too high	Lower saddle
Iliotibial band friction syndrome	Cleats too internally rotated	Adjust cleats to neutral or slight external rotation
	Saddle too far back	Move saddle forward
	Saddle too high	Lower saddle so that knee flexes 30°-35° at bottom of pedal stroke to decrease contact of iliotibial band with lateral femoral condyle
Low-back pain	Excessive vibration	Use wider tires and/or lower inflation pressure; consider adding or adjusting front suspension
	Incorrect reach	Check upper-body position; consider decreasing reach if cyclist is too far forward or if pain is related to extension on physical examination; increase reach if upper body is crowded or if pain is related to flexion on exam
	Incorrect saddle position	Ensure proper saddle position
	Low-back inflexibility	Raise handlebar or change to upright handlebar

Back to the Slopes

The rapid evolution of the mountain bike and off-road cycling in recent years suggests that veteran and new participants share a remarkable enthusiasm for their sport. Healthcare professionals who understand the nature of the sport and the types of injuries mountain bikers may sustain can help return injured off-road cyclists confidently to the trails.

Table 22.2. Common Mountain Biking Overuse Injuries, Bicycle-Related Causes, and Suggested Adjustments (continued from previous page)

Injury or Symptom	Possible Cause	Suggested Adjustments
Neck pain	Excessive neck extension	Raise handlebar or change to a shorter stem; consider upright handlebars
	Excessive vibration	Try wider tires, lower inflation pressure, and padded gloves and grips; consider adding or adjusting front suspension
	Incorrect riding position	Unlock elbows; change hand, head, and neck positions frequently
Patellar tendinitis, patellofemoral pain, quadriceps tendinitis	Saddle too low and/or too far forward	Raise saddle and/or move saddle back
Pes anserine bursitis	Saddle too high	Lower saddle
Pudendal neuropathy	Saddle compresses nerve against pubic bone	Check saddle position; use padded cycling shorts; consider changing saddle tilt or changing to wider or more padded saddle
Ulnar or median neuropathy	Excessive vibration	Use wider tires, lower inflation pressure, and padded gloves and grips; consider adding or adjusting front suspension
	Incorrect frame size	Ensure correct frame size
	Handlebars too low	Raise handlebars; add bar ends; change hand position frequently
	Reach too long	Use a shorter and/or more upright stem

228

References

1. 1997 NORBA Demographics. Colorado Springs, National Off-Road Bicycle Association, 1997.

2. Wilber RL, Zawadzki KM, Kearney JT, et al: Physiological profiles of elite off-road and road cyclists. *Med Sci Sports Exerc* 1997;29(8):1090-1094.

3. Chow TK, Bracker MD, Patrick K: Acute injuries from mountain biking. *West J Med* 1993;159(2):145-148.

4. Pfeiffer RP: Injuries in NORBA pro/elite category off-road bicycle competitors. *Cycling Sci* 1993;5(1):21-24.

5. Pfeiffer RP: Off-road bicycle racing injuries: the NORBA pro/elite category. *Clin Sports Med* 1994;13(1):207-218.

6. Kronisch RL, Rubin AL: Traumatic injuries in off-road bicycling. *Clin J Sport Med* 1994;4(4):240-244.

7. Pfeiffer RP, Kronisch RL: Off-road cycling injuries, an overview. *Sports Med* 1995;19(5):311-325.

8. Kronisch RL, Chow TK, Simon LM, et al: Acute injuries in off-road bicycle racing. *Am J Sports Med* 1996;24(1):88-93.

9. Kronisch RL, Pfeiffer RP, Chow TK: Acute injuries in cross-country and downhill off-road bicycle racing. *Med Sci Sports Exerc* 1996;28(11):1351-1355.

10. Rivara FP, Thompson DC, Thompson RS, et al: Injuries involving off-road cycling. *J Fam Pract* 1997;44(5):481-485.

11. Barnett B: More on mountain biking, letter. *West J Med* 1993;159(6):708.

12. Lovell ME, Brett M, Enion DS: Mountain bike injury to the abdomen, transection of the pancreas and small bowel evisceration. *Injury* 1992;23(7):499-500.

13. Le Bescond Y, Lebeau J, Delgove L, et al: Mountain sports: their role in 2200 facial injuries occurring over 4 years at the University Hospital Center in Grenoble. [in French] *Rev Stomatol Chir Maxillofac* 1992;93(3):185-188.

14. Chow TK, Corbett SW, Farstad DJ: Do conventional bicycle helmets provide adequate protection in mountain biking? *Wilderness Environ Med* 1995;6(4):385-390.

15. Thompson DC, Rivara FP, Thompson RS: Effectiveness of bicycle safety helmets in preventing head injuries. *JAMA* 1996;276(24):1968-1973.

16. Thompson DC, Nunn ME, Thompson RS, et al: Effectiveness of bicycle safety helmets in preventing serious facial injury. *JAMA* 1996;276(24):1974-1975.

17. Holmes JC, Pruitt AL, Whalen NJ: Cycling knee injuries. *Cycling Sci* 1991;3(2):11-15.

18. Holmes JC, Pruitt AL, Whalen NJ: Cycling injuries, in Nicholas JA, Hershman EB (eds): *The Lower Extremity and Spine in Sports Medicine*, ed 2. St Louis, Mosby-Year Book, 1995, pp 1559-1576.

19. Mellion MB: Neck and back pain in cycling. *Clin Sports Med* 1994;13(1):137-164.

20. Richmond DR: Handlebar problems in bicycling. *Clin Sports Med* 1994;13(1):165-174.

21. Weiss BD: Clinical syndromes associated with bicycle seats. *Clin Sports Med* 1994;13(1):175-186.

Additional Information

Robert L. Kronisch, MD
San Jose State University, Student Health Center
1 Washington Square
San Jose, CA 95192
Tel: 408-925-6120
Website: www.sjsu.edu/depts/Student_Health
E-mail to kronisch@email.sjsu.edu.

—Dr. Kronisch is a staff physician and sports medicine consultant at the San Jose State University student health center in San Jose, California. He is a member of the American College of Sports Medicine and the American Medical Society for Sports Medicine.

Chapter 23

Exercise-Related Injuries

Contents

Section 23.1

Civilian and Military Studies

"Exercise-Related Injuries Among Women: Strategy Prevention from Civilian and Military Studies," by Julie Gilchrist, M.D., Bruce H. Jones, M.D., M.P.H., David A. Sleet, Ph.D., and C. Dexter Kimsey, Ph.D., M.S.E.H. Report prepared by Stephen B. Thacker, M.D., M.Sc. and Christine Branche, Ph.D. Published in *MMWR*, March 31, 2000/49(RR02); pp.13-33.

In 1996, the U.S. Surgeon General's report on physical activity brought together for the first time current knowledge regarding the health benefits of regular physical activity.[1] The report concluded that persons who are inactive can improve their current and future health by becoming moderately active on a regular basis. In addition, the report indicated that activity does not need to be strenuous to achieve some health benefits, but that greater health benefits can be achieved by increasing the amount (frequency, duration, or intensity) of physical activity. Although many studies have documented the hazards of inactivity, few have assessed the adverse effects of increased physical activity (e.g., injury). Increased physical activity increases the risk for injury. Although opportunities for women to participate in sports and organized fitness activities have increased substantially during the preceding century, little is known about the risks for injuries associated with increased physical activity and exercise for women. This report reviews key military and civilian research studies regarding musculoskeletal injury associated with common weight-bearing exercise (e.g., running, walking, and aerobics) and provides general recommendations for preventing exercise-related injuries among women.

Public health reports have reviewed the scientific evidence supporting the association between physical activity and several health benefits.[1,2] Documented health benefits of regular physical activity include reducing the risk for coronary heart disease, noninsulin-dependent diabetes, hypertension, colon cancer, osteoporosis, and other disorders.[1] Physical activity decreases the symptoms and might reduce episodes of anxiety and depression.[1] In addition, regular physical activity improves physical fitness (e.g., cardiorespiratory endurance and muscle strength); reduces body fat; and builds and maintains healthy bones, joints, and muscles.[1] Physical activity enhances strength, balance, and coordination.[1] These benefits might be particularly important in preventing falls and maintaining independence in older adults. As a consequence of these health benefits, regular physical activity is highly recommended for women and men of all ages.[1]

The U.S. Surgeon General's report indicated that approximately 60% of adult women in the United States did not engage in the recommended amount of physical activity, and 25% did not participate in physical activity during their leisure time.[1] Physical inactivity is more common in women than men.[1,3] To help increase the proportion of persons engaged in regular physical activity, two of the Healthy People 2010 objectives are to a) reduce to <20% the proportion of persons aged >18 years who engage in no leisure-time physical activity (objective 22-1), and b) increase to >30% the proportion of persons aged >18 years who engage in regular, preferably daily, moderate physical activity for at least 30 minutes per day (objective 22-2). Because regular physical activity is considered essential to health, it has been included as one of the leading health indicators for health promotion and disease prevention in the United States.[4]

Although physical activity has many health benefits, exercise has corresponding injury risks. Participants are at risk for exercise-related traumatic or overuse injuries. Some of the consequences of these injuries can be long-term (e.g., osteoarthritis and adverse health effects resulting from inactivity because of an injury). Injury causes many persons to stop participating in exercise.[2,5] Efforts to increase physical activity and exercise in women must also be balanced with efforts to prevent injury.

Because lifestyles have become more sedentary and work has become less physically demanding, planned physical activity intended to improve physical fitness has become more important. Consequently, many adults choose to participate in exercise programs or sports. Health-related exercise programs and sports are excellent ways for women to increase their physical activity.

Opportunities for young women to participate in sports have substantially increased in recent decades. Since passage of the 1972 Title IX legislation that prevented sex discrimination in educational settings, the number of young women who participate in high school athletics has increased from approximately 300,000 during the early 1970s to nearly 2.7 million (one in three high school women) in the 1998-99 school year.[6,7] This increased participation in high school athletics has fostered increased participation in college and elite athletics as well. Women now comprise approximately one third of all college athletes and 37% of U.S. Olympic athletes.[7]

Many adult women participate in recreational aerobic activities. The National Sporting Goods Association reported that an estimated 37.4 million women participate more than twice a week in common aerobic activities (i.e., aerobic dance, cycling, exercise walking, exercising with equipment, calisthenics, swimming, and running).[8] Walking is the most prevalent physical activity among adults in the United States.[1,9] If trends of increased participation in women's sports expand to include increased participation in recreational and other physical activities, the number of exercise-related injuries can also be expected to increase.

Injuries occur in association with physical activity, exercise, and sports,[10-13] but the incidence and underlying causes of such injuries are not well understood. At the peak of the fitness boom in the 1980s, researchers knew little about exercise-related injuries and injury rates, even for common activities (e.g., walking and running).[12] During that period, researchers were only beginning to study the epidemiology of and risk factors for exercise-related injuries.[12,14] Today, injury risk factors for physically active men remain poorly defined, and the specific risks for women who exercise are even less understood.

Studies of runners have provided the most thorough examination of injury incidence and some related risk factors in civilian populations.[5,12,14-17] Studies of military populations provide sex-specific information on injury risks associated with physical training and exercise; activities are controlled, and complete and detailed health records, physical examinations, and physical fitness assessments are available.[18,19] Studies of basic combat training, which occurs in all branches of the military and involves running, marching, and other weight-bearing aerobic activities, can often provide information relevant to civilian populations. Uniformity of training within military units provides unique control for the variability observed in exercise routines in the civilian population. Examination of military studies provides some data on exposure risks [18,20] and intrinsic risk factors (e.g., sex, previous injuries, health behaviors, sports participation, physical fitness, and anatomic factors).[19-24]

This report describes civilian and military research related to weight-bearing aerobic exercise and injuries. Aerobic exercises (e.g., running, walking, and aerobic dance) are highlighted in this report because they are popular and commonly prescribed activities. Military studies of training-related injuries are presented to identify shared and sex-specific intrinsic risk factors. Risks for men will be discussed briefly for comparative purposes. This report focuses on modifiable risk factors, which underlie the recommendations for prevention and future research.

Definitions

In this report, distinctions between the terms "physical activity," "exercise," and "physical training" are important. Physical activity has been defined as movement created by skeletal muscle contractions, resulting in energy expenditure. Exercise is a type of physical activity that is planned, repetitive, and designed to improve or maintain at least one of the health-related components of physical fitness.[25] Physical training (as used in the military) is organized exercise intended to enhance fitness. The terms exercise and physical training are used interchangeably. Physical fitness can be categorized into five health-related components: a) cardiorespiratory endurance (aerobic fitness), b) muscle endurance, c) strength, d) flexibility, and e) body composition.[1,25] The focus of this report is on exercise for women aimed at enhancing cardiorespiratory endurance (aerobic fitness). When discussing research results from cited literature, the terms "significant" and "not significant" refer to a documented p-value of <0.05 or >0.05, respectively, unless otherwise stated.

Musculoskeletal injuries related to exercise can be classified as either traumatic (acute) injuries (e.g., sprains and fractures) or overuse injuries (e.g., tendinitis, bursitis, and stress fractures). A distinction is also made between extrinsic and intrinsic risk factors for musculoskeletal injury. Extrinsic risk factors refer to the parameters of training (e.g., frequency, duration, and intensity) and the conditions associated with the environment in which the exercise takes place. Intrinsic risk factors refer to the personal and internal characteristics of the participant.

Findings from Civilian Studies

The incidence of exercise-related injury among women in the civilian population is not well documented. Civilian studies of male and female exercise participants provide some indication of the frequency of such injuries. Surveys demonstrate that the incidence of self-reported running-related injury is high. Annually, approximately 25%-65% of male and female runners report being injured to the extent that they reduced or stopped training.[5,13,15-18,26] In addition, 14%-50% of these injured runners seek medical care for their injuries,[5,13,15-18] representing substantial healthcare costs for treatment and rehabilitation. Prospective studies that incorporated follow-up of injury among runners and other persons involved in vigorous physical activities suggest that the incidence of injuries might be even higher.[11,27-29]

In an 18-month study of runners training for a marathon, 85% experienced >1 injury, and 174 injuries were reported among the 73 participants (159 injuries per 100 runners per year).[27] In a 12-week study of aerobic dancers, 200 (49%) of 411 participants reported complaints associated with aerobics, and approximately 25% had to modify or stop participation because of an injury.[28] In a study of participants engaged in several recreational sporting activities, 475 injuries occurred among 986 participants during a 12-week period (192 injuries per 100 participants per year).[11] In a 6-month study of walkers who averaged 14 miles per week, 21% stopped walking for >1 week because of injury.[29] Although injuries during fitness activities are common, few studies of women or men who participate in recreational fitness activities are available to quantify risk or identify modifiable risk factors.

Findings from Military Studies

Many civilian fitness activities (e.g., walking and jogging) have corollaries in military physical training (e.g., marching and running). The incidence of injury and related intrinsic risk factors for these activities have been more thoroughly studied in military populations than in civilians. Because physical fitness is required for military readiness, recruits undergo a vigorous basic training (BT) course, and substantial research has been devoted to methods of enhancing fitness and understanding the causes of training-related injuries. Studies from the U.S. Army 8-week BT have documented cumulative injury rates from 42% to 67% among women during the course of training.[19,20,30] Of women in the U.S. Air Force, 33% incurred an injury during the 6-week BT.[20] Similarly, 22% of women in the U.S. Navy sustained an injury during the 9-week BT, and 49% of women in the U.S. Marine Corps were injured during the 11-week BT.[20] The range of injury incidence (22%-67%) among women in the different services and over time might be explained by differences in the duration and intensity of BT.

Most of the injuries to both women and men engaged in military BT are overuse injuries (e.g., achilles tendinitis, patellar-femoral syndrome, plantar fasciitis, and stress fractures). Most injuries occur to the lower extremities. Studies during Army BT indicate that 60%-80%

of BT injuries are related to overuse, and 80%-90% occur to the lower extremities.[21,22,30]

Injuries in the military have substantial effects on training and combat readiness because they require greater rehabilitation and recovery time than illnesses. Approximately 50% of healthcare visits in these young, vigorously active military populations are injury-related.[20] The rate ratios of injury-to-illness sick call visits for women in the Army, Marine Corps, and Air Force are 1.0, 1.0, and 0.8, respectively. Furthermore, the rates of limited duty days (i.e., days when a trainee cannot fully function on duty) are often substantially higher from an injury than from illness.[20,24] In one Army study, women were assigned 129 injury-related limited duty days per 100 female trainees per month compared with 6 illness-related limited duty days per 100 trainees per month. The rate ratio between injury and illness limited-duty days was 22, even though 50% of sick-call visits were for illnesses.[20] Among men, the rates of limited duty for injury were five times higher than the rates of limited duty for illness. In the physically active and generally healthy military populations, injury can be expected to account for a substantial proportion of morbidity, healthcare costs, and rehabilitation time in comparison with illnesses. The burden of injuries among physically active civilian populations might reflect a similar pattern.

Risk Factors for Exercise-Related Injuries

Risk factors for exercise-related injuries can be either extrinsic or intrinsic to the participant. This report focuses on extrinsic training factors, perhaps the most important factors in determining injury risks, and addresses selected intrinsic factors. The association between training parameters and injury risks in civilian and military populations will be examined first because they are potentially the most important.

Extrinsic Training Factors

The same training parameters that are modified to achieve a training effect (i.e., frequency, duration, and intensity of exercise) are also the most important factors related to injury. Several surveys of distance runners indicate a relation between a higher number of miles run per week and a higher incidence of injury in both women and men.[5,10,13,15,26] Several studies have demonstrated that the relative risk (RR) of injury among civilian women and men is a function of the miles run per week.[5,15,26] One classic study indicated that as the average weekly training mileage increased in 10-mile increments from <10 miles per week to >50 miles per week, the incidence of injury for women increased from 29% to 57%. The incidence of injury for men increased in a similar manner.[5] Two additional studies reported similar sex-specific trends.[15,26] The annual incidence of injury among female and male runners was approximately the same, and the RRs of injury for both sexes increased with increasing miles run. These and other studies suggest that, for weight-bearing exercise (e.g., running), injury rates increase as the amount of training increases in a dose-response manner.

In a study that examined the benefits of aerobic fitness and injury risks associated with increased duration or frequency of training among men, injury rates increased with duration of exercise (when frequency and intensity remained constant). Participants received limited additional aerobic fitness benefits when they exercised 45 minutes compared with 30 minutes. As duration of running increased from 15 minutes to 30 minutes to 45 minutes per workout, injury rates increased from 22% to 24% to 54%, respectively, whereas aerobic fitness (measured by maximal oxygen uptake) improved only 9%, 16%, and 17%, respectively. Although a plateau in fitness occurred, more exercise increased the incidence of injury. This study also demonstrated that frequency of exercise (number of training sessions per week), although positively related to aerobic fitness, was also positively related to injury.[31]

A similar study of male walkers and joggers demonstrated that injury rates were more related to total mileage walked and jogged than to the intensity of exercise. This study controlled the total amount of activity in two groups of participants during a 6-month period. Both groups exercised the same duration per day (30 minutes); however, the walkers exercised more frequently (more days per week) than the joggers to accumulate approximately the same mileage. The walkers averaged 120 minutes of exercise per week, and the joggers averaged 90 minutes per week; however, the total distance accumulated by both groups was approximately the same (13.7 km per week and 14.7 km per week, respectively). At the end of the 6-month study period, the two groups had similar injury rates: 21% of the walkers and 25% of the joggers had sustained injuries sufficiently severe to require terminating their activity for >1 week.[29] Studies such as these indicate that the total amount of training is an important determinant of injury risk. These studies were conducted with men, and similar studies of women are needed.

Studies of military populations have also examined the relation between training frequency and duration, gains in cardio-respiratory fitness, and injury risk. As mileage during physical training increases, both aerobic fitness and the risk of injury increases. Similar to the findings in civilian populations,[31] military studies have documented thresholds in physical training, above which increased training does not improve fitness levels but continues to increase the likelihood of injury.[18-20] These studies of military populations examined the association between training parameters and injury risk among men only. Additional studies among women are needed.

Intrinsic Training Factors

Military BT provides a unique opportunity to study some intrinsic risk factors for exercise-related injuries. Unlike civilian fitness participants, regimentation in military training requires that trainees do the same type and amount of training. Researchers studying military populations have systematically examined several intrinsic factors and their relation to musculoskeletal injury risk. The most consistently identified intrinsic risk factors have been a) sex, b) age, c) history of previous injury, d) adverse health behaviors (e.g., smoking tobacco), e) previous physical activity (e.g., sedentary lifestyle), and f) current level of physical fitness.

Sex has consistently been identified as a risk factor for injury in military BT. In studies from the 1980s to 1997 that examined women and men at the same training site who performed essentially the same physical training, incidences of injuries for women were 1.7-2.2 times higher than those for men.[19,20,21,30,32,33]

In addition, rates of some specific injuries during military training (e.g., stress fractures) are higher for women than men.[20,24,30,33,34] In Army training, RR for stress fractures is 210 times higher for women than men engaged in the same training regimen.[20,21,30,34-36] In the Marine Corps recruit training, the risk for stress fractures is 3.7 times higher for women than men.[20]

Some specific injuries (e.g., anterior cruciate ligament tears in the knee) occur more frequently in female athletes.[37] However, in studies comparing civilian runners (the most extensively studied civilian recreational fitness activity), the overall rates of exercise-related injury are similar among women and men. Researchers suggest that female civilian runners have the same injury rates as men because they can modulate their training frequency, duration, and intensity (unlike military trainees) to accommodate their fitness levels and the minor overuse injuries that might occur.[10] Injury studies among military populations suggest that without controlling for physical fitness, at any fixed level of activity, women will be at greater risk for injury than men.

Age. Results of military studies regarding the effects of age on training and injuries have been inconsistent. Some studies have revealed that during BT, female[38] and male trainees aged >23 years are at greater risk for injury.[22,38,39] Other military studies have indicated no statistically significant difference in injury risk by age.[20,36,40] Studies of civilian runners have also had inconsistent results. Some studies have demonstrated that age is not an important risk factor, whereas others have demonstrated that rates of injury decrease with age.[10,13,15,16,26] Among civilian women, older age was not associated with elevated risk.[10] Unlike military trainees, older participants in civilian studies might have been able to decrease their risk by modulating the frequency, duration, or intensity of their personal training regimens.[10] Alternatively, a "survivor effect" might exist, whereby persons who have sustained injury change activities or cease participation and thus are unavailable for inclusion in studies.[10] Data from military and civilian studies suggest that among adults aged <45 years, age alone is not a strong predictor of injury in exercise.

History of Previous Injury. A history of previous musculoskeletal injury has also been reported as a risk factor for injury in both civilian and military studies. In a systematic review of the literature regarding the prevention of ankle sprains in sports, the most commonly identified risk factor for an ankle sprain was a previous ankle sprain.[41] Overuse injuries occurred twice as frequently in trainees with a previous history of ankle sprain.[19] A previous ankle sprain is also a risk factor for injuries among male trainees in Army BT.[22] In addition, data from the Marine Corps suggest that previous injuries pose a risk for future injury.[20,40] These findings are consistent with civilian studies of female and male distance runners, in which RR for an injury in a person who has had an injury during the preceding year was 1.8-2.4 for women and 1.7-2.7 for men.[15,26]

Health-Related Behaviors. Health behaviors engaged in before entry into military service (e.g., smoking tobacco and participating in regular physical activity) can influence a woman's injury risk during BT.

Smoking. Both female and male smokers who participate in Army or Marine Corps BT are at a significantly higher risk for injury than nonsmokers.[20] Women who were smokers on entry into the Army were 25% more likely to be injured in BT; injury rates were 77% for smokers and 62% for nonsmokers.[20] Similarly, the risk for injury among women in the Marine Corps who smoked before beginning BT was 1.7 times higher than for those who were nonsmokers.[20] Male smokers in Army and Marine Corps BT were 1.9 times and 2.3 times more likely to have an injury, respectively, than their nonsmoking male counterparts.[20,22] Studies have not indicated whether civilian athletes or exercise participants who smoke tobacco are at greater risk for injury. However, in a literature review of the potential association between smoking and injuries, researchers estimated that smokers were two times more likely than nonsmokers to sustain unintentional injuries in the workplace, although some of these injuries might not be related to physical activity.[42] Data from these studies suggest that women who smoke are at a higher risk for training-related injuries than women who do not smoke.

Previous Physical Activity. Although some health behaviors (e.g., smoking) might increase injury risk, previous regular physical activity might be protective against injury. This protective effect has been documented in men in the Army and Marine Corps.[20-22,32,39] Among male trainees in the Army, running before entry into the service might be protective. For military women, the association between previous regular physical activity and injury risk has not been documented.[20,32,36] Researchers documented that, for men, more years of participating in running was protective against injury; however, for women, more years of participating in running might be associated with higher risk for injury.[15] These results are difficult to interpret because of possible survivor effects (e.g., injured runners cease to run). Because no comparable data in civilian populations of women exist, no conclusions can be drawn regarding the influence of previous regular physical activity as a protective factor against injury among women. Further research is needed regarding the influence of previous physical activities and exercise-related injury risk among women and men in both military and civilian populations.

Current Level of Physical Fitness. A person's current level of physical fitness has been one of the most important predictors of injury in military studies.[19-21,24,32,33,40] Of the five health-related components, low levels of aerobic fitness and, to a lesser extent, low muscular endurance have consistently been associated with injury risk during BT. Other factors (e.g., body composition and strength) demonstrated weaker and less consistent associations with injury risk.

Aerobic fitness, as measured by timed performance of 1- to 2-mile runs during Army or Marine Corps physical fitness entry tests, has been the single most consistently and strongly associated intrinsic risk factor for subsequent training-related injury. During Army BT, women who scored in the slowest quartile on the initial entry physical fitness test experienced 1.5-1.7 times greater injury risk than women in the fastest quartile.[21,36] Findings were similar for women in Marine Corps BT: women in the slowest quartile experienced 2.4 times greater risk for injury than women in the fastest quartile. Women and men with the slowest run times (i.e., least aerobically fit) were consistently at greater risk for injury than those with the fastest run times (i.e., most aerobically fit). Comparable trends were documented among female Army cadets at West Point Academy, New York.[24] Among men, the inverse relation of aerobic fitness and injury risk is similar to that of women. Male trainees with slower run times were at greater risk for injury than those who ran the fastest.[20,36]

In addition to being at greater risk for injury, women who had the slowest run times experienced 2.5 times the risk of stress fractures and stress reactions compared with women who had faster run times.[20,32] Similar findings were documented among women in Marine Corps BT.[20,40] Researchers demonstrated that the least aerobically fit and least physically active trainees were 3.5 times more likely than persons who were the most fit and most active to sustain a stress fracture.[23]

A prospective study of Army trainees in BT demonstrated an association between maximal oxygen consumption (ml O_2 per kg body weight per minute), which is a measure of aerobic fitness, and subsequent risk for injury. Maximal oxygen consumption (VO_2 max) was measured in trainees running on a treadmill before the start of BT. For women in successive tertiles of VO_2 max, risk for injury increased from 39% in the highest tertile to 50% in the middle tertile, to 55% in the lowest. Similarly, men with the lowest VO_2 max were at greatest risk for injury.[36] Prospective studies among civilians examining the association between aerobic fitness and injury are not available. Military research suggests that higher levels of baseline physical fitness is protective, at least at the start of a training program. Further research is needed to determine the degree and duration of this protection.

Higher levels of muscular endurance and strength can also be protective against injury in military BT. For both women and men, greater muscular endurance (measured by the number of push-ups completed in 2 minutes) was associated with fewer training-related injuries.[20] When categorized into quartiles, risk for injury decreased for women who could do more push-ups. The cumulative incidence of injury was 57% for women who completed the least number of push-ups in 2 minutes and 38% for women who did the most push-ups. Similarly, Army women who could not lift >34 kg had RR for injury of 1.4 compared with women who could lift >46 kg.[20]

The relation of body composition to exercise-related injury risk is complex. Some studies indicate no association between body composition and exercise-related injury risk.[20,36] When an association between measures of body fat and injury incidence for women in Army BT has been identified, the relation has been bimodal (U-shaped). Women with the least and the most body fat were at greater risk for injury.[21,32,40] Among women in Army BT, the risk for injury varies by body mass index (BMI). To obtain BMI, weight in kilograms is divided by height in meters squared (weight [kg]/[height squared [m^2]). The cumulative incidence of injuries in successive quartiles of increasing BMI were 56% (lowest quartile), 46%, 38%, and 63% (highest quartile). The corresponding RRs were 1.5, 1.2, 1.0, and 1.6, respectively. BMI for women ranged from 18 kg/m^2 to 27 kg/m^2.[32] A study of civilian male distance runners demonstrated a statistically significant bimodal relation between BMI and injury.[16] A study of civilian female runners indicated a statistically not significant but also bimodal relation between BMI and injury.[15] Additional research is needed to better determine the relation between body fat, BMI, and incidence of injury; these studies should control for physical fitness and previous physical activity.

The Relation Between Sex and Level of Physical Fitness

The observation that low levels of physical fitness on entry into BT is related to injuries during BT is particularly relevant to the issue of injuries among women. The incidence of injuries among women in Army BT is consistently 1.6-2.1 times higher than the incidence for men in Army BT. However, several studies also document that on entry into the Army, women are less physically fit than men.[20,21,32,35,43] On average, women have slower run times, perform fewer push-ups, and have a higher percentage of body fat than men.

What would be the effect of controlling for level of fitness when making comparisons between men and women? In several studies, injury risks were stratified by quartiles or quintiles of run times to enable comparison of groups of women and men who performed similarly on the initial-entry physical training test.[20,32,35,43] In these studies,

243

initial RRs of injury for women were higher than for men, with RRs ranging from 1.6 to 2.1. However, when stratified by aerobic fitness (run times), the stratum-specific risk ratios all approached 1.0, and the summary risk ratios declined (range = 0.9-1.2). In a logistic regression model that controlled for physical fitness (i.e., run times, numbers of push-ups and sit-ups, and strength), age, and race, the odds ratio for women versus men was 1.1.[20,43] Slower run times were the only component of fitness associated with increased odds of injury. Odds of injury progressively increased for successive quintiles of run time from fastest to slowest: 1.0, 1.4, 1.5, 2.5, and 3.2, respectively. In another logistic regression model, female sex was initially a risk factor, with an odds ratio of 2.5 for women compared with men, until run time was entered into the model. When corrected for run times, the odds ratio for females declined to 1.0; however, run time remained a significant predictor.[32] These findings suggest that the most important underlying risk factor for injuries among military trainees engaged in vigorous aerobic weight-bearing activities (e.g., running and marching) is aerobic fitness level and not female sex.[33,43] Studies that compare injury risks between men and women with similar fitness levels have not been conducted in civilian populations.

Because the findings in this report are derived from studies of special populations (e.g., runners and military trainees), they might not be able to be generalized to other U.S. populations. A review of the studies in these special populations provides guidance toward establishing general principles that will be valuable in preventing injuries and guiding research in the general population.

Recommendations for Prevention of Exercise-Related Injury in Women

Scientific research regarding injuries related to physical training and exercise has focused on men rather than women, on military trainees rather than physically active civilians, and on competitive rather than recreational athletes. In addition, the studies of military populations generally involve a young, healthy population. Studies of recreational athletes in the civilian population are difficult to conduct and might not be able to completely control for the frequency, duration, and intensity of activity, as is possible in studies of military populations. In addition, measures of current physical fitness might be difficult to obtain.

Based on the limited scientific research regarding physical activity, exercise, and injuries among women and generally agreed on "best practices," the following recommendations are made to reduce the risk of exercise-related injury among women:

- Although most healthy women do not need to visit their physician before starting a moderate-intensity exercise program, women aged >50 years or women who have either a chronic disease or risk factors for a chronic disease should consult their physician to ensure that their exercise program is safe and appropriate.

- The choice of an exercise program should be tailored to a woman's current physical fitness level. Resources that include examples of activities categorized by exercise intensity levels are available and can aid women in choosing activities based on their respective physical fitness levels.

- Decisions regarding the frequency, duration, and intensity of exercise should be individualized, based on the woman's current level of physical fitness, history of physical activity, and history of injury.

- Women, particularly those with lower fitness levels, should begin participating in exercise at a lower level of training (frequency, duration, and intensity) and progress slowly. Women who are sedentary and start a new exercise program or activity might need to begin with intervals of activity as short as 5-10 minutes of light-intensity activity and gradually increase to the desired intensity and/or duration of participation.

- Participants should be aware of early signs of potential injury (i.e., increasing muscle soreness, bone and joint pain, excessive fatigue, and performance decrements). Coaches, personal trainers, and instructors should be alert to these signs among the women they are supervising.

- When a participant senses any of the warning signs (i.e., increasing muscle soreness, bone and joint pain, excessive fatigue, performance decrements, or current injury), she should incrementally decrease training (i.e., reduce frequency, duration, or intensity) until symptoms diminish or cease participation temporarily, depending on the severity of injury.

- Women who sustain a musculoskeletal injury should allow sufficient recovery and rehabilitation time and take precautions to prevent reinjury.

- Women who smoke should be informed that smoking might increase their risk for exercise-related injury. They should make every effort to stop smoking, not only to reduce their risk for injury, but also to enhance their long-term overall health.

- Women should be realistic in setting their exercise goals by balancing the desire for measurable weight reduction, increases in endurance or strength, or other health-related fitness benefits with the risk for injury.

Conclusion

Persons who participate in vigorous exercise might incur a higher number of musculoskeletal injuries than more sedentary persons. However, several intrinsic and extrinsic factors interact to modify the risk for incurring an exercise-related injury. For activities other than running and military training, little data are available regarding the incidence or risk factors for such injuries. The data suggest that a combination of factors (e.g., sex, current level of fitness, previous exercise experience, smoking, previous injury, and body composition) might affect the risk for exercise-related injury in women. However, how these factors act singly and in combination to influence injury risk is not well understood. The following conclusions might help in the development of further research regarding the relation between exercise and the risk for injury:

- The most important risk factors for exercise- or training-related injuries are the frequency, duration, and intensity of the physical training activity. The total amount of exercise (e.g., the frequency, duration, and intensity) is the most consistently identified predictor for injury risk.

- Physical fitness is inversely related to injury risk; as physical fitness level increases, risk for injury decreases. Men and women who participate in the same activities and have the same physical fitness levels generally have similar incidences of injury. Thus, physical fitness rather than female sex is the underlying risk factor.

- A dose-response relation exists between the amount of weight-bearing exercise performed and the risk of injury for both women and men.

- A training threshold exists, above which increased training does not appreciably increase fitness but will substantially increase risk for injury. This threshold might be different for each person.

- Although higher current amounts of exercise or physical activity are risk factors for injury because of increased exposure, at any fixed amount of activity, men with a history of higher amounts of physical activity are at lower risk for injury. For women, the relation is unclear.

- At any given amount of aerobic weight-bearing activity, women and men who have the highest aerobic fitness levels can be expected to have lower subsequent injury rates.

- The combined findings of research regarding the association of training, previous physical activity, and current physical fitness levels suggest that tailoring exercise to accommodate a person's current level of fitness and previous physical activity reduces injury rates. Changes in frequency, duration, or intensity of exercise can have cumulative effects on injury risk. These findings are particularly important for persons who are the least fit or most sedentary because they are at the greatest risk for injury when initiating physical activity.

- The protective effect against injury of higher levels of aerobic fitness provides an incentive to become more physically active. It suggests that incremental increases in fitness are beneficial in terms of increasing health benefits and decreasing injury risks.

- The relation between previous injuries and higher risk for subsequent exercise-related injuries provides some indication of the importance of a) recovery and rehabilitation, and b) consideration of the history of previous injuries when planning exercise programs.

- The association between smoking tobacco and higher exercise-related injury risks suggests another possible reason to discourage smoking, both for injury reduction in the short-term and increased overall health benefits in the long-term.

- Although the association of body composition with exercise-related injury risks is not completely clear, the bimodal relation that exists suggests that proper maintenance of body weight in the normal range (i.e., BMI 18.5 kg/m^2-24.9 kg/m^2) is important not only for health and appearance but also to reduce risks for injury.

Further research is needed to answer many of the remaining epidemiologic questions and to help develop exercise programs for women that improve health while reducing the risk for injury.

References

1. US Department of Health and Human Services. *Physical activity and health: a report of the Surgeon General.* Atlanta, GA: US Department of Health and Human Services, CDC, National Center for Chronic Disease Prevention and Health Promotion, 1996.

2. Pate RR, Pratt M, Blair SN, et al. Physical activity and public health: a recommendation from the Centers for Disease Control and Prevention and the American College of Sports Medicine. *JAMA* 1995;273:402-7.

3. CDC. Behavioral Risk Factor Surveillance System, 1998 data tape. Atlanta, GA: US Department of Health and Human Services, CDC, National Center for Chronic Disease Prevention and Health Promotion, 1998.

4. US Department of Health and Human Services. *Healthy people 2010: understanding and improving health* [Conference ed.; two vols.]. Washington, DC: US Department of Health and Human Services, 2000.

5. Koplan JP, Powell KE, Sikes RK, Shirley RW, Campbell CC. An epidemiologic study of the benefits and risks of running. *JAMA* 1982;248:3118-21.

6. National Federation of State High School Associations. *High school athletics reaches all-time high* [News release]. Kansas City, MO: National Federation of State High School Associations, September 1999. Available at http://www.nfhs.org/1999-part-index.htm. Accessed February 10, 2000.

7. President's Council on Physical Fitness and Sports. *Physical activity and sport in the lives of girls.* Washington, DC: President's Council on Physical Fitness and Sports, 1997.

8. National Sporting Goods Association. *Sports participation in 1998*, series I. Mt. Prospect, IL: National Sporting Goods Association, 1999.

9. CDC. *1996 Behavioral Risk Factor Surveillance System Summary Prevalence Report*. Atlanta, GA: US Department of Health and Human Services, CDC, National Center for Chronic Disease Prevention and Health Promotion, 1996.

10. Macera CA. Lower extremity injuries in runners: advances in prediction. *Sports Med* 1992;13:50-7.

11. Requa RK, DeAvilla LN, Garrick JG. Injuries in recreational adult fitness activities. *Am J Sports Med* 1993;21:461-7

12. Koplan JP, Siscovick DS, Goldbaum GM. The risks of exercise: a public health view of injuries and hazards. *Public Health Rep* 1985;100:189-95.

13. Van Mechelen W. Running injuries: a review of the epidemiological literature. *Sports Med* 1992;14:320-35.

14. Powell KE, Kohl HW, Caspersen CJ, Blair S. An epidemiological perspective on the causes of running injuries. *Physician and Sports Medicine* 1986;14:100-14.

15. Macera CA, Pate RR, Powell KE, Jackson KL, Kendrick JS, Craven TE. Predicting lower-extremity injuries among habitual runners. *Arch Intern Med* 1989;149:2565-8.

16. Marti B, Vader JP, Minder CE, Abelin T. On the epidemiology of running injuries: the 1984 Bern Grand-Prix Study. *Am J Sports Med* 1988;16:285-94.

17. Marti B. Benefits and risks of running among women: an epidemiologic study. *Int J Sports Med* 1988;9:92-8.

18. Jones BH, Cowan DN, Knapik JJ. Exercise, training and injuries. *Sports Med* 1994;18:202-14.

19. Jones BH, Knapik JJ. Physical training and exercise-related injuries: surveillance, research, and injury prevention in military populations. *Sports Med* 1999;27:111-25.

20. Jones BH, Shaffer RA, Snedecor MR. Injuries treated in outpatient clinics: surveys and research data. In: Jones BH, Amoroso PJ, Canham ML, Weyandt MB, Schmitt JB, eds. Atlas of injuries in the U.S. Armed Forces. *Mil Med* 1999;164(suppl):6-1-6-89.

21. Jones BH, Bovee MW, Harris JMcA, Cowan DN. Intrinsic risk factors for exercise-related injuries among male and female Army trainees. *Am J Sports Med* 1993;21:705-10.

22. Jones BH, Cowan DN, Tomlinson JP, Robinson JR, Polly DW, Frykman PN. Epidemiology of injuries associated with physical

training among young men in the Army. *Med Sci Sports Exerc* 1993;25:197-203.

23. Shaffer RA, Brodine SK, Almeida SA, Williams KM, Ronaghy S. Use of simple measures of physical activity to predict stress fractures in young men undergoing a rigorous physical training program. *Am J Epidemiol* 1999;148:236-42.

24. Bijur PE, Horodyski M, Egerton W, Kurzon M, Lifrak S, Friedman S. Comparison of injury during cadet basic training by gender. *Arch Ped Adolesc Med* 1997;151:456-61.

25. Caspersen CJ, Powell KE, Christenson GM. Physical activity, exercise, and physical fitness: definitions and distinctions for health-related research. *Public Health Rep* 1985;100;126-31.

26. Walter SD, Hart LE, McIntosh JM, Sutton JR. The Ontario Cohort Study of Running-Related Injuries. *Arch Intern Med* 1989;149:2561-4.

27. Bovens AMP, Janssen GME, Vermeer HGW, Hoeberigs JH, Janssen MPE, Verstappen FTJ. Occurrence of running injuries in adults following a supervised training program. *Int J Sports Med* 1989;10:S186-S190.

28. Garrick JG, Gillien DM, Whiteside P. The epidemiology of aerobic dance injuries. *Am J Sports Med* 1986;14:67-72

29. Suter E, Marti B, Gutzwiller F. Jogging or walking—comparison of health effects. *Ann Epidemiol* 1994;4:375-81.

30. Deuster PA, Jones BH, Moore J. Patterns and risk factors for exercise-related injuries in women: a military perspective. *Mil Med* 1997;162:649-55.

31. Pollock ML, Gettman LR, Milesis CA, Bah MD, Durstine L, Johnson RB. Effects of frequency and duration of training on attrition and incidence of injury. *Med Sci Sports Exerc* 1977;9: 31-6.

32. Jones BH, Bovee MW, Knapik JJ. Associations among body composition, physical fitness, and injury in men and women Army trainees. In: Marriott BM, Grumstrup-Scott J, eds. *Body composition and physical performance*. Washington, DC: National Academy Press, 1992: 141-72.

33. Institute of Medicine. *Assessing readiness in military women: the relationship of body composition, nutrition, and health.* Washington, DC: National Academy Press, 1998:77,243.

34. Jones BH, Harris JMcA, Vinh TN, Rubin C. Exercise-induced stress fractures and stress reactions of bone: epidemiology, etiology, and classification. In: Pandolf KB, ed. *Exercise and sport sciences reviews.* Vol 17. Baltimore, MD: Williams and Wilkins, 1989.

35. Canham ML, Knapik JJ, Smutok MA, Jones BH. Training, physical performance, and injuries among men and women preparing for occupations in the Army. In: Kumar S, ed. *Advances in occupational ergonomics and safety: proceedings of the XIII*th *Annual International Occupational Ergonomics and Safety Conference*, 1998. Washington, DC: IOS Press,1998:711-4.

36. Knapik JJ, Sharp MA, Canham ML, et. al. Injury incidence and injury risk factors among U.S. Army basic trainees (including fitness training unit personnel, discharges, and newstarts). Aberdeen Proving Ground, MD: US Army Center for Health Promotion and Preventive Medicine, 1998. *Epidemiological Consultation Report 1999*; report no. 29-HE-8370-98.

37. Arendt E, Dick R. Knee injury patterns among men and women in collegiate basketball and soccer: NCAA data and review of literature. *Am J Sports Med* 1995;23:694-701.

38. Brudvig TJS, Gudger TD, Obermeyer L. Stress fractures in 295 trainees: a one-year study of incidence as related to age, sex, and race. *Mil Med* 1983;148:666-7.

39. Gardner LI, Dziados JE, Jones BH, et al. Prevention of lower extremity stress fractures: a controlled trial of a shock absorbent insole. *Am J Public Health* 1988;78:1563-7.

40. Kimsey Jr CD. The epidemiology of lower extremity injuries in United States Marine Corps recruits [Dissertation]. Columbia, SC: University of South Carolina, 1993.

41. Thacker SB, Stroup DF, Branche CM, Gilchrist J, Goodman RA, Weitman EA. The prevention of ankle sprains in sports: a systematic review of the literature. *Am J Sports Med* 1999;27: 753-60.

42. Sacks JJ, Nelson DE. Smoking and injuries: an overview. *Prev Med* 1994;23:515-20.

43. Bell NS, Mangione TW, Hemenway D, Amoroso PJ, Jones BH. High injury rates among female Army trainees: a function of gender? *Am J Prev Med* 2000;18(suppl 3):S141-S146.

Section 23.2

Fitness and Bone Health: The Skeletal Risk of Overtraining

"Fitness and Bone Health: The Skeletal Risk of Overtraining,"
Osteoporosis and Related Bone Diseases—National Resource Center,
National Institutes of Health, revised 3/1/00.

Are you exercising too much? Eating too little? Have your periods become irregular or stopped? If so, you may be putting yourself at high risk for several serious health problems that could affect your health, your ability to remain active, and your risk for injuries. You also may be putting yourself at risk for developing osteoporosis, a disease in which bone density is decreased, leaving your bones vulnerable to fracture (breaking).

Why Is Missing My Period Such a Big Deal?

Some athletes see amenorrhea (the absence of menstrual periods) as a sign of appropriate levels of training. Others see it as a great answer to a monthly inconvenience. And some young women accept it blindly, not stopping to think of the consequences. But missing your menstrual periods is often a sign of decreased estrogen levels. And lower estrogen levels can lead to osteoporosis, a disease in which your bones become brittle and more likely to break.

Usually, bones become brittle and break when women are much older, but some young women, especially those who exercise so much that their periods stop, develop brittle bones and may start to have fractures at a very early age. Some 20-year-old female athletes have been described as "having the bones of an 80-year-old woman." Even if bones don't break when you're young, low estrogen levels during the peak years of bone building, the pre-teen and teen years, can affect bone density for the rest of your life. And studies show that bone growth lost during these years may not ever be regained.

Broken bones don't just hurt—they can cause lasting deformities. Have you noticed that some older women and men have a stooped posture? This is not a normal sign of aging. Fractures from osteoporosis have left their spines permanently altered.

By the way, missing periods isn't the only problem. Not eating adequate amounts of calcium and vitamin D (among other nutrients) can also cause bone loss, and may lead to decreased athletic performance, decreased ability to exercise or train at desired levels of intensity or duration, and increased risk of injury.

Who Is at Risk for These Problems?

Girls and women who may be trying to lose weight by restricting their eating and/or engaging in rigorous exercise regimes are at risk for these health problems. This may include serious athletes, "gym rats" (who spend considerable amounts of time and energy working out), and/or girls and women who believe "you can never be too thin."

How Can I Tell if Someone I Know, Train with, or Coach May Be at Risk for Bone Loss, Fracture, and Other Health Problems?

Here are some signs to look for:

- missed or irregular menstrual periods
- extreme and/or unhealthy-looking thinness
- extreme or rapid weight loss
- frequent dieting behaviors such as:
  - eating very little
  - not eating in front of others
  - trips to the bathroom following meals
  - preoccupation with thinness or weight

- focus on low-calorie and diet foods
- possible increase in the consumption of water and other no- and low-calorie foods and beverages (possible increase in gum chewing, as well)
- limiting diet to one food group or eliminating a food group

- frequent intense bouts of exercise such as:
  - continuous exercise or training sessions (e.g., taking an aerobics class, then running five miles, then swimming for an hour, followed by weight-lifting, etc.)
  - an "I can't miss a day of exercise/practice" attitude
  - an overly anxious preoccupation with an injury
  - exercising in spite of conditions that might lead others to take the day off, including illness, inclement weather, injury, etc.

- high levels of self-criticism and/or self-dissatisfaction
- high levels of psychological or physical stress, such as:
  - depression
  - anxiety or nervousness
  - inability to concentrate
  - low levels of self-esteem
  - feeling cold all the time
  - problems sleeping
  - fatigue
  - injuries
  - talking about weight constantly

How Can I Make Necessary Changes in the Interest of My Bone Health?

If you recognize some of these signs in yourself, the best thing you can do is to begin eating a more healthful diet, including enough calories to support your activity level. It's best to check with a doctor to make sure your missed periods aren't a sign of some other problem, and to get his or her help as you work toward a more healthy balance of food and exercise. Also, a doctor can help you take steps to protect your bones from further damage.

What Can I Do if I Suspect a Friend May Have Some of These Signs?

First, be supportive. Approach your friend or teammate carefully and sensitively. She probably won't appreciate a lecture about how she should be taking better care of herself. But maybe you could share this chapter with her, or suggest that she talk to a trainer, coach, or doctor about the symptoms she's experiencing.

My Friend Drinks a Lot of Diet Sodas. She Says That This Helps Keep Her Trim.

Often, girls and women who may be dieting will drink diet sodas rather than much-needed milk. (Milk and other dairy products are a good source of calcium, an essential ingredient for healthy bones.) Drinking sodas instead of milk can be a problem, especially during the teen years when peak bone growth occurs. If you (or your friend) find yourself addicted to sodas, try drinking half as many sodas each day, and gradually add more milk and dairy products to your diet. A frozen yogurt shake can be an occasional low fat, tasty treat. Or try a fruit smoothie made with frozen yogurt, fruit, and/or calcium-enriched orange juice!

For Fitness Instructors and Trainers

It's important for you to be aware of problems associated with bone loss in today's active young women. As an instructor or trainer, you are the one who sees, leads, and perhaps even evaluates the training sessions and performances of your clients. You may know best when something seems to be amiss. You also may be best for the role of helping a zealous female exerciser, who may be putting herself at risk for bone loss and other health problems, to recognize the risks of her behaviors and to help her establish new goals.

Trainers and instructors should also be aware of the implicit or explicit messages they send to their clients. An emphasis on health, strength, and fitness should be stressed, rather than an emphasis on thinness. Use caution when advising female clients to lose weight, and if such a recommendation is deemed necessary, education and assistance regarding proper, safe weight management should be offered by knowledgeable personnel. As an instructor or trainer, it's best to maintain a professional rapport with your clients, so they can feel comfortable approaching you with concerns about their exercise training programs, appropriate exercise goals and time lines, body image and nutrition issues, as well as more personal problems regarding eating practices and menstruation.

My Coach and I Think I Should Lose Just a Little More Weight. I Want to Be Able to Excel at My Sport!

Years ago, it was not unusual for coaches to encourage athletes to be as thin as possible for many sports (dancing, gymnastics, figure skating, swimming, diving, running, etc.). However, many coaches are realizing that being too thin is unhealthy and can negatively affect performance. It is important to exercise and watch what you eat. However, it's also important to develop and maintain healthy bones and bodies. Without these, it will not matter how fast you can run, how thin you are, or how long you exercise each day. Balance is the key!

I'm Still Not Convinced. If My Bones Become Brittle, so What? What's the Worst Thing That Could Happen to Me?

Brittle bones may not sound as scary as some other fatal or rare disease. The fact is, osteoporosis can be very painful. It can cause disability. Imagine having so many spine fractures that you've lost inches in height and walk bent over. Imagine looking down at the ground everywhere you go because you can't straighten your back. Imagine not being able to find clothes that fit you. Imagine having difficulty breathing and eating because your lungs and stomach are compressed into a smaller space. Imagine having difficulty walking, let alone exercising, because of pain and deformity. Imagine constantly having to be aware of what you are doing and having to do things so slowly and carefully because of a very real fear and dread of a fracture—a fracture that could lead to a drastic change in your life—including pain, loss of independence, loss of mobility, loss of freedom, and more.

But osteoporosis isn't just an older person's disease. Young women also experience fractures. Imagine being sidelined because of a broken bone and not being able to get those good feelings you get from regular activity.

Eating for Healthy Bones: How Much Calcium Do I Need?

It is very important to your bone health that you receive adequate daily amounts of calcium, vitamin D, phosphorus, and magnesium. These are the vitamins and minerals that are most influential in building bones and teeth. Table 23.1 will help you decide how much calcium you need.

Table 23.1. Recommended Calcium Intakes (mg/day)

Ages	Amount
9-19	1300
14-18	1300
19-30	1000

Source: National Academy of Sciences, 1997

Where Can I Get Calcium and Vitamin D?

Dairy products are the primary food sources of calcium. Choose milk, yogurt, cheeses, ice cream, or products made or served with these choices to fulfill your daily requirement. Three servings of dairy products per day should give you at least 900 milligrams of calcium. Green vegetables are another source. A cup of broccoli, for example, has about 136 milligrams of calcium. Sunlight is one important source of vitamin D, but when the sun isn't shining, milk is also a good source of vitamin D.

Milk and Dairy Products

There are many great snack and meal items that contain calcium. With a little planning and know how, you can make meals and snacks calcium-rich!

- Milk

Wouldn't a tall, cold glass of this refreshing thirst quencher be great right now? If you're concerned about fat and calories, you can drink 1% or skim milk. You can drink it plain, or with a low/no-fat syrup or flavoring, such as chocolate syrup, vanilla extract, hazelnut flavoring, cinnamon, etc.

- Cheese is another winner

Again, you can choose the low/no fat varieties. Use all different types of cheese for sandwiches, bagels, omelets, vegetable dishes, pasta creations...or as a snack by itself!

- Puddings (prepared with milk)

You can now purchase (or make your own from a mix) a variety of flavors with little or no fat. Rocky road, butterscotch, vanilla, chocolate, or pistachio.

- Yogurt

Add fruit. Eat it plain. Add a low/no fat sauce or syrup. No matter how you choose to eat this calcium-rich food, it remains a quick, easy, and convenient choice. It's also available in a variety of flavors. Try mocha-fudge-peppermint-swirl for the more adventurous at heart, and vanilla for the more traditional yogurt snacker!

- Frozen yogurt (or fat free ice cream)

Everybody loves ice cream. And now, without the unnecessary fat grams, you can enjoy it more often! Mix yogurt, milk, and fruit to create a breakfast shake. Have a cone at lunchtime or as a snack. A scoop or two after dinner can be cool and refreshing.

What Are Other Sources of Calcium?

Many foods you already buy and eat may be calcium-fortified. Try calcium-fortified orange juice or calcium-fortified cereal. Check food labels to see if some of your other favorite foods may be good sources of calcium. You can also take calcium supplements if you think you may not be getting enough from your diet.

Additional Information

NIH Osteoporosis and Related Bone Diseases—National Resource Center
1232 22nd Street, N.W.
Washington, DC 20037-1292
Toll-Free: 800-624-BONE (2663)
Tel: 202-223-0344
TTY: 202-466-4315
Fax: 202-293-2356
Website: www.osteo.org
E-mail: orbdnrc@nof.org

National Osteoporosis Foundation
1232 22nd Street, N.W.
Washington, D.C. 20037-1292

Tel: 202-223-2226
Website: www.nof.org
E-mail: patientinfo@nof.org

Section 23.3

Athletes and Asthma

"Athletes and Asthma: Coaches, athletes need to know the warning signs of an asthma attack," Press Release Monday, August 6, 2001, © American Academy of Allergy, Asthma and Immunology, reprinted with permission.

Coaches, Athletes Need to Know the Warning Signs of an Asthma Attack

In August 2001, at Northwestern University in Milwaukee, Wisconsin, starting safety Rashidi Wheeler died of an asthma attack. Wheeler collapsed during practice after running sprints. Wheeler had a history of asthma and team officials were aware of his condition. There are 10 other asthmatics on the Northwestern football team.

"It is critical that we screen athletes for asthma and educate athletes and coaches about asthma," Christopher Randolph, MD, FAAAAI, Chair of the American Academy of Allergy, Asthma and Immunology (AAAAI) Sports Medicine Committee said. "The tragic story of Rashidi highlights the Academy's concern over preventable deaths due to asthma. Proper diagnosis and management can prevent most, if not all deaths."

Asthmatic Athletes

Whether you play in a community softball league or on an NFL football team, chances are some of your teammates are asthmatic. Twenty years ago, a diagnosis of asthma meant the end of a sports career, but medical advancements allow asthmatic athletes to compete at a high level, according to the AAAAI.

A study in the November 1998 *Journal of Allergy and Clinical Immunology* showed that one in six athletes representing the United States in the 1996 summer Olympics in Atlanta had asthma. Thirty percent of the asthmatic athletes took home team or individual medals.

They fared as well as athletes without asthma (28.7%) who took earned team or individual medals.

"Yes, athletes who have asthma can compete at high levels," Randolph said. "However, in order for these athletes to remain healthy and competitive, they must be diagnosed with asthma and take proper steps to control their condition."

What Is Exercise Induced Asthma (EIA)?

Approximately 7% of the population, or about 18 million Americans, are reported to suffer from asthma. With strenuous physical exercise, most of these individuals experience asthma symptoms. In addition, many non-asthmatic patients (about 11%), often those who have allergies or a family history of allergy, experience asthma associated with exercise.

"People with exercise induced asthma (EIA) have airways that are overly sensitive to sudden changes in temperature or humidity," Randolph said. "During strenuous activity, people tend to breathe through their mouths, allowing the cold or dry air to reach the lower airways without passing through the warming, humidifying effect of the nose. In addition to mouth-breathing, air pollutants, high pollen counts, and viral respiratory tract infections can also increase the severity of wheezing with exercise."

Symptoms of EIA can include:

- Breathing difficulty within 5-20 minutes after exertion begins
- Prolonged shortness of breath, often beginning 5-10 minutes after brief exercise
- Wheezing
- Chest tightness
- Coughing
- Chest pain

"It is crucial for coaches and referees at all levels of competition to be on the look out for these symptoms," Randolph said.

Managing Asthma in Athletes

Most asthmatics, whether athletes or not, take two medications. One is a daily, long acting, medication that controls the bronchial inflammation at the root of asthma. The other is an inhaled, short-acting (reliever) medication. This medication relieves acute asthma symptoms.

"It is important for asthmatics to take their medications as prescribed, especially if one of those medications is a long acting medication," Randolph said. "Asthmatics also must be able to recognize their acute symptoms and take the appropriate reliever medication at the onset of symptoms. Taking a break from practice to take your reliever medication may not be a macho thing to do, but it may save your life."

Inhaled medications taken prior to exercise are helpful in controlling and preventing exercise-induced bronchospasm, according to Randolph. The medication of choice in preventing EIA symptoms is a short-acting *beta 2 agonist bronchodilator* spray used 15 minutes before exercise. These medications are effective in 80 to 90 percent of patients, have a rapid onset of action, and last for up to four to six hours.

In addition to medications, a warm-up period of activity before exercise may lessen the chest tightness that occurs after exertion. A cool-down period, including stretching and jogging after strenuous activity, may prevent air in the lungs from changing rapidly from cold to warm, and may prevent EIA symptoms that occur after exercise.

Athletes should restrict exercising when they have viral infections, when temperatures are extremely low, or—if they are allergic—when pollen and air pollution levels are high, according to Randolph.

"If you suspect you have asthma that is triggered by exercise, it is important that you see an allergist," Randolph said. "Allergists can diagnose your condition and work to develop a management plan that will keep you healthy and on the playing field."

Additional Information

American Academy of Allergy, Asthma and Immunology
611 E. Wells Street
Milwaukee, WI 53202-3889
Toll-Free Physician Referral and Information Line: 800-822-2762
Tel: 414-272-6071
Website: www.aaaai.org
E-mail: info@aaaai.org

Chapter 24

Risks Associated with Inline Skates and Skateboards

Each year, more than 100,000 people are treated in hospital emergency departments for injuries related to in-line skating, and nearly 40,000 seek emergency treatment for skateboarding injuries. The majority of these patients are under age 25. Many injuries can be prevented if skaters wear proper safety gear and avoid risky skating behavior.

Who Is Affected?

Millions of people in the U.S.—the majority of them under age 25— take part in in-line skating and skateboarding as a form of recreation and exercise. But these sports can be dangerous, especially when safety precautions are ignored. Each year, more than 100,000 skaters are injured seriously enough to need medical care in hospital emergency departments, doctors' offices, clinics, and outpatient centers. Most of these injuries occur when skaters lose control, skate over an obstacle, skate too fast, or perform a trick.

While most skating injuries are minor or require only outpatient care, 36 fatalities have been reported since 1992. Thirty-one of those skating deaths were from collisions with motor vehicles. Among all

"Skates and Skateboards Safety," SafeUSA™, Centers for Disease Control and Prevention (CDC), updated March 25, 2002; and Abstract of "Skatepark Injuries and Skatepark Design," by Worth W. Everett, *Academic Emergency Medicine* Volume 8, Number 5, 457-458, © 2001 Society for Academic Emergency Medicine, reprinted with permission.

age groups, 63 percent of skating injuries are fractures, dislocations, sprains, strains, and avulsions (tears). More than one-third of skating injuries are to the wrist area, with two-thirds of these injuries being fractures and dislocations. Approximately 5 percent are head injuries. Safety gear has been shown to be highly effective in preventing injuries among skaters. Pads can reduce wrist and elbow injuries by about 85 percent and knee injuries by 32 percent. Although studies have not determined the degree to which helmets reduce head injuries among skaters, helmets have been shown to be highly protective among bicyclists.

Despite the proven safety benefits and relative low cost of helmets and pads, many skaters don't wear them. Nearly two-thirds of injured in-line skaters and skateboarders were not wearing safety gear when they crashed. One study found that one-third of skaters wear no safety gear, and another one-third use only some of the recommended safety equipment. Teens are least likely to wear all the safety gear. Nine out of ten beginning skaters wear all the safety gear, but studies have shown that many skaters shed the helmet and pads as they gain experience.

Skatepark Injuries and Skatepark Design Study

Commercial skateparks (SPs) provide a controlled setting where ideal conditions and equipment requirements exist for purported safer skateboard and rollerblade activity.

Objectives: To describe injury patterns in a local SP. The two hypotheses that significant differences in 1) the number of people injured, and 2) the total number of injuries occurring between each of the three unique physical designs (half-pipe, gullies, and ramps/bars {RB}) within the SP were tested.

Methods: A one-year (7/99-6/00) prospective consecutive case series of subjects presenting to an urban university ED after injury at a local SP (any type of activity). Chisquare analysis was used.

Results: 102 of 106 eligible subjects enrolled (98% male, average 19) and sustained 107 injuries: 62 fx/dislocations (58% of total, 76% upper/24% lower extremity), 18 head/face (17%), 24 sprain/lacerations (22%), 1 pulmonary contusion, and splenic fracture. Skateboard (75%) predominated over in-line skate (17%) and bike (8%) injuries. Significantly more people were injured in the RB region (p=0.001); more total injuries occurred in the RB region (p=0.003). The admission rate was 9%. Protective gear was nearly uniform (helmet 98%, knee 94%, and elbow 91%).

Conclusions: Substantial and significant injuries occurred at the Skatepark, despite controlled conditions. SP design may significantly influence injury patterns. Further study is needed to elucidate safer and better SP designs to minimize injuries.

Injury Prevention Tips for In-line Skaters and Skateboarders

To help your child avoid injuries while in-line skating and skate-boarding, follow these safety tips from the American Academy of Pediatrics, the Centers for Disease Control and Prevention (CDC), the U.S. Consumer Product Safety Commission, and other sports and health organizations. (Note: Adult skaters should heed this advice, too.)

- Make sure your child wears all the required safety gear every time he or she skates. All skaters should wear a helmet, knee and elbow pads, and wrist guards. If your child does tricks or plays roller hockey, make sure he or she wears heavy-duty gear.

- Check your child's helmet for proper fit. The helmet should be worn flat on the head, with the bottom edge parallel to the ground. It should fit snugly and should not move around in any direction when your child shakes his or her head.

- Choose in-line skates or a skateboard that best suits your child's ability and skating style. If your child is a novice, choose in-line skates with three or four wheels. Skates with five wheels are only for experienced skaters and people who skate long distances.

- Choose a skateboard designed for your child's type of riding— slalom, freestyle, or speed. Some boards are rated for the weight of the rider.

- Find a smooth skating surface for your child; good choices are skating trails and driveways without much slope (but be careful about children skating into traffic). Check for holes, bumps, and debris that could make your child fall. Novice in-line skaters should start out in a skating rink where the surface is smooth and flat and where speed is controlled.

- Don't let your child skate in areas with high pedestrian or vehicle traffic. Children should not skate in the street or on vehicle parking ramps.

- Tell your child never to skitch. Skitching is the practice of holding on to a moving vehicle in order to skate very fast. People have died while skitching.

- If your child is new to in-line skating, lessons from an instructor certified by the International In-line Skating Association may be helpful. These lessons show proper form and teach how to stop. Check with your local parks and recreation department to find a qualified instructor.

- If your child gets injured while skating, see your doctor. Follow all the doctor's instructions for your child's recovery, and get the doctor's approval before your child starts skating again.

Safety Resources

American Academy of Pediatrics (AAP)
141 Northwest Point Boulevard
Elk Grove Village, IL 60007-1098
Tel: 847-434-4000
Fax: 847-434-8000
Website: www.aap.org
E-mail: kidsdocs@aap.org

American Academy of Orthopaedic Surgeons
6300 North River Road
Rosemont, IL 60018-4262
Toll-Free: 800-346-2267
Tel: 847-823-7186
Fax: 847-823-8125
AAOS Fax on Demand: 800-999-2939
Website: www.aaos.org
E-mail: custserv@aaos.org

Brain Injury Association
Toll-Free: 800-444-6443
Website: www.biausa.org

U.S. Consumer Product Safety Division
Toll-Free: 800-638-2772
Website: www.cpsc.gov/kids/skate.html

National Pediatric Trauma Registry
Website: www.nemc.org/rehab/factshee.htm

National SAFE KIDS Campaign
1301 Pennsylvania Ave N.W., Suite 1000
Washington, DC 20003
Tel: 202-662-0600
Fax: 202-393-2072
Website: www.safekids.org
E-mail: info@safekids.org

National Youth Sports Safety Foundation
One Beacon Street, Suite 3333
Boston, MA 02108
Tel: 617-277-1171
Fax: 617-722-9999
Website: www.nyssf.org
E-mail: nyssf@aol.com

References

American Academy of Orthopaedic Surgeons. *Injuries from in-line skating*. Position statement. Available at www.aaos.org/wordhtml/papers/position/inline.htm. Accessed July 8, 1999.

American Academy of Pediatrics. In-line skating injuries in children and adolescents. *Pediatrics* 1998;101(4):720-721.

CDC. Toy safety–United States, 1984. *Morbidity and Mortality Weekly Report* 1985;34(5):755-6, 761-2.

National Pediatric Trauma Registry. *Falls while skating or skateboarding*. NPTR fact sheet #9. April 1999. Available at www.nemc.org/rehab/factshee.htm. Accessed July 7, 1999.

Schieber R, Branche-Dorsey C, Ryan G. Comparison of in-line skating injuries with rollerskating and skateboarding injuries. *JAMA* 1994;271(23):1856-1858.

Schieber R, Branche C. In-line skating injuries: Epidemiology and recommendations for prevention. *Sports Medicine* 1995;19(6):427-432.

U.S. Consumer Product Safety Commission. *CPSC projects sharp rise in in-line skating injuries*. News release, June 21, 1995. Available at www.cpsc.gov/cpscpub/prerel/prhtml95/95135.html. Accessed July 12, 1999.

U.S. Consumer Product Safety Commission. *Safety commission warns about hazards with in-line roller skates: Safety alert*. CPSC document #5050. Available at www.cpsc.gov/cpscpub/pubs/5050.html. Accessed July 12, 1999.

U.S. Consumer Product Safety Commission. *Holiday skateboard and rollerskates safety*. Available at www.cpsc.gov/kids/skate.html. Accessed July 12, 1999.

Chapter 25

Ice Hockey Can Hurt

Ice hockey is a popular winter sport in the United States, with more than 500,000 registered amateur players. But injuries in this sport are common and can be severe. Many injuries can be prevented if players wear all their safety gear and avoid dangerous moves like body checking (using the hip and shoulder to slow or stop an opponent who has the puck).

Who Is Affected?

More than 500,000 amateur athletes in the U.S. play ice hockey, a game that carries significant risk of injury for players of all ages. Ice hockey is the second leading cause of winter sports injury among children. The most common types of injuries are sprains and contusions (bruises) to the thigh, knee, and ankle. Lower extremity injuries account for about one-third of the injuries in ice hockey. A high rate of facial lacerations and head injuries (including concussions) is also associated with this sport. Cases of paralysis and death resulting from head and spinal cord injuries have been reported, but these catastrophic injuries are rare.

Body checking is the most commonly reported cause of injury and is associated with the more severe injuries. Many of the players injured by body checking collide with goal posts and the boards. Contact between opponents, usually in the form of body checking, is associated with 46 percent of all minor injuries and 75 percent of major injuries.

"Ice Hockey Safety," SafeUSA™, Centers for Disease Control and Prevention (CDC), updated 2002.

Safety gear and changes in the rules of play have significantly reduced both the number and severity of injuries related to ice hockey. Many head injuries have been prevented by the use of helmets and the elimination of body checking. A reduction in eye injuries has occurred through the addition of full face guards on helmets and the stricter enforcement of penalties for high sticking. Neck guards have reduced the number of both soft tissue and spinal injuries. Currently, most youth leagues and some high school leagues require these safety measures. Other leagues recommend these measures, but are lax on enforcement. A much greater reduction in injuries could be achieved if all amateur and professional leagues mandated these safety practices.

Tips for Preventing Ice Hockey Injuries

To help your child avoid injury while playing ice hockey, follow these safety tips from the American Academy of Pediatrics, the American Academy of Orthopaedic Surgeons, USA Hockey, and other sports and health organizations. (Note: Adults should follow this guidance, too.)

- Before your child starts a training program or plays competitive ice hockey, take him or her to the doctor for a physical exam. The doctor can help assess any special injury risks your child may have.

- Make sure your child wears all the required safety gear every time he or she plays and practices. All youth, high school, and college ice hockey leagues require players to wear the following gear: a helmet with foam lining and full face mask; a mouth guard; pads for the shoulders, knees, elbows, and shins; and gloves. Some leagues recommend neck guards. All equipment should be certified by the HECC (Hockey Equipment Certification Council), the CSA (Canadian Standards Association), or the ASTM (American Society for Testing and Materials).

- Make sure your child's equipment fits properly. The helmet should fit snugly with a strap that gently cradles the chin when it's fastened.

- Insist that your child warm-up and stretch before playing. Exercises that strengthen the neck and increase flexibility may help prevent injuries.

- Teach your child not to play through pain. If your child gets injured, see your doctor. Follow all the doctor's orders for recovery, and get the doctor's approval before your child returns to play.

- Make sure first aid is available at all games and practices.

- Talk to and watch your child's coach. Coaches should enforce all the rules of the game, encourage safe play, and understand the special injury risks that young players face. Coaches should limit body checking (some youth leagues prohibit it). Checking from behind should never be allowed. This move, which is an illegal play, has been associated with a high rate of injury.

- Teach your child to avoid head contact with the boards or other players. Serious head and neck injuries can occur from this kind of contact.

- Above all, keep ice hockey fun. Putting too much focus on winning can make your child push too hard and risk injury.

Safety Resources

American Academy of Orthopaedic Surgeons
6300 North River Road
Rosemont, IL 60018-4262
Toll-Free: 800-346-2267
Tel: 847-823-7186
Fax: 847-823-8125
AAOS Fax on Demand: 800-999-2939
Website: www.aaos.org
E-mail: custserv@aaos.org

National Athletic Trainers Association
2952 Stemmons Freeway
Dallas, TX 75247-6916
Toll-Free: 800-879-6282
Tel: 214-637-6282
Fax: 214-637-2206
Website: www.nata.org
E-mail: natanews@nata.org

National Youth Sports Safety Foundation
One Beacon Street, Suite 3333
Boston, MA 02108
Tel: 617-277-1171
Fax: 617-722-9999
Website: www.nyssf.org
E-mail: nyssf@aol.com

National Pediatric Trauma Registry
Website: www.nemc.org/rehab/factshee.htm

USA Hockey
Toll-Free: 800-667-0781
Website: www.usahockey.com
E-mail: comments@usahockey.org

References

Caine D, Caine C, Lindner K, editors. Epidemiology of Sports Injuries. Champaign, IL: *Human Kinetics*, 1996:247-267.

McCabe M, Roose B. Hockey neck guards made mandatory. *Detroit Free Press* 1999 May 13.

National Foundation of State High School Associations. *Focus on the rules: Ice hockey*.

National Pediatric Trauma Registry. *Sports injuries on snow and ice*. NPTR fact sheet #3. October 1993.

USA Hockey. *Heads Up Hockey: Safer, smarter, better*. Colorado Springs: USA Hockey.

Chapter 26

Sledding Risks

Overview

Objectives: Sledding is a common recreational activity in northern communities. The objective of this study was to examine the frequency and nature of sledding injuries (SIs) in patients presenting to emergency departments (EDs).

Methods: The data were derived from a cohort of patients treated at all five EDs in an urban Canadian health region over a two-year period. Following chart review, consenting patients were interviewed by telephone about their sledding activities and the circumstances surrounding the injury.

Results: Three hundred twenty-eight patients were correctly coded as having SIs, with 212 patients (65%) reached during the follow-up survey. The median age of those with SIs was 12 years (IQR = 8, 21), and 206 (59%) were male. Injury rates peaked in the 10-14-year age group (87/100,000) for boys and in the 5-9-year age group (75/100,000) for girls. Most patients stated they were drivers (75%), fewer than half were thrown from the sled (42%), and fewer than half

"Sledding Injuries in Patients Presenting to the Emergency Department in a Northern City," by Donald C. Voaklander, PhD, Karen D. Kelly, PhD, BScN, Nina Sukrani, BSc, Andy Sher, BSc and Brian H. Rowe, MD, MSc, *Academic Emergency Medicine* Volume 8, Number 6 629-635, © 2001 Society for Academic Emergency Medicine, reprinted with permission.

(44%) were sledding on community-designated sledding hills at the time of injury. Injuries to the lower extremity (32%), upper extremity (31%), and head (13%) were most common. Thirty-seven (11%) patients with SIs were admitted to hospital vs. 4% of patients with other sports/recreation injuries (p < 0.05).

Conclusions: Sledding injuries are common and potentially serious wintertime injuries in northern communities, involving primarily younger patients, with a large pre-adolescent group. However, older sledders (>20 years) have poorer outcomes (hospitalization, lost time from work/school) than their younger counterparts. The SIs treated in the ED appear to lead to hospitalization more frequently than other types of sport/recreation injury, and injury prevention strategies appear warranted.

Introduction

Snow sledding is a common recreational activity among youth during the winter months in northern regions such as Canada. Gliding across snow-covered slopes, slicing through the crisp winter air, and succumbing to gravity can be exhilarating for participants. While there is public perception that sledding is a safe activity, research has indicated that sledding injury is common, and may result in serious injury, hospitalization, and even death.[1,2,3]

A number of sled types are used in this recreational activity, including traditional toboggans, GT-type steerable sleighs, circular flying saucers, and simple plastic mats. These sled options offer various levels of control, with the GT-type sleighs being the most maneuverable, followed by wooden or plastic toboggan types. Snow disks or flying saucers as well as inflated inner tubes offer almost no control over the path of the sled. There are numerous public sledding hills in most northern Canadian cities as well as other places where children simply use an available hill or incline.

Despite the high frequency and severity of sledding injury, little information concerning these injuries that is population-based and/or comprehensive is available in the medical literature. In addition, few studies have focused on the behaviors leading to sledding injury [4,5,6,7] and, to the best of our knowledge, none have been conducted in western North America. The objective of this study was to examine the frequency and nature of sledding injury (SIs) in patients presenting to the emergency department (ED).

Discussion

To the best of our knowledge, this is the first study to generate population-based ED data regarding sledding injury in a Canadian Center. Using a standardized database, the results suggest that this problem is a relatively common sports/recreation trauma presentation in these linked EDs. Males were found to have significantly higher risk of presenting to the ED with SI in most age groupings; however in the 5-9 year age group, the risks of SI were similar between males and females. Additionally, there was no statistically significant difference in risk of SI for those aged 30 years and more. Others have found males to be at excess risk; [4,5,6,7,10] however, comparison by specific age and gender groupings has not been reported prior to this study. In age groupings where risks are similar, it is likely that a smaller exposure differential exists between males and females.

Several other study findings are noteworthy. First, one of the important findings of the study was the relationship between age and increased use of health services as a result of injury. Those who were hospitalized were significantly older than those discharged from the ED. Additionally, there was a significant positive correlation between time lost from work/school and age. This is an important finding because much of the sledding injury research has focused on the pediatric population. In the present study, those aged 20 years and over accounted for almost one-third of the injuries treated, even though their reported exposure was significantly less than that of younger age groups. It also appears that the circumstances of injury are different for the adult sledding enthusiast. Many of the older persons treated were injured while being thrown from the sled or by landing hard on the sled after traveling over a jump or bump.

Hedges and Greenberg[10] found a relationship between age and severity of sledding injury in a review of ED records in Philadelphia. Paradoxically, in the only Canadian study that included adult patients, it was found that none of the persons over the age of 20 years were admitted to hospital.[4] Other studies in which adults with SIs were included did not report any apparent age-severity relationship.[11,12]

Researchers have hypothesized that older sledders are less resilient than their younger counterparts,[10] while others have described scenarios where adults are injured in efforts to protect young children with whom they are sledding.[3] However, given the age of the seriously injured sledders in this study, there are likely three issues at play. First, serious injury in the older sledder is a likely a consequence of the physical forces involved. The force generated by a 160-pound adult at the same velocity is substantially greater (4 times) than for a 40-pound child. In an equivalent event with the potential for injury, this excess of force would result in a much larger transfer of mechanical energy for the larger person, putting high load points such as the extremities at potentially higher risk of injury. For example, the 160-pound adult being thrown from a sled traveling at 30 feet/second (20.4 miles/hour) would have about 2,250 foot-pounds of energy, while the 40-pound child would have about 562.5 foot-pounds.

When these individuals come to a sudden stop (hitting the ground), this energy must be dissipated into the sled, the environment, or the individual. Clearly, all else being equal, the person with the larger mass has a greater potential for injury. In addition, many of these older injured sledders were drivers of their sled, and observation suggests that their risk-taking behaviors (e.g., jumps, standing while riding, running starts) are different from those of the young child (Rowe BH, unpublished observations, 2000). Further, older sledders may also be under the influence of drugs or alcohol.[13] Consequently, their speed and behavior may create more opportunity for injury.

The rate of hospitalization observed is comparable to what has been reported in the literature from countries other than Canada.[5,6,10,11,12,14,15] These range from 5% to as high as 24%. Canadian studies by Wynne et al.[4] and Lee et al.[7] reported 7% and 11%, respectively; however, the latter work did not include adults. External comparisons of hospitalization rates are problematic as admission threshold, health insurance, and available health services can vary greatly between hospitals, regions, provinces, and countries. Internally, the use of health services by those reporting with SIs was found to be significantly greater than that of other types of sport/recreation activity assessed and treated in these Canadian EDs. This is reflected by a higher hospital admission rate as well as the more frequent use of an ambulance as a mode of transport to the ED for SI when compared with other sports/recreation injury. This indicates that injury control efforts are warranted for sledding in reducing the overall severity of sport and recreation injury.

The anatomic and diagnostic distributions of injury observed in this study are consistent with the published literature.[5,6,10,11,12,14,15] It is not surprising that the extremities appear to be at highest risk; the legs and/or arms are often used in efforts to brake or steer the sled.[13] Additionally, when multiple individuals use a single sledding device, the extremities can get caught under other persons falling or flying off, providing excessive stress to bones and joints. Consistent with Wynne et al.,[4] the majority of injuries to the back and coccyx were caused by individuals going over bumps and jumps and landing with impact

276

either back on the sled or on the ground. Additionally, more than half of the clavicle fractures were caused by being thrown from the sled. These fractures are most likely the result of individuals attempting to break the impact with their arms, which can lead to excessive loading on the clavicle.[16]

Numerous individuals surveyed indicated there is little community information available on safe sledding practices, in contrast to programs that promote safe cycling or swimming. One role of the ED in the prevention of sledding injury could be in providing educational material to children and their parents regarding safe sledding practices. However, emergency staff have been shown to be equivocal about their ability to impact injury through patient education.[17] More likely, with their knowledge of the serious consequences of sledding injury, ED staff could provide referent support to programs or individuals working to reduce sledding injury at the community level. Mass media campaigns have also been found to be effective, if seasonally relevant to the injury issue being addressed.[18]

Limitations and Future Questions

The major limitation of this study is that it is a retrospective survey of injured patients. While the ED records are prospectively coded, our contact with the patient was up to two years after the event. The potential for recall bias exists. However, since the event had led to

Table 26.1. Male and Female Injury Rates

Age Group	Male (Annual Rate per 100,000)	Female (Annual Rate per 100,000)	Odds Ratio (95% Confidence Interval)
4 years or younger	28.0	13.9	2.0 (1.1,2.9)*
5-9 years	85.2	74.5	1.1 (0.7, 1.5)
10-14 years	86.6	57.4	1.5 (1.1, 1.6)*
15-19 years	52.7	32.1	1.6 (1.0, 2.2)*
20-29 years	59.9	26.0	2.3 (1.7, 2.9)*
30-39 years	13.0	17.9	0.7 (0.1, 1.4)
40 years or more	3.0	2.4	1.3 (0.4, 2.2)

*p<0.05.

Table 26.2. Diagnostic Distribution of Sledding Injuries

Injury	Percentage
Other	7.8
Superficial	1.4
Dislocation	2.3
Concussion	4.0
Laceration	11.5
Sprain/Strain	14.4
Contusion	21.9
Fracture	36.6

Table 26.3. Anatomic Distribution of Sledding Injuries

Body Region	Percentage
Not Specified	13.5
Multiple	1.4
Neck	2.3
Torso/Back	11.6
Head	12.4
Upper Extremity	28.8
Lower Extremity	30.0

Table 26.4. Mechanism of Sledding Injuries

Mechanism	Percentage
Other	16.2
Collision with Person	4.4
Collision with other Sled	10.8
Collision with Fixed Object	27.2
Thrown from Sled (includes those suffering impact from going over jumps)	41.5

an ED visit, we suggest that such an important life event results in limited recall bias influence on the study results. In addition, only a crude attempt was made to measure exposure. This is a limitation of many retrospective studies as this information is often not available or detail is lacking through memory decay or proxy responses. The response rate to the follow-up survey was also not optimal at 65%. However, no systematic differences were noted between the respondents and the nonrespondents with regard to age and gender, and we believe that this nonresponse rate did not influence the results of the study.

Calculated rates are likely an underestimate, for two reasons. Sledders who were treated at other health services, such as walk-in clinics, family physicians' offices, and physical therapists' offices, were not counted. Strains/sprains and contusions have a greater likelihood of being treated at physicians' offices than EDs.[19,20] Second, coders may have not have identified all SIs due to a lack of chart-based information. It is unknown what the cumulative effect of these are on the injury rates; however, the authors are sure that most acute serious injuries would have been reported to one of the five EDs in the region.

Finally, at the time of the study, no direct measure of severity was available for all ED cases; therefore, the study was limited to using health service utilization (ambulance, inpatient admission) when comparing SIs with other sports and recreation injuries.

Notwithstanding the above limitations, the study does have some important strengths. For example, the population-based estimates of injury are unique, and the use of the ED system database to identify sport/recreation participants is an important research/surveillance advance. In addition, this comprehensive and relatively complete follow-up survey adds information that would not generally be available. Future study should include analytic studies comparing those injured with a suitable comparison group. This has been done with playground injuries and has been useful in identifying play areas with substantially greater injury potential.[21] Studies of this type can assist community planners in identifying high-risk hills that may need to be either closed or modified.

Conclusions

Based on these data, several recommendations can be made regarding sledding injury prevention. The first relates to participants. Older sledders should be warned about traveling over bumps and jumps. It appears they are at increased risk for injury from this mechanism. This is likely due to a combination of large impact forces and less resilience of the adult joint and bone system. Risk-taking behavior in this group may also be a factor.

Numerous individuals were seriously injured in collisions with fixed objects. Sledders and their parents or supervisors should take care to ensure that sledding is conducted in obstruction-free areas with sufficient run out. Administrators should conduct annual audits of sanctioned and unsanctioned hills where sledding takes place to ensure the risks are minimized and dangerous hills have restricted access.

One third of injuries occurred at dusk or after dark, while 78% of the subjects reported never or rarely sledding in darkness. Half of these injuries occurred at hills where artificial light was available. It is likely that decreased vision at dark or poorly lighted hills contributes to injury. Sledders would have less time to react to both fixed objects and other sledders. Additionally, after dark, many bumps or obstructions may not be visible from the top of the hill, leading to unforeseen incidents. Community hills either should have lighting of sufficient quality to provide a safe environment or should be closed to sledders at dusk. Parents should not allow their children to sled at unlit hills after dark.

Notes

Presented at the American College of Emergency Physicians annual meeting, Las Vegas, NV, October 1999, and at the Fifth World Injury Prevention Conference, New Delhi, India, March 2000.

Supported in part by a grant from the Canadian Association of Emergency Physicians. The Department of Rural Health, University of Melbourne, is supported by a grant from the Commonwealth Department of Health and Aged Care, Canberra, Australia.

References

1.   Bernardo LM, Gardner MJ, Rogers KD. Pediatric sledding injuries in Pennsylvania. *J Trauma Nurs*. 1998;5 (2): 34-40. [Medline]

2.   Rowe BH, Bota GW. Sledding deaths in Ontario. *Can Fam Physician*. 1994; 40:68-72. [Medline]

3. Fiennes A, Melcher G, Ruedi TP. Winter sports injuries in a snowless year: skiing, ice skating, and tobogganing. *Br Med J.*1990; 300:659-61.

4. Wynne AD, Bota GW, Rowe BH. Sledding trauma in a northeastern Ontario community. *J Trauma*. 1994; 37:820-5. [Medline]

5. Bjornstig U, Tordai P. Tobogganing and sledging accidents. *Scand J Soc Med*. 1986; 14:83-6. [Medline]

6. Shuggerman RP, Rivara FP, Wolf ME, Schneider CJ. Risk factors for childhood sledding injuries: a case—control study. *Pediatr Emerg Care*. 1992; 8:283-6. [Medline]

7. Lee F, Osmond MH, Vaidyanathan CP, Sutcliffe T, Klassen TP. Descriptive study of sledding injuries in Canadian children. *Inj Prev*. 1999; 5:198-202. [Medline]

8. Kahn HA, Sempos CT. *Statistical Methods in Epidemiology*. New York: Oxford University Press, 1989.

9. SPSS. SPSS Base 9.0 Syntax Reference Guide. Chicago: SPSS Inc., 1999.

10. Hedges JR, Greenberg MI. Sledding injuries. *Ann Emerg Med*. 1980; 9:131-3. [Medline]

11. Major CP, Guest DP, Smith LA, Barker DE, Burns RP. Sledding injuries in the southern United States. *South Med J.*1999; 92:193-6. [Medline]

12. Lewis LM, Lasater LC. Frequency, distribution, and management of injuries due to an ice storm in a large metropolitan area. *South Med J*. 1994; 87:74-8. [Medline]

13. Larkin M. Sliding into sledding injuries. *Physician Sportsmed*. 1991; 19(1):91-102.

14. Dershewitz R, Gallagher SS, Donahoe P. Sledding-related injuries in children. *Am J Dis Child*. 1980; 144:1071-73.

15. Landsman IS, Knapp JF, Medina F, Sharma V, Wasserman GS, Walsh I. Injuries associated with downhill sledding. *Pediatr Emerg Care.*1987; 3:277-80. [Medline]

16. Arnheim DD. *Modern Principles of Athletic Training*. St. Louis: C. V. Mosby, 1985.

17. Cummings G, Voaklander DC, Vincenten J, Polichio C, Borden K. Emergency staff opinion on their role in pediatric injury prevention education. *J Emerg Med*. 2000;18:299-303. [Medline]

18. Cochrane Library. *Mass media interventions: effects on health services utilisation* [monograph on CD-ROM]. Grilli R, Freemantle N, Minozzi S, Domenighetti G, Finer D. Oxford Software Cochrane Library, Version 2, 2000.

19. Voaklander DC, Saunders LD, Quinney HA, Macnab RBJ. Epidemiology of recreational and old-timer ice hockey injuries. *Clin J Sports Med*. 1996; 6:15-21.

20. Dryden DM, Francescutti LH, Rowe BH, Spence JC, Voaklander DC. Epidemiology of women's recreational ice hockey injuries. *Med Sci Sports Exerc*. 2000; 32:1378-3. [Medline]

21. Mowat DL, Wang F, Pickett W, Brison RJ. A case—control study of risk factors for playground injuries among children in Kingston and area. *Inj Prev*. 1998; 4:39-43. [Medline]

Chapter 27

Snowboarders Risk Bones and Ligaments

Snowboarding is a popular winter sport that involves riding a single board down a ski slope or on a half-pipe snow ramp. Compared with injuries resulting from traditional alpine skiing, snowboarding injuries occur more frequently in the upper extremities and ankles and less frequently in the knees. Different types of snowboard equipment, rider stance, and snowboarding activity tend to result in different types of injury. Snowboarder's ankle, a fracture of the lateral talus, must be considered in a snowboarder with a severe ankle sprain that has not responded to treatment. Risk of injury may be lowered by using protective equipment such as a helmet and wrist guards.

Snowboarding is an increasingly popular winter sport in which participants ride an epoxy-fiberglass board (resembling a large skateboard) down a ski slope or on a half-pipe ramp, a specialized snow structure used for performing tricks. Introduced in the United States in 1965 when Sherman Poppen bolted two skis together, snowboarding became popular with the introduction of commercial snowboards in the late 1970s. Today, with more than 3.4 million participants, snowboarding is the fastest growing winter sport in the United States.

"Snowboarding Injuries," by Craig C. Young, M.D., and Mark W. Niedfeldt, M.D. Reprinted with permission from *American Family Physician*, January 1999, Vol. 59, No. 11 © American Academy of Family Physicians Family. All Rights Reserved. Also, "Upper Extremity Snowboarding Injuries: Ten-Year Results from the Colorado Snowboard Injury Survey," by Jan R. Idzikowski, *American Journal of Sports Medicine,* Nov, 2000, © American Orthopaedic Society for Sports Medicine, reprinted with permission

Snowboarders now make up 20 percent of the visitors to U.S. ski resorts. The National Sporting Goods Association estimates that since 1988, the number of snowboarders has increased 77 percent, whereas the number of skiers has fallen 25 percent. The popularity of snowboarding was further boosted after its introduction as an Olympic sport at the 1998 Winter Games in Nagano, Japan.

In the 1980s, most snowboarders were young males. Recent surveys have shown that females and older persons are increasingly more apt to take up this sport. For example, the male-to-female participant ratio dropped from 9 to 1 in 1989 to 3 to 1 in 1995.[1,2]

Snowboarding differs from downhill skiing in many respects. The most important difference is that snowboarders ride with both feet affixed by non-releasable bindings to a single board. Unlike downhill skiers, snowboarders stand perpendicular to the long axis of their boards. Furthermore, snowboarders do not use ski poles, but use their hands and arms for balance, much like skateboarders or surfers.

Equipment

Snowboards

Knowing the type of equipment used and the rider's position on the board is important in evaluating injuries. Traditional snowboards are symmetric, allowing the snowboarder to travel backward easily, that is, lead with the tail of the board (a move called a *fakie* by snowboarders). Asymmetric boards that enhance freestyle, slalom, and giant slalom events are more recent introductions. Traditionally, snowboard riders use their left foot as the forward foot and face toward the right side of the board (known as the frontside). Occasionally, snowboarders ride in a reverse position, called goofy-footed.

A fall that occurs while a snowboarder is waiting in line for a ski lift is likely to cause a knee injury, resulting from the torque force on the locked leg.

Boots

Snowboarding boots come in three styles: soft, hard, and hybrid. Traditionally, snowboarders use soft boots. The current soft snowboard boot is made of leather or synthetic material that allows moderate stability yet is balanced by moderate flexibility. The advantages of soft boots are increased maneuvering ability and comfort. Sorrel-type soft boots are worn by 75 to 90 percent of recreational snowboarders. Some beginners wear moon boots or hiking boots, both of which lack stability and may lead to a higher injury rate. These types of boots should not be used for snowboarding.

Hard boots provide greater ankle support and increased control, and are primarily worn by racers.

The increasingly popular hybrid boots are relative newcomers to the snowboarding scene. This classification includes boots that are constructed with a soft leather or synthetic outer shell and a stiff inner boot. Another design is constructed with a hard shell base and a soft upper component. This combination balances the increased comfort and maneuvering ability of soft boots with the increased stability of hard boots. Since each boot style places the body under different stresses, knowing the type of boot worn is important in determining the risk of injury.

Bindings and Safety Equipment

Most snowboard bindings are non-releasable. Soft bindings are molded plastic shells with buckle systems that are used with soft boots and include a high back to give extended Achilles tendon support. The plate-type bindings consist of a steel and plastic base plate with heel and toe clips and are typically used with hard boots. Safety equipment includes helmets, face guards, goggles, forearm guards and wrist guards. Unfortunately, *safety equipment is rarely used by recreational snowboarders.*

Injury Patterns

Although advanced snowboarders may try more dangerous maneuvers such as jumps and other aerial tricks, beginning snowboarders are the most frequently injured. Almost one-quarter of snowboarding injuries occur during a person's first experience,[1,3,4] and almost one-half occur during the first season of snowboarding.[2-8] A typical first snowboarding experience consists of a cycle of brief rides followed by falls; since falling is the leading cause of snowboarding injuries, the beginning snowboarder is at high risk for injury.[3]

Jumps are the second most common cause of injuries and may be associated with head, facial, spinal, and abdominal injuries.[4] Collisions are associated with 5 to 10 percent of injuries.[3,4,8] Severe injuries that require referral to a tertiary trauma center are rare. The most common cause of severe injury is collision with a tree. Severe injuries usually involve the head (54 percent), abdomen (32 percent), bones (32 percent), and thorax (16 percent).[9]

Four to 8 percent of snowboarding injuries take place while the person is waiting in ski-lift lines or entering and exiting ski lifts.[8,10] Snowboarders push themselves forward with a free foot while in the ski-lift line, leaving the other foot (usually that of the lead leg) locked on the board at a 45- to 90-degree angle, placing a large torque force on this leg and predisposing the person to knee injury if a fall occurs. Equipment failures rarely cause injuries (0.5 to 1.2 percent).[8,10]

Although early studies showed that approximately one-half of snowboarding injuries were located in the lower extremities, this pattern has changed with the evolution of snowboard boots and bindings. Currently, fewer than one-third of snowboarding injuries are to the lower extremities (Table 27.1).[1,3-8,10,11] The lead leg, which is at greatest risk, accounts for almost three-quarters of such injuries.[1,5,8] Injury location is related to boot type. Hard boots place the snowboarder at risk for fractures of the tibia and fibula at the level of the boot top, called boot-top fractures.[2,6]

Table 27.1. Summary of Snowboard Injury Studies

Study	Number of injuries	Upper extremity injuries (%)	Lower extremity injuries (%)	Wrist injuries (%)	Knee injuries (%)	Ankle injuries (%)
Pino and Colville, 1989[1]	110	29.1	52.7	7.3	11.8	26.4
Abu-Laban, 1991[5]	132	25.9	49	16	16	28
Ganong, et al., 1992[3]	415	44	43	23.9	18.1	16.9
Bladin, et al., 1993[6]	276	30	57		23	23
NEISS, 1993[11]	565	47	31.8	20.4	12	12.8
Warme, et al., 1995[7]	47				17	21
Calle and Evans, 1995[10]	487	38	34.1	19.9	15	12.5
Davidson and Laliotis, 1996[8]	931	40	38	19	17	16
Chow, et al., 1996[4]	355	58	16	20.3*	2.8	3.1

*Only fractures were included.
Information from references 1, 3-8, 10 and 11.

Table 27.2. Average Distribution of Snowboarding Injuries*

Location	Percentage	Location	Percentage
Wrist	23.0	Shoulder	8.3
Ankle	16.7	Trunk	7.8
Knee	16.3	Other	6.5
Head	9.2	Elbow	4.4

*Table percentage values do not equal 100 percent because of varying methods of measurement used in the studies from which the information was compiled. Information sources: references 1, 3-8, 10 and 11.

Knee injuries, especially sprains, account for approximately 16 percent of all snowboarding injuries (Table 27.2).[1,3-8,10,11] Hard boots give the snowboarder approximately twice the risk of a knee injury compared with soft boots.[6]

Ankle Injuries

On the other hand, soft boots give the snowboarder approximately twice the risk of ankle injury compared with hard boots.[1,3,6] Ankle injuries account for almost 17 percent of snowboarding injuries. Almost 50 percent of the ankle injuries are fractures, which are usually easily diagnosed.[3,4] However, snowboarder's ankle, a fracture of the lateral process of the talus, may be difficult to see on a standard ankle x-ray series [12,13] This fracture may comprise up to 15 percent of those ankle injuries in snowboarders that require medical evaluation. Physicians should maintain a high index of suspicion for snowboarder's ankle in a snowboarder with a severe ankle sprain that is persistently painful, has limitation of motion, and fails to improve with appropriate management[2] (Table 27.3). The mechanism of injury is a forcing of the ankle into dorsiflexion and inversion, which may occur during a landing from an aerial maneuver or a jump, especially when the landing has been over-rotated.

Classification of Ankle Injuries

Snowboarder's ankle injuries are classified by degree of severity. A type 1 fracture is an articular process chip fracture of the talus with no extension into the talofibular joint. A type 2 fracture is a single large fragment extending from the talofibular joint to the subtalar joint. A type 3 fracture is a comminuted fracture of the entire lateral process. A lateral plain ankle x-ray with the ankle in 10 to 20 degrees of inversion may be better than standard ankle views for viewing the fracture.[12,13] Other diagnostic tests, such as computed tomographic scanning or magnetic resonance imaging, may be useful in evaluating these injuries.

Treatment of Ankle Injuries

Treatment for a nondisplaced or minimally-displaced fracture (less than 2 mm) is a short-leg, partial weight bearing cast for six weeks. Patients with large displaced fractures and comminuted fractures should be referred to an orthopedic surgeon for possible open reduction and internal fixation, and/or excision of the fragments.

- Compared with hard boots, soft boots place a snowboarder at approximately twice the risk for incurring an ankle injury.

Upper Extremity Injuries

Upper extremity injuries make up an increasing proportion of the total number of snowboarding injuries, rising from approximately one-quarter of all injuries in the early 1990s to almost one-half of all injuries today. The lead upper arm appears to be slightly more vulnerable to injury.[1,8] The wrist is the most common site of injury, accounting for almost one-quarter of snowboarding injuries (Table 27.2) and for one-half of all fractures.[3-5,10] Other common fracture sites are the clavicle and the elbow.[3,4] The shoulder is the most common site of dislocation, accounting for almost two-thirds of dislocations, followed by the elbow, which accounts for almost one-quarter of total dislocations.[3,4]

- Snowboarders are more likely than alpine skiers to have upper extremity injuries but are less likely to have knee injuries.

Compared with skiers, snowboarders have a much higher risk of wrist injuries (23 percent versus 4 percent) and ankle injuries (17 percent versus 5 percent), but a lower risk of knee injuries (16 percent versus 38 percent).[1,3-8,10,11] Despite the lack of releasable bindings, snowboard-related knee injuries tend to be less severe than those experienced by downhill skiers. This lower risk may be related to features that are unique to snowboarding:

1.   the shorter length of the board results in a smaller potential lever arm and lower forces during twisting injuries, and

2.   a single board decreases the number of edges that can get caught, thereby decreasing the chance of a twisting crash or of the knees rotating in different directions.

Injury Prevention

Although most snowboarders do not wear protective equipment, some snowboarders wear wrist guards similar to those worn by in-line skaters. These wrist guards have been shown to be very effective in preventing wrist injuries in in-line skaters.[14] Although protective equipment decreases the overall incidence of injury by reducing the force of impact, it may actually place the areas proximate to the device at increased risk, by shifting the distribution of impact forces. For example, skiers and snowboarders who wear hard boots are at greater risk for boot top fractures, and in-line skaters are at greater risk for wrist guard top fractures.[15,16] This effect is illustrated in a survey that included 21 snowboarders who had been injured while wearing wrist guards: although none of these persons had a wrist injury, six had a shoulder injury and four had radial shaft fractures.[4] Novice snowboarders who refuse to wear wrist guards are advised to keep their hands in a "closed-fist" position while snowboarding. This hand position minimizes the temptation of snowboarders to check themselves with an open hand when falling, since falling on a hyperextended wrist increases the risk of injury. Falling backward was the mechanism of injury in almost three-quarters of wrist injuries in one series.[8] Since beginners are most likely to lose their balance and fall backward, they are most likely to benefit from wearing wrist guards. Some instructors have their beginning students use ski poles to decrease the frequency of falling.

Head Injuries

Another frequent impact area in beginning snowboarders is the back of the head. Fortunately, the force load on the head is usually relatively mild since most of the force is first absorbed by the buttocks, back, and upper extremities, and impact usually results only in headache. Many instructors recommend that beginning snowboarders wear a helmet during their initial attempts at the sport to prevent or reduce the severity of head injuries.

Table 27.3. Types of Snowboarding Injuries

Degree of injury	Head	Shoulder	Elbow	Wrist and hand	Trunk	Knee	Ankle
				Location of injury			
Common, less serious injuries	Soft tissue injuries*	Sprain	Soft tissue injuries*	Sprain Fracture Soft tissue injuries*		ACL sprain MCL sprain	Sprain Fracture
Less common, more serious injuries	Concussion Closed head injury	Dislocation Fracture	Dislocation Fracture	Dislocation Fracture	Clavicle fracture	Fracture Internal injuries	Fracture

ACL=anterior cruciate ligament; MCL=medial collateral ligament.

* Includes abrasions, contusions and lacerations.

References

1. Pino EC, Colville MR. Snowboard injuries. *Am J Sports Med* 1989;17:778-81.

2. Bladin C, McCrory P. Snowboarding injuries. An overview. *Sports Med* 1995;19:358-64.

3. Ganong RB, Heneveld EH, Beranek SR, Fry P. Snowboarding injuries: a report on 415 patients. *Physician Sportsmed* 1992;20:114-21.

4. Chow TK, Corbett SW, Farstad DJ. Spectrum of injuries from snowboarding. *J Trauma* 1996;41: 321-5.

5. Abu-Laban RB. Snowboarding injuries: an analysis and comparison with alpine skiing injuries. *Can Med Assoc J* 1991; 145:1097-103.

6. Bladin C, Giddings P, Robinson M. Australian snowboard injury data base study. A four-year prospective study. *Am J Sports Med* 1993;21:701-4.

7. Warme WJ, Feagin JA Jr, King P, Lambert KL, Cunningham RR. Ski injury statistics, 1982 to 1993, Jackson Hole Ski Resort. *Am J Sports Med* 1995;23:597-600.

8. Davidson TM, Laliotis AT. Snowboarding injuries, a four-year study with comparison with alpine ski injuries. *West J Med* 1996;164:231-7.

9. Prall JA, Winston KR, Brennan R. Severe snowboarding injuries. *Injury* 1995;26:539-42.

10. Callé SC, Evans JT. Snowboarding trauma. *J Pediatr Surg* 1995;30:791-4.

11. U.S. Consumer Product Safety Commission. NEISS: National Electronic Injury Surveillance System. Washington, D.C.: U.S. Consumer Product Safety Commission, 1997.

12. Nicholas R, Hadley J, Paul C, James P. "Snowboarder's fracture": fracture of the lateral process of the talus. *J Am Board Fam Pract* 1994;7:130-3.

13. McCrory P, Bladin C. Fractures of the lateral process of the talus: a clinical review. "Snowboarder's ankle." *Clin J Sport Med* 1996;6:124-8.

14. Schieber RA, Branche-Dorsey CM, Ryan GW, Rutherford GW Jr, Stevens JA, O'Neil J. Risk factors for injuries from in-line skating and the effectiveness of safety gear. *N Engl J Med* 1996;335: 1630-5.

15. Cheng SL, Rajaratnam K, Raskin KB, Hu RW, Axelrod TS. "Splint-top" fracture of the forearm: a description of an in-line skating injury associated with the use of protective wrist splints. *J Trauma* 1995;39:1194-7.

16. Hoflin F, van der Linden W. Boot top fractures. *Orthop Clin North Am* 1976;7:205-13.

Ten-Year Results from the Colorado Snowboard Injury Survey

The popularity of snowboarding continues to burgeon. Each year a growing number of ski resorts open their slopes to snowboarders, accommodating their special interests by creating snowboard parks with half-pipes, rails, and jumps. The 1994 to 1995 National Ski Association of America Kottke National Business Survey indicated that 14% of the 54 million ski area visits in the United States in that season were by snowboarders.[17] We conducted a 10-year survey of snowboarding injuries in Colorado to assess injury patterns, to compare results with previous studies, to identify trends or changing injury patterns associated with newer equipment technology, and to determine the efficacy of protective equipment. This section describes the findings on upper extremity snowboarding injuries.

Materials and Methods

The survey period spanned 10 snowboarding seasons (1988 through 1998). An optically scannable questionnaire was completed by injured snowboarders seeking medical care at 47 medical facilities near Colorado ski areas, which have an estimated 5 to 6 million skier/snowboarder days annually. The questionnaire evaluated 20 variables including stance, equipment used, mechanism of injury, and experience level. The treating physician completed the portion concerning diagnosis. Characteristics of injured snowboarders were compared with those of a non-injured population of snowboarders obtained from the 1995 and 1996 Ski Industries of America Snowboard Survey (N = 1640),[17] and the Canadian Ski Council 1994 National Snowboard Survey (N = 642).[6] Both surveys evaluated age, sex, snowboard ability distributions, behaviors, and attitudes of non-injured snowboarders who completed questionnaires at destination resort ski areas in various geographic areas of Canada and the United States. In addition, a control group of 825 non-injured snowboarders at five Colorado ski resorts was used during the 1997 to 1998 season. Participants completed a questionnaire similar to the injured snowboarders questionnaire excepting mechanism of injury data.

Previous studies have demonstrated a relatively high incidence of wrist injuries to snowboarders;[1,2,7,10-12] therefore, attention was focused on these injuries and the possible effect of the use of protective wrist guards on the incidence of wrist injury. Univariate and logistic regression statistical analyses were performed on all data using SPSS statistical software (SPSS, Inc., Chicago, Illinois). For the analyses, P values of [is less than] 0.05 were considered significant.

Not all patients answered all the questions of each survey; therefore, response rates differ for certain diagnoses and cross-tabulations, and not all tabulations may add up. To minimize possible confusion, the number and percentages is given for all cross-tabulations presented in the text, tables, and figures. In all instances, unless otherwise stated, the reference point is the number of injuries.

Also, it is well understood that a certain number of injured skiers/snowboarders do not seek medical attention. Up to 40% of injuries go unreported,[7] and during the 1996 to 1997 season at one Colorado resort, 31% of skiers and 29% of snowboarders refused medical attention after an encounter with the ski patrol (personal communication with ski patrollers at Copper Mountain Resort, Colorado, 1997).

Results

A total of 7,430 snowboarding injuries were seen. There were 3,645 injuries to the upper extremity, which were 49.06% of all snowboarding injuries. The majority of injuries to the upper extremity were fractures (56.43%, N = 2057), followed in frequency by sprains (26.78%, N = 976), dislocations (9.66%, N = 352), contusions (6.36%, N = 232), lacerations (0.44%, N = 16), and miscellaneous (0.33%, N = 12). The wrist accounted for 44% (N = 1604) of all upper extremity injuries. The shoulder and clavicle were injured 33.09% (N = 1206) of the time, followed by the hand (8.37%, N = 305), the elbow (7.79%, N = 284), the forearm (5.49%, N = 200), and the humerus (1.26%, N = 46).

Injured snowboarders in this survey were primarily young men. Most injuries (89.1%) occurred in snowboarders 30 years or younger. The average age of injured snowboarders was 22.5 years (range, 7 to 71). Nineteen percent of injuries occurred in skeletally immature snowboarders. For 7,415 injuries, the sex of the person was known; 74.1% of injuries (N = 5,494) occurred in men and 25.9% (N = 1,921) in women. The average age of the injured snowboarder population increased from 20 to 24 years during the study period. The average age and sex distributions of the control groups were similar to those of the study group (Table 27.4).

Skill level was self-reported by the snowboarders. Of 6,504 injuries where the skill level of the person was known, in 45.2% (N = 2,938) the injured snowboarders considered themselves beginners, whereas in 31.4% (N = 2,042) the injured person considered themselves intermediate, and in 23.4% (N = 1,524) they considered themselves expert riders. When skill level and sex were cross-tabulated, we found that significantly more injured men reported higher skill levels than did injured women. When the skill levels of injured and non-injured populations were compared, a significantly greater percentage of injured snowboarders were beginners, while a larger proportion of non-injured snowboarders reported more advanced skill levels (P = 0.0001).

Eighty-one percent of all snowboarding injuries (N = 6,018) were the result of a fall, with about 9% from a collision with a tree or skier and the remainder from a twist or lift mishap. However, 92% (N = 3,354) of upper extremity injuries were due to a fall. Of these, 53.6%

occurred during a forward fall (toe-side) and 46.4% during a backward fall (heel-side). The direction of the fall was predictive of the anatomic site injured. Shoulder injuries were more often associated with a forward fall, and wrist injuries were more commonly the result of a backward fall. Neither sex nor experience level correlated with the direction of the fall.

Table 27.4. Characteristics of the Control Groups and the Study Groups

Characteristics	Ski Industries America[17]		Canadian Ski Council[6]
	1996	1995	
No. of subjects	749	891	642
Average age	24	22	22
Women (%)	30	24	28
Men (%)	70	76	72

	Current Survey		
Characteristics	10-year	Controls	1998
No. of subjects	7430[a]	825	1263
Average age	22	23.14	22.56
Women (%)	26	24.50	27.7
Men (%)	74	75.50	72.3

[a] Number of injuries.

The mechanism of injury varied with ability level, age, and sex. A higher percentage of beginners and those aged 10 to 19 years injured themselves from a fall or lift mishap than did those of more advanced ability and older age (Table 27.5). Ninety percent of collisions with trees and other objects were seen in 20- to 29-year-old male intermediate and expert riders.

Aerial maneuvers are the domain of intermediate and expert riders. Injuries of greater severity resulted when a poor landing of an

Table 27.5. Mechanism of Snowboarding Injury by Experience and Sex

Mechanism of injury	Beginner (%)		Intermediate(%)		Expert (%)	
	Male	Female	Male	Female	Male	Female
Fall	89.1	86.2	80.1	81.3	72.0	67.2
Twist	5.5	8.2	7.0	8.9	7.2	9.8
Getting off lift	0.4	0.6	0.2	1.6	0.2	0.0
Getting on lift	1.5	3.2	1.9	0.8	1.4	4.9
Collide with tree	2.7	0.6	9.1	5.7	16.7	13.1
Collide with skier	0.8	1.2	1.7	1.6	2.5	4.9

aerial maneuver was a component of the injury mechanism. For instance, 63% of elbow dislocations (45 of 72), 60% of acromioclavicular sprains (231 of 385), and all of the wrist dislocations (N = 20) occurred at the conclusion of an aerial maneuver.

Some sex-specific differences were noted (Table 27.6). Men were more likely to injure their shoulders (dislocation, acromioclavicular separations, and clavicle fractures) and elbows and to sustain more severe injuries than women. Women, on the other hand, sustained more wrist fractures, excluding scaphoid fractures, and sprains than expected from sex distribution alone. When sex-related variance in reported ability level was factored in, these differences in injury rates were eliminated in the injured beginner group only. A persistent sex difference emerged among the intermediate and expert men, who were more likely to experience upper extremity injuries than women with the same ability (46% and 39% for intermediate-skill men and women, respectively, and 40% and 30% for expert men and women, respectively, P = 0.0001). Particularly apparent was the predisposition for shoulder injuries and perilunate dislocations among the male snowboarders.

There was no correlation between hand dominance and side of upper extremity injury.

The Wrist

There were 1,604 wrist injuries in the series, making the wrist the most common anatomic site of injury to snowboarders (21.6% of all

Table 27.6. Selected Snowboarding Injuries by Sex

Injury	Male (74% expected) N (%)	Female (26% expected) N (%)	Total
Wrist			
Fracture	744 (62)	455 (38)	1199
Dislocation	19 (95)	1 (5)	20
Sprain	160 (52.7)	144 (47.3)	304
Scaphoid fracture	36 (76.6)	11 (23.4)	47
Elbow			
Fracture	64 (81)	15 (19)	79
Dislocation	52 (72.2)	20 (27.8)	72
Forearm fracture	60 (65.2)	32 (34.8)	92
Shoulder			
Fracture	38 (70.4)	16 (29.6)	54
Dislocation	199 (87.7)	28 (12.3)	227
Acromioclavicular joint	352 (91.4)	33 (8.6)	385
Clavicle fracture	262 (94)	17 (6)	279
Hand fracture	126 (78.3)	25 (21.7)	161

snowboarding injuries). Wrist injuries represented 44% of all upper extremity injuries. Nearly 78% of wrist injuries were fractures (Table 27.7); 8.61% of wrist fractures were growth plate injuries and buckle fractures in skeletally immature riders. Fifty percent of distal radius fractures were in the 10- to 19-year-old age group. Those in the 1st and 2nd decades of life were twice as likely to sustain a wrist injury than older groups (34% versus 14% to 17%). Wrist fractures, except to the scaphoid, and sprains occurred predominantly in beginner snowboarders. Thirty-four percent of all injuries in beginners (those who listed experience as none or beginner) were to the wrist, mostly wrist fractures. Intermediate and expert riders sustained the majority of scaphoid fractures and suffered more severe fractures than beginners.

Ninety-six percent of wrist injuries (1,540 of 1,604) were caused by a fall. Distal radius fractures were nearly twice as likely to be the result of a backward fall than a forward fall.

Table 27.7. Wrist Injuries in Snowboarding

Injury	N	(%)
Fractures	1243	(77.5)
Distal radius	1064	
Distal radius/buckle	107	
Scaphoid	48	
Styloids	12	
Carpal	12	
Dislocations	24	(1.5)
Sprains	304	(18.9)
Contusions	27	(1.68)

There were 24 perilunate or lunate fracture-dislocations. All but one of the wrist dislocations in this series were sustained by intermediate or expert male riders, the other by an expert female rider. Seventy-five percent of wrist dislocations (18 of 24) resulted from a backward fall and all of them were preceded by an aerial maneuver.

In 6,725 snowboarding injuries we were able to determine whether the rider had used protective wrist guards. Overall, in 5.6% of injuries (N = 377) the snowboarders wore protective wrist guards of some fashion. Women, older, and less-experienced injured riders were more likely to use wrist protection than their counterparts (Table 27.8). The Ski Industries of America and Canadian Ski Council control surveys did not evaluate wrist guard use. As a result, wrist guard use could not be discerned in that non-injured population. In comparing the control group with the 1997 to 1998 injured population, it was found that of 825 control riders, 8.4% (N = 69) wore wrist guards, compared with 6.2% of the injured group (78 of 1,263). This difference did not reach statistical significance.

Injured snowboarders in this survey who wore wrist guards were about half as likely to be seen for a wrist injury than those who did not wear guards (P = 0.0001). It could not be determined if those who used wrist guards and sustained a wrist fracture had different fracture patterns or severity (or both) from those who did not wear them. A significant change was not detected in the expected incidence of injury to other anatomic sites with wrist guard use.

Table 27.8. Who Wore Wrist Guards

Group	No.	Yes (%)	No (%)
Overall	6725	5.6	94.4
Female	1681	7.3	92.7
Male	4681	5.0	95.0
Age 10-19	2102	3.2	96.8
Age 20-29	3581	5.7	94.3
Age 30-39	592	10.1	89.9
Age 50-59	56	21.4	78.6
No experience	834	6.1	93.9
Beginner	1721	6.2	93.8
Intermediate	1873	6.4	93.6
Expert	1400	4.1	95.9

The Shoulder

Thirty-three percent (N = 1206) of the upper extremity snowboarding injuries in this survey were to the shoulder, as opposed to 10% reported for alpine skiers.[12] Twenty-nine percent (N = 348) of the shoulder injuries were fractures, mostly to the clavicle (N = 280), 19.82% were dislocations of the glenohumeral joint (N = 239), and 32.09% were acromioclavicular separations (N = 387). There was a higher incidence of certain shoulder injuries in intermediate and expert snowboarders than in beginners. Of 294 shoulder fractures, intermediate riders sustained 44.21% (N = 130), compared with 11.22% in those with no experience, 27.21% in beginners, and 17.35% in expert riders. Of 186 glenohumeral dislocations, 67.72% were sustained by intermediate and expert riders while 32.26% were in beginner snowboarders. There was no correlation between experience and acromioclavicular sprains.

Shoulder injuries were more often the result of a forward than of a backward fall. In fact, 88.8% (182 of 205) of clavicle fractures and 84.6% (242 of 286) of acromioclavicular separations were sustained during forward falls.

There were 46 fractures to the humeral shaft. These accounted for 1.26% of the upper extremity injuries.

The Hand

There were 305 hand injuries in the study (8.37% of upper extremity injuries). Almost 50% (49.83%, N = 152) of hand injuries were fractures, 31.47% (N = 96) were sprains, and 5.57% (N = 17) were dislocations. Hand injuries occurred predominantly in intermediate and expert riders of either sex (73%, N = 223), and almost half (49.8%, N = 152) of the injuries were in the expert group.

Injuries to the ulnar collateral ligament of the thumb were relatively rare (N = 65). Ulnar collateral injuries of the thumb are the most common upper extremity injury in alpine skiers, accounting for as many as 80% of injuries,[18] but they accounted for only 1.78% of upper extremity snowboarding injuries evaluated in our survey.

The Elbow

Elbow injuries comprised 7.79% (N = 284) of the upper extremity injuries and 3.8% of all snowboarding injuries in this study. By comparison, 1% of alpine ski injuries are to the elbow.[12] Forty-seven percent (N = 133) were fractures and 25% (N = 72) were dislocations, nearly all the result of a fall. The direction of the fall did not correlate with the incidence of elbow injuries. Intermediate and expert riders were more likely to dislocate their elbows than beginners (81% of elbow injuries versus 19%, respectively).

The Forearm

There were 200 forearm injuries, or 5.49% of upper extremity snowboarding injuries; the majority were fractures (72%, N = 144). Of those, 56.94% (N = 82) were fractures of both the radius and ulna. Relatively uncommon forearm injuries were Galeazzi fracture/dislocations (3%, N = 6) and Monteggia fracture/dislocations (2%, N = 4). There was no correlation between forearm injuries and sex, ability, or direction of fall.

Discussion

This survey produced findings similar to those of other studies in that 1) there were one and a half to two times more upper extremity injuries in snowboarding than in alpine skiing, and 2) the wrist was the most common site of injury in snowboarders.[3-17]

In addition, it was determined from the data that injured snowboarders, as a group, were more likely to be beginners than intermediate or expert riders. Mechanism of injury and type and severity of injury varied significantly with age, sex, and ability level. More shoulder, hand, and elbow injuries, as well as more severe injuries, were sustained by advanced and male snowboarders, suggesting that they had more aggressive riding styles than other groups. Male snowboarders seemed to ride more aggressively than female snowboarders at all levels of ability. It is interesting to note that in the Ski Industries of America and Canadian Ski Council surveys, snowboarders ranked "risk of injury" ninth of their perceived negative aspects of snowboarding, superseded by "getting stuck in the flats" (ranked first), lift problems, falling, the cold, the snowboarding stigma, bindings, and expense.

It is presumed that all snowboarding injuries that occurred at the ski areas during the study period were not surveyed. Those snowboarders with minor injuries would not have sought immediate treatment, and those with extreme injuries, requiring evacuation to Level 1 trauma centers, for example, were unable to complete questionnaires, so the injured study population was biased to more moderate injuries.

A weakness in the study design was that a control group of non-injured snowboarders was not obtained for all years of the survey, so the prevalence of wrist guard use in non-injured snowboarders throughout the study period could not be ascertained. Although the comparison groups of non-injured snowboarders were somewhat diverse in year and location, the similarities in age, sex, and ability levels for all the control groups were striking.

Because of the questionnaire design, there was a certain degree of vagueness regarding the severity of injury. For instance, the written diagnosis "distal radius fracture" could encompass a wide spectrum or injuries from minor, nondisplaced fractures treated with simple immobilization to severely comminuted and displaced intra-articular fractures requiring open reduction and internal fixation. As a result, the severity of some injuries could not be graded, especially wrist fractures, in snowboarders who wore wrist guards to compare it with the severity of these injuries in snowboarders who did not wear wrist guards.

Furthermore, the rating of snowboarding level of experience in this study was self-reported and, therefore, subjective. Specific and uniform criteria for the level of experience for snowboarders are needed for comparison studies.

The wrist was the most common site of injury in snowboarders in this survey. Significant, independent predictors of wrist injury were younger age ($P = 0.0001$), less experience ($P = 0.0001$), and not using wrist guards ($P = 0.006$). The most promising preliminary finding of this study was that injured snowboarders who wore protective wrist guards were about half as likely to sustain a wrist injury as those who did not wear wrist guards. This is further supported by the fact that, in the survey, those who wore wrist guards were more likely to be younger, less-experienced female snowboarders, groups that otherwise had the highest incidence of wrist injuries. The survey results, however, could not detect whether wrist guards affected the severity of fractures in those who used wrist guards and suffered a fracture or if use of wrist guards increased the incidence of injury to other anatomic sites. Although we cannot state that wrist guards will prevent 50% of snowboarding wrist injuries, we can deduce from this data that wrist guards provide a significant protective effect.

A number of biomechanical analyses have evaluated the protective efficacy of wrist guards. Giacobetti et al.[8] conducted a cadaver study testing commercially available in-line skating wrist guards using a quasistatic loading model. They found no significant difference in the force required to produce fracture with or without wrist guards. They concluded that, other than preventing palmar abrasions, the tested wrist guards would not protect against wrist fracture. Greenwald and associates,[9] however, testing newer, high-density thermoplastic wrist guards and, using a unique testing model that simulated a fall onto a snowy surface, revealed that significantly more force was needed to produce a fracture in wrists with wrist guards than in those without them. They suggested that the reason their results differed from those of Giacobetti et al. lies in the testing model. Greenwald et al. concluded that "wrist guards may have a prophylactic effect during low energy dynamic impact situations."

With the continued growth of snowboarding, a correspondingly growing number of snowboarding injuries will be treated. In light of the relatively high prevalence of wrist injuries in snowboarders, especially in beginners and skeletally immature riders, and the apparent protective effect of wrist guards, we strongly advocate the use of protective wrist guards constructed from high-density, thermoplastic materials for all snowboarders.

References

1. Abu-Laban RB: Snowboarding injuries: An analysis and comparison with alpine skiing injuries, *CMAJ* 145:1097-1103, 1991

2. Bladin C, Giddings P, Robinson M: Australian snowboard injury data base study. A four-year prospective study. *Am J Sports Med* 21: 701-704, 1993

3. Bladin C, McCrory P: Snowboarding injuries: An overview. *Sports Med* 19: 358-364, 1995

4. Cadman R, Macnab AJ: Age and gender; Two epidemiological factors in skiing and snowboarding injury, in Mote CD Jr, Johnson RJ, Hauser W, et al. (eds): Skiing Trauma and Safety. Volume 10. ASTM STP 1266. Philadelphia, *ASTM*, 1996, pp 58-65

5. Calle SC, Evens JT: Snowboarding trauma. *J Pediatr Surg* 30: 791-794, 1995

6. Canadian Ski Council National Snowboard Rider Survey of 1994. Mississauga, Ontario, Canada, Canadian Ski Council, 1994

7. Ganong RB, Heneveld EH, Beranek SR, et al: Snowboarding injuries: A report of 415 patients. *Physician Sportsmed* 20(12): 114-122, 1992

8. Giacobetti FB, Sharkey PF, Bos-Giacobetti MA, et al: Biomechanical analysis of the efficacy of in-line skating wrist guards for preventing wrist fractures. *Am J Sports Med* 25: 223-225, 1997

9. Greenwald RM, Janes PC, Swanson SC, et al: Dynamic impact response of human cadaver forearms using a brace. *Am J Sports Med* 26: 825-830, 1998

10. Janes PC, Finken GT: Snowboarding injuries, in Johnson RJ (ed): Skiing Trauma and Safety. Volume 7. AST STP 1182. Philadelphia, *ASTM*, 1993, pp 255-261

11. Lamont MK: Ski field injuries: The snowboarders, in Mote CD Jr, Johnson RJ, Hauser W, et al. (eds): Skiing Trauma and Safety. Volume 10. ASTM STP 1266. Philadelphia, *ASTM*, 1996, pp 82-86

12. Molinari M, Bertoldi L, Zucco P: Epidemiology of skiing injuries in a large Italian ski resort during 1988-1992, in Mote CD Jr, Johnson RJ, Hauser W, et al. (eds): Skiing Trauma and Safety. Volume 10. ASTM STP 1266. Philadelphia, *ASTM*, 1996, pp 87-97

13. Pino EC, Colville MR: Snowboard injuries. *Am J Sports Med* 17: 778-781, 1989

14. Prall JA, Winston KR, Brennan R: Severe snowboarding injuries. *Injury* 26: 539-542, 1995

15. Shealy JE: Snowboard vs. downhill skiing injuries, in Johnson RJ (ed): Skiing Trauma and Safety. Volume 7. ASTM STP 1182. Philadelphia, *ASTM,* 1993, pp 75-81

16. Shealy JE, Ettlinger CF: Gender related injury patterns in skiing, in Mote CD Jr, Johnson R J, Hauser W, et al. (eds): Skiing Trauma and Safety. Volume 10. ASTM STP 1266. Philadelphia, *ASTM*, 1996, pp 45-57

17. SIA National Snowboarder Survey. McLean, VA, SnowSports Industries America, October 1996

18. Van Dommelen BA, Zvirbulis RA: Upper extremity injuries in snow skiers. *Am J Sports Med* 17: 751-754, 1989

Chapter 28

Water-Related Injuries

Unintentional Drowning in the United States

- In 1998, 4,406 people drowned, including 1,003 children younger than 15 years old.[1]

- According to the U.S. Coast Guard, 734 people died in recreational boating incidents in 1999.

- In 1992, the U.S. Coast Guard received reports of 6,000 crashes involving recreational boats that resulted in 3,700 injuries and 816 deaths.[2]

- Alcohol use is involved in about 25% to 50% of adolescent and adult deaths associated with water recreation. It is a major contributing factor in up to 50% of drownings among adolescent boys.

- Nearly three-quarters of boating-related deaths were due to drowning; 89% of people who drowned were not wearing personal flotation devices.

This chapter includes "Drowning Prevention," National Center for Injury Prevention and Control (NCIPC), reviewed October 27, 2000; and "Water-Related Injuries," *Injury Fact Book, 2001-2002*, National Center for Injury Prevention and Control (NCIPC), 2002.

High Drowning Risk

Children

Drowning is the second leading cause of injury-related death for children (aged 1 through 14 years), accounting for 940 deaths in 1998.[1] In 1998, more than 1,300 children and young people ages 0-18 died from drowning.

- For every child who drowns, another four are hospitalized and 16 receive emergency department care for near-drowning.

- Among children ages 1 to 4, most drownings occur in residential swimming pools. Most children who drowned in pools were last seen in the home, had been out of sight less than five minutes, and were in the care of one or both parents at the time.

- African American children ages 5 to 19 drowned at 2.5 times the rate of white children in this age group in 1998.

Males

In 1998, males comprised 81% of people who drowned in the United States.[1]

Blacks

In 1998, the overall age-adjusted drowning rate for blacks was 1.6 times higher than for whites. Black children ages 5 through 19 years drowned at 2.5 times the rate of whites.[1] Black children ages 1 through 4 years had a lower drowning rate than white children, largely because drownings in that age group typically occur in residential swimming pools, which are not as accessible to minority children in the United States.[1,3,4]

Where Do Childhood Drownings Occur Most Often?

Most children drown in swimming pools. According to the U.S. Consumer Product Safety Commission (CPSC), emergency departments reported that among children younger than 5 years old, about 320 fatal drownings in 1991 and nearly 2,300 non-fatal near-drownings in 1993 occurred in residential swimming pools. Between 60-90% of drownings among children aged 0-4 years occur in residential pools; more than half of these occur at the child's own home. Compared with in-ground pools without four-sided fencing, 60% fewer drownings occur in in-ground pools with four-sided isolation fencing.[5]

How Often Is Alcohol Use Involved in Drownings?

Alcohol use is involved in about 25-50% of adolescent and adult deaths associated with water recreation. It is a major contributing factor in up to 50% of drownings among adolescent boys.[6,7]

Table 28.1. States with the Highest Rates of Unintentional Drowning per 100,000 population* (1998)[1]

State	Number of people drowned	Rate per 100,000 persons (1996)
Alaska	47	7.41
Mississippi	95	3.47
Louisiana	129	3.03
Idaho	34	2.90
Florida	396	2.64
Alabama	112	2.60
Arkansas	59	2.53
Hawaii	33	2.53
South Carolina	92	2.49
Oregon	76	2.38
United States	4,406	1.65

*Ranking based on age-adjusted rate. Source: NCHS 2000 Vital Statistics System

What Can Government Agencies Do to Prevent Drownings?

- Mandate and enforce legal limits for blood alcohol levels during water recreation activities.

307

- Provide public service announcements about the danger of combining alcohol with water recreation.

- Eliminate advertisements that encourage alcohol use during boating.

- Restrict the sale of alcohol at water recreation facilities.

CDC Study Results

Report Assesses Lifeguards for Drowning Prevention

A 2001 report by CDC's Injury Center assesses lifeguards as a strategy for preventing drowning and water-related injuries. The report is the product of a meeting of experts and a review of data from the United States Lifeguard Association (USLA) and other sources. Data show that during 1988–1997, more than three-quarters of drownings at USLA sites occurred when beaches were unguarded and that the chance of drowning at a beach protected by lifeguards trained under USLA standards were more than 1 in 16 million. This report will help communities, local government officials, and owners of private water recreational areas make informed decisions about whether to begin, retain, or discontinue lifeguarding services.

Survey Assesses Swimming Ability

Injury Center researchers analyzed data collected during the first Injury Control and Risk Survey to assess how well American adults thought they could swim. They found

- More than one-third of the adult population reported that they were unable to swim at least one pool length or 24 yards.

- Self-reported swimming ability declined as age increased; it increased as level of education increased.

- African Americans reported the most limited swimming ability.

- More women than men reported limited ability, despite much lower drowning rates among women.

These data, published in the journal *Public Health Reports*, will help public health practitioners identify groups at greater risk for drowning and better target water safety messages and swimming education efforts.

Pool Fencing Not Enough to Prevent Drowning Among Young Children

The majority of drownings among the youngest Americans would not have been prevented if all pools in the U.S. had adequate fencing. In a CDC-funded study, researchers estimated that proper pool fencing would have prevented about one-fifth of drownings among children under 5. This finding suggests that additional strategies (e.g., pool covers, alarms, community education) are needed to prevent drowning.

Injuries from Boat Propellers Highlight Need for Education

Injuries from boat propellers can result in permanent scarring, significant blood loss, broken bones, amputation, or death. Injury Center scientists worked with Texas public health professionals and the Texas Parks and Wildlife Department to characterize injuries from boat propellers in that state. During the three-month study of four Texas lakes, researchers identified 13 people who had been injured by boat propellers. Three of them died; those non-fatally injured sustained lacerations and broken bones. The results of the study, published in CDC's *Morbidity and Mortality Weekly Report*, indicate that severe boat propeller-related injuries may be more common than previously reported, underscoring a need to increase public awareness of safety measures and to improve tracking of such injuries.

Injuries Associated with Personal Water Craft

As sales of personal water craft (e.g., jet skis) skyrocketed in the early 1990s, so did associated injuries, Injury Center researchers found in a 1997 study. Of the estimated 33,000 people treated in hospital emergency departments between 1990 and 1995 for injuries related to personal water craft (PWC), nearly three-quarters were males. Most injuries were blunt trauma to the legs, lower torso, and head. Researchers recommended that PWC users receive specific training, that parents or other adult caregivers supervise children and teens who use PWCs, and that PWCs not be used where people are swimming or wading. Use of personal flotation devices (e.g., life jackets, life vests) can also reduce injuries among PWC users.

How Can People Guard Against Drowning?

You can greatly reduce the chances of you or your children becoming drowning or near-drowning victims by following a few simple safety tips:

- Whenever young children are swimming, playing, or bathing in water, make sure an adult is constantly watching them. By definition this means that the supervising adult should not read, play cards, talk on the phone, mow the lawn, or do any other distracting activity while watching children.

- Never swim alone or in unsupervised places. Teach children to always swim with a buddy. Keep small children away from buckets containing liquid—5-gallon industrial containers are a particular danger. Be sure to empty buckets when household chores are done. Never drink alcohol during or just before swimming, boating, or water skiing.

- Never drink alcohol while supervising children. Teach teenagers about the danger of drinking alcohol and swimming, boating, or water skiing.

- To prevent choking, never chew gum or eat while swimming, diving, or playing in water.

- Learn to swim. Enroll yourself and/or your children aged 4 and older in swimming classes. Swimming classes are not recommended for children under age 4.

- Learn CPR (cardio-pulmonary resuscitation). This is particularly important for pool owners and individuals who regularly participate in water recreation.

- *Do not* use air-filled swimming aids (such as water wings) in place of life jackets or life preservers with children. These can give parents and children a false sense of security and increase the risk of drowning.

- Check the water depth before entering. The American Red Cross recommends 9 feet as a minimum depth for diving or jumping.

If you have a swimming pool at your home:

- Install a four-sided, isolation pool fence with self-closing and self-latching gates around the pool. The fence should be at least

4 feet tall and completely separate the pool from the house and play area of the yard.

- Prevent children from having direct access to a swimming pool.

- Install a telephone near the pool. Know how to contact local emergency medical services. Post the emergency number, 911, in an easy to see place.

- Learn CPR.

Additional Tips for Open Water

- Know the local weather conditions and forecast before swimming or boating. Thunderstorms and strong winds can be extremely dangerous to swimmers and boaters.

- Restrict activities to designated swimming areas, which are usually marked by buoys.

- Be cautious, even with lifeguards present.

- Use U.S. Coast Guard-approved personal flotation devices (life jackets) when boating, regardless of distance to be traveled, size of boat, or swimming ability of boaters.

- Remember that open water usually has limited visibility, and conditions can sometimes change from hour to hour. Currents are often unpredictable—they can move rapidly and quickly change direction. A strong water current can carry even expert swimmers far from shore.

- Watch for dangerous waves and signs of rip currents—water that is discolored, unusually choppy, foamy, or filled with debris.

- If you are caught in a rip current, swim parallel to the shore. Once you are out of the current, swim toward the shore.

References

1. National Center for Health Statistics (NCHS). National Mortality Data, 1998. Hyattsville (MD): NCHS 2000.

2. US Coast Guard Boating Statistics, 1992. Washington, DC: US Department of Transportation (COMDTPUB P16754.8).

3. Branche CM. What is happening with drowning rates in the United States? In: JR Fletemeyer and SJ Freas (eds). *Drowning:*

New perspectives on intervention and prevention. Boca Raton, Florida: CRC Press LLC, 1999.

4. Branche-Dorsey CM, Russell JC, Greenspan AI, Chorba TC. Unintentional injuries: the problems and some preventive strategies. In: IL Livingston (ed). *Handbook of Black American Health: The mosaic of conditions, issues, policies and prospects*. Westport, CT: Greenwood Publishing Group, 1994.

5. US Consumer Product Safety Commission Clearinghouse, Washington DC, (301) 504-0424.

6. National Safety Council, 1993. *Accident Facts*, 1993 Ed. Itasca, Illinois: Author.

7. Howland J, Hingson R. Alcohol as a risk factor for drowning: a review of the literature (1950-1985). *Accident Analysis and Prevention* 1988;20:19-25.

Additional Information

National Center for Injury Prevention and Control
Mailstop K65
4770 Buford Highway N.E.
Atlanta, GA 30341-3724
Tel: 770-488-1506
Fax: 770-488-1667
Website: www.cdc.gov/ncip
E-mail: OHCINFO@cdc.gov

Centers for Disease Control and Prevention
6525 Belcrest Road
Hyattsville, MD 20782-2003
Tel: 301-458-4636
Website: www.cdc.gov/healthyswimming

Healthy Swimming has information about reducing the spread of recreational water illnesses.

SafeUSA™
P.O. Box 8189
Silver Springs, MD 20907-8189
Toll-Free: 888-252-7751

Website: www.cdc.gov/safeusa
E-mail: sainfo@cdc.gov

U.S. Consumer Product Safety Commission Clearinghouse
4330 East-West Highway
Bethesda, MD 20814-4408
Toll-Free: 800-638-2772
Tel: 301-504-0990
Fax: 301-504-0124 and 301-504-0025
Website: www.cpsc.gov
E-mail: info@cpsc.gov

For information about pool-related drownings and injuries.

U.S. Coast Guard, Office of Recreational Boating Safety
2100 Second St. S.W.
Washington DC 20593
Toll-Free Infoline: 800-368-5647 (Monday-Friday, 8 a.m.-4 p.m.)
Tel: 202-267-1077
Website: www.uscgboating.org/default.asp
E-mail: uscginfoline@gcrm.com

For information about boating-related drownings

The United States Lifesaving Association (USLA)
P.O. Box 366
Huntington Beach, CA 92648
Website: www.usla.org
E-mail: guard4life@aol.com

USLA works to reduce the incidence of death and injury in the aquatic environment through public education, national lifeguard standards, training programs, promotion of high levels of lifeguard readiness, and other means.

Chapter 29

Horse-Related Injuries in Pediatric Patients

Background

The American Horse Council reported 258,400 youth were involved in 4-H horse and pony programs in 1994. In 1999, 13,390 youth were members of the United States Pony Club. The actual number of youth participating in equestrian activities is greater since many youth are not members of equestrian organizations. Horseback riding tends to be more popular among girls than boys. Horses can weigh up to 1100 pounds and travel up to 40 m.p.h.

What Is the Injury Experience of Youth Involved in Horse-Related Activities?

Non-Fatal and Fatal Injuries

- Nationwide in 1999, an estimated 15,000 horse-related emergency department visits were made by youth under 15 years old.

- In 1998 and 1999, youth under 15 years represented roughly 20% of all horse-related emergency room visits nationwide.

- The most frequent types of injury include fractures, soft tissue, and head injuries.

"Horses and Children: Fact Sheet," Copyright December 2001, Marshfield Clinic. All Rights Reserved. Reprinted with permission from Marshfield Clinic.

- The most frequent body parts injured, in order, include arms, legs, and head/face.

- The most frequent cause of death and serious injury for mounted and dismounted horse activities is head injury.

- A 2000 study of U.S. horse-related pediatric trauma events revealed 36% occurred at the youth's home, 23% at a recreational area, 19% on a farm, and 5% at school.

- In a U.S. study of youth sports and recreational injuries, the highest proportion of injury events involving multiple injuries were due to riding animals—a higher proportion than bicycling, in-line skating, or sports-related falls.

- A population-based study in rural Wisconsin revealed the horse-related injury rate for youth under 16 years to be 5.6 injuries per 10,000 per year compared to 3.9 per 10,000 for adults.

Dismounted and Mounted Injuries

- Studies indicate roughly 20-30% of horse-related injuries occur while dismounted such as leading, grooming, or playing around a horse.

- Mounted injuries most often involve a youth falling off or being thrown from a horse. Dismounted injuries most often involve a youth being kicked or trodden by a horse.

- One Australian study found that youth injuries sustained while dismounted were more likely to require hospitalization than mounted injuries (42% vs. 30%).

Helmet Use

- Reliable and current information on helmet use among horse riders is not available. Studies suggest helmet use is more common among girls than boys and English riders than Western riders. Youth using horses to perform work are less likely to wear a helmet.

What Factors Are Associated with Horse-Related Injuries to Youth?

- Female gender

- 10-19 years

- No helmet use

- Immature judgment, risk taking, motor skills or technique

- More experienced riders (5+ years)

- Riding English style

- Riding 15-24 hours per month

- Horse being "spooked" by another animal, car, etc.

What Developmental Factors Must a Youth Possess to Participate in Horse-Related Activities?

- Physical size, strength, balance, and coordination to ride a horse

- Cognitive capacity to look for and react to potential hazards and follow directions

- Good judgment to not act impulsively or take excessive risks while riding

- Physically and mentally disabled youth should be evaluated by appropriate medical personnel to determine if therapeutic riding is a suitable and appropriate activity.

What Strategies Promote Safe Youth Participation in Horse-Related Activities?

- Evidence demonstrates that consistent use of a secured equestrian helmet that meets the ASTM* standard and is SEI** certified will prevent head injury.

- The American Academy of Pediatrics (AAP) recommends young riders:
    - wear a helmet that meets the ASTM standard and is SEI certified while riding horses
    - should be supervised based on skill level
    - be matched with horses appropriate for their levels of cognitive development and riding ability

- New York state and Plantation, FL have enacted legislation requiring helmet use for youth under 14 and 16 years (respectively) mounted on a horse. The effectiveness of these laws in preventing horse-related injuries is unknown.

*American Society of Testing Materials, ASTM F-1163-99

**Safety Equipment Institute, SEI

Additional Information

National Children's Center for Rural and Agricultural Health and Safety

National Farm Medicine Center
1000 North Oak Avenue
Marshfield, WI 54449
Toll-Free: 888-924-SAFE (7233)
Fax: 715-389-4996
Website: http://research.marshfieldclinic.org/children/Resources/
Equestrian/FactSheet.htm
E-mail: nccrahs@mfldclin.edu

Chapter 30

Playground Injuries

How Large Is the Problem of Playground-Related Injuries?

- Each year in the United States, 200,000 preschool and elementary school children visit emergency departments for care of injuries sustained on playground equipment (about 1 injury every 2½ minutes).[1]

- About 35% of all playground-related injuries are severe (e.g., fractures, internal injuries, concussions, dislocations, amputations, crushes).[1]

- Public playgrounds account for about 70% of injuries related to playground equipment.[1]

- In schools, most injuries to students between the ages of 5 and 14 years occur on playgrounds.[2]

Which Playground Equipment Causes the Most Injury?

- Most injuries occur when children fall off swings, monkey bars, climbers, or slides.[1]

- Falls off of playground equipment to the ground account for more than 60% of all playground-related injuries.[1,3]

"Playground Injuries," National Center for Injury Prevention and Control (NCIPC), reviewed January 27, 2000.

How Many Injuries Require Hospitalization?

- Slightly less than 3% of all playground injuries require hospitalization.[1]

How Many Children Die Each Year Because of Playground-Related Injuries?

- Each year, nearly 20 children die from playground-related injuries. More than half of these deaths result from strangulation and about one-third result from falls.[2]

What Costs Are Associated with Playground-Related Injury?

- In 1995, the costs were $1.2 billion for children younger than 15 years old.[2]

What Is CDC Doing to Prevent Playground-Related Injuries?

- The National Center for Injury Prevention and Control, CDC, funds the National Program for Playground Safety (NPPS), which works to prevent playground-related injuries and the attendant suffering and costs. This program is based at the University of Northern Iowa in Cedar Falls, Iowa.

What Are the Goals of NPPS?

- To implement a national plan for the prevention of playground-related injuries.

- To maintain a clearinghouse of materials on playground safety and make those materials available to anyone who requests them.

- To provide an information hotline on preventing playground-related injury.

- To hold training programs for teachers and playground safety inspectors.

- To research the impact attenuation characteristics of playground surfaces under a variety of conditions.

References

1. Consumer Product Safety Commission (CPSC). *National Electronic Injury Surveillance System 1990-94*. Washington (DC): CPSC.

2. Office of Technology Assessment. *Risks to students in school*. Washington (DC): U.S. Government Printing Office, 1995.

3. U.S. Consumer Product Safety Commission (CPSC). *Handbook for public playground safety*. Washington, DC: author, 1997. Publication No. 325.

Additional Information

National Program for Playground Safety
School for Health, Physical Education and Leisure Services
WRC 205
University of Northern Iowa
Cedar Falls, IA 50614-0618
Toll-Free: 800-554-PLAY
Tel: 319-273-2416
Fax: 319-273-7308
Website: www.uni.edu/playground
E-mail: playground-safety@uni.edu

Brochures available from NPPS:
- Inspection Guide for Parents
- A Blueprint for Increasing Playground Safety
- Supervision Means…
- All Children Should Play on Age-Appropriate Equipment
- Falls to Surface Should Be Cushioned
- Equipment Should Be Safe
- Planning a Play Area for Children
- The National Action Plan for Playground Safety
- Funding Tips for Playgrounds
- SAFE Playground Resources

Videos available from NPPS:
- ABC's of Supervision (training for elementary school supervisors)

- America's Playgrounds—Make Them Safe (NPPS overview)
- Sammy's Playground (for grades K-3)
- SAFE Playgrounds—General Description of SAFE Playgrounds

  Other Materials available from NPPS
- Summary Report for NPPS
- SAFE Playground Workbook
- SAFE Playground Handbook

National Center for Injury Prevention and Control
Mailstop K65
4770 Buford Highway NE
Atlanta, GA 30341-3724
Tel: 770-488-1506
Fax: 770-488-1667
Website: www.cdc.gov/ncipc
E-mail: OHCINFO@cdc.gov

SafeUSA™
P.O. Box 8189
Silver Springs, MD 20907-8189
Toll-Free: 888-252-7751
Website: www.cdc.gov/safeusa
E-mail: sainfo@cdc.gov

U.S. Consumer Product Safety Commission
4330 East-West Highway
Bethesda, MD 20814-4408
Toll-Free: 800-638-2772
Tel: 301-504-0990
Fax: 301-504-0124 and 301-504-0025
Website: www.cpsc.gov
E-mail: info@cpsc.gov

Chapter 31

Scooter Injuries Soar

Non-Powered Scooters Injury Data

- Injuries associated with non-powered scooters increased dramatically since 2000.

- From January 2000 through December 31, 2000, CPSC estimates there were about 40,500 emergency room treated injuries associated with scooters.

- In November 2001, CPSC estimated there were more than 84,400 emergency room treated injuries relating to scooters for January 2001 through September 2001.

- About 85% of the injuries were to children less than 15 years old.

- Two-thirds of the injuries are to males.

- Most common injuries are fractures.

Motorized Scooter Injury Data

- CPSC reported that 2,870 emergency room treated injuries relating to motorized scooters were reported for the first 9 months of 2001. There were 2,760 injuries reported in the same period in 2000.

"Scooter Data," U.S. Consumer Product Safety Commission, 2001.

- There were 4,390 total injuries reported in 2000 associated with motorized scooters and 1,330 in 1999.

- 39 percent of the injuries occurred to children under 15 years of age. The most common injuries were fractures. Most injuries were to the arms, legs, faces, and heads.

Non-Powered Scooter Death Data

The following is the latest CPSC update on non-powered scooter-related deaths. CPSC has reports of 16 deaths relating to non-powered scooters through November 19, 2001.

- A man riding a scooter down an Albuquerque, NM, roadway at night was struck and killed by a pickup truck on January 25, 2001.

- A 12-year-old boy from Spring Hill, FL, died January 20, 2001, after both he and his twin brother were hit by a car while riding their scooters.

- A 10-year-old boy from Forest, OH, died January 6, 2001, after a fall from a scooter.

- An 8-year-old boy from Stockton, CA, died March 26, 2001, after being hit by a car.

- A 13-year-old boy from Mount Sterling, KY, died April 3, 2001, after being struck by a car.

- A 10-year-old boy from San Leandro, CA, died April 9, 2001, when he lost control of his scooter on a steep hill and fell.

- A 9-year-old boy from Miami, FL, died April 23, 2001, when he was struck by a van while riding his scooter out of his driveway.

- A man from Augusta, GA, reportedly died of head trauma relating to a scooter incident. The date of the incident was not given.

- An 8-year old boy from Detroit, MI, died when he was struck by a car on June 17. An 18-year old male from Harpers Ferry, WV, died when the scooter he was riding swerved in the path of an on-coming pickup truck.

- A 12-year-old boy from Harpers Ferry, WV, died when the scooter he was riding collided with a garbage truck in July 2001.

- A man, 57, from Temecula, CA, died on July 31, 2001 when he fell off a scooter and struck his head.

- A boy, 10, from San Diego, CA, died on July 31, 2001 when he was riding a scooter down a hill at a high rate of speed and struck by a car.

- A man, 66, from Lebanon, PA, died on August 8, 2001 when he fell from a scooter and struck his head against the curb.

- A 50-year-old New Jersey man died August 22 after losing control of a scooter at Elk Neck State Park, MD, according to the Department of Natural Resources.

- A 9-year-old boy from Altamonte Springs, FL, died on September 12, 2001 when he was struck by the van driven by his father, after he lost grip or let go of the side view mirror he was holding onto.

Motorized Scooter Deaths Data

The following is the latest CPSC update on motorized scooter-related deaths. CPSC has reports of three deaths relating to motorized scooters so far in 2001.

- A 27-year-old male in Phoenix, AZ, died on July 24 when he was struck by a van.

- A 45-year-old woman died in July 2001 from head injuries sustained after falling from a motorized scooter near Escanaba, MI.

- In September 2001, a 13-year-old boy died after being struck by a car while riding a motorized scooter in St. Petersburg, FL.

Safety Recommendations

- Wear a helmet, knee pads, and elbow pads. (Wrist guards may make it difficult to grip the handle and steer the scooter.)

- Children under age 8 should not use non-powered scooters without close adult supervision.

- Children under 12 should not ride motorized scooters.

- Avoid gravel and uneven pavement, which can cause falls.

- Don't ride scooters in traffic.

- Don't ride scooters at night—riders can't see where they're going or be seen by others.

- Wear sturdy shoes.

- Owners of scooters should check with local authorities for local laws regarding scooters.

Chapter 32

BB Gun Injuries

Each year in the United States, approximately 30,000 persons with BB and pellet gun*-related injuries are treated in hospital emergency departments (EDs).[1] Most (95%) injuries are BB or pellet gunshot wounds (GSWs); 5% are other types of injuries (e.g., lacerations sustained inadvertently while cleaning or shooting a gun or contusions resulting from being struck with the butt of a gun).[1] Most (81%) persons treated for BB and pellet GSWs are children and teenagers (aged less than or equal to 19 years). To assist in developing strategies for preventing these injuries, CDC analyzed data from an ongoing special study of nonfatal gun-related injuries conducted using the National Electronic Injury Surveillance System (NEISS) of the U.S. Consumer Product Safety Commission; this study has characterized the epidemiology of BB and pellet GSWs among children and teenagers in the United States during June 1992-May 1994.[2] This report summarizes the circumstances of six cases of BB and pellet gun-related injuries identified through NEISS and presents the findings of the analysis of NEISS data.

NEISS includes a probability sample of 91 hospitals selected from all hospitals with at least six beds and that provide 24-hour emergency service.[2] Data were weighted to provide national estimates of injuries treated in hospital EDs in the United States and its territories.[1]

"BB and Pellet Gun-Related Injuries–United States, June 1992-May 1994," *MMWR Weekly*, December 15, 1995/ 44(49); 909-13, reviewed May 2001.

Case Reports

- A 9-year-old boy was struck by a BB beneath his lower left eyelid after he stepped from behind a board at which other children were shooting. The children had been left unsupervised following a youth club target practice session.

- A 16-year-old boy sustained a severe midbrain injury from a self-inflicted combination BB/pellet gun GSW through the roof of his mouth.

- A 9-year-old girl incurred a pellet injury to the back of her right ankle after four boys fired a pellet gun at her from a passing car while she was walking on a sidewalk.

- A 10-year-old boy sustained injuries to his neck and trachea after being struck by a BB from a gun that had been fired unintentionally by an unspecified person.

- A 13-year-old boy was shot in the neck with a BB gun while he and a friend were playing in a house. The friend, who believed the gun was unloaded, had aimed the gun at the 13-year-old and pulled the trigger.

- A 16-year-old boy sustained a penetrating injury to his right eye after being struck by a BB that ricocheted from a gun fired by a friend.

Summary of NEISS Data

During June 1992-May 1994, a total of 959 BB and pellet GSWs among children and teenagers were reported through NEISS. Based on these reports, an estimated 47,137 (95% confidence interval {CI} = 39,746-54,528) children and teenagers were treated for BB or pellet GSWs in hospital emergency departments (ED) during this period (an average of 23,600 per year or 65 per day) (Table 32.1). The incidence of BB or pellet gun-related injuries was highest for males (53.5 per 100,000 population) and children aged 10-14 years (66.6 per 100,000 population) (Table 32.1), and the sex- and age group-specific rate was highest for males aged 10-14 years (114.3 per 100,000 population {95% CI=94.1-134.5}).

Although most (64%) persons with GSWs were transported to EDs by private vehicles, 8% of those treated were taken to EDs by emergency medical services (Table 32.2). Injuries to the eye, face, head, and neck accounted for 31% of all injuries. Hospitalization was required for 5% of cases; of these, 37% were associated with severe injury to the eye.

Data on victim-shooter relationship were complete for 71% of cases (Table 32.2). Based on these data, 31% of injuries were self-inflicted, and 33% were caused by friends, acquaintances, or relatives. Data on 76% of the incidents indicated the type of injury: although most (66%) resulted from unintentional shootings, approximately 10% were assaults; suicide attempts were rare (0.1%). Locale of the injury incident was known for approximately 55% of cases; approximately 45% of injuries occurred in and around a home, apartment, or condominium.

Reported by: Office of Statistics and Programming, Div. of Violence Prevention and Div. of Unintentional Injury Prevention, National Center for Injury Prevention and Control, CDC.

Table 32.1. Characteristics of Children and Teenagers Aged ≤19 Years Treated in Hospital Emergency Departments for BB and Pellet Gun-Related Injuries–United States, June 1992-May 1994

Characteristic	No. *	(%)	Rate +	(95% CI &)
Sex				
Male	40,605	(86.1)	53.5	(45.1-61.9)
Female	6,532	(13.9)	9.0	(6.7-11.3)
Age (yrs)				
0-4 @	1,040	(2.2)		
5-9	8,033	(17.0)	21.6	(16.5-26.7)
10-14	24,400	(51.8)	66.6	(54.9-78.3)
15-19	13,664	(29.0)	39.6	(31.8-47.4)
Total	47,137	(100.0)	31.8	(26.8-36.8)

*Based on weighted data from 959 BB and pellet gunshot injuries reported through the National Electronic Injury Surveillance System.

+ Annualized rate per 100,000 population.

& Confidence interval.

@ Rate was not calculated because of the small number (21) of cases in this age group; interpret estimate with caution.

Table 32.2. BB and Pellet Gun-Related Injuries Treated in Hospital Emergency Departments (EDs) for Children and Teenagers Aged ≤19 Years, by Selected Characteristics–United States, June 1992-May 1994 (continued on next page)

Characteristic	No.*	(%)
Mode of transport to ED		
Private vehicle	30,298	(64.3)
Walked in	7,788	(16.5)
Emergency medical service/		
Fire rescue/Ambulance	3,742	(8.0)
Police vehicle	468	(1.0)
Other/Not stated	4,841	(10.2)
Primary body part injured		
Extremity	25,453	(54.0)
Trunk	7,276	(15.4)
Face	6,788	(14.4)
Head/Neck	4,747	(10.1)
Eye	2,839	(6.0)
Other	34	(0.1)
ED Discharge Disposition		
Not hospitalized	44,759	(95.0)
Hospitalized	2,378	(5.0)
Victim-Shooter relationship		
Self	14,636	(31.0)
Friend/Acquaintance	9,280	(19.7)
Relative	6,445	(13.7)
Stranger	1,260	(2.7)
Other/Shooter not seen	1,821	(3.9)
Not Stated	13,695	(29.1)
Type of Injury		
Unintentional	30,960	(65.7)
Assault	4,903	(10.4)
Suicide attempt	34	(0.1)
Not stated	11,240	(23.8)

Table 32.2. BB and Pellet Gun-Related Injuries Treated in Hospital Emergency Departments (EDs) for Children and Teenagers Aged ≤19 Years, by Selected Characteristics–United States, June 1992-May 1994 (continued from previous page)

Characteristic	No.*	(%)
Locale of injury incident		
Home/Apartment/Condominium	21,413	(45.4)
Street/Highway	1,821	(3.9)
Other property	1,389	(2.9)
School/Recreation area	1,104	(2.3)
Farm	90	(0.2)
Not stated	21,320	(45.2)
Total	47,137	(100.0)

*Based on weighted data from 959 BB and pellet gunshot injuries reported through the National Electronic Injury Surveillance System.

An estimated 3.2 million nonpowder guns are sold in the United States each year; 80% of these have muzzle velocities greater than 350 feet per second (fps) and 50% have velocities from 500 fps to 930 fps (AC Homan, US Consumer Product Safety Commission, unpublished data, 1994). Most of these guns are intended for use by persons aged 8-18 years. At close range, projectiles from many BB and pellet guns, especially those with velocities greater than 350 fps, can cause tissue damage similar to that inflicted by powder-charged bullets fired from low-velocity conventional firearms.[3] Injuries associated with use of these guns can result in permanent disability or death;[4] injuries from BBs or pellets projected from air guns involving the eye particularly are severe.[5] For example, based on data from the National Eye Trauma System and the United States Eye Injury Registry—a system of voluntary reporting by ophthalmologists—projectiles from air guns account for 63% of reported perforating eye injuries that occur in recreational settings.[6]

Despite the large number of BB and pellet gun-related injuries treated in hospital EDs each year,[1] there are no nationally specified safety standards for nonpowder guns. Although voluntary industry standards were established in 1978 and revised in 1992,[7] the effectiveness of these standards for preventing injuries has not been determined. These voluntary standards specify two types of warning labels, including one on the gun itself ("Warning: Before using read Owner's Manual available free from {company name}"), and one on the packaging ("Warning: Not a toy. Adult supervision required. Misuse or careless use may cause serious injury or death. May be dangerous up to {specific distance} ** yards ({specific distance} meters).").[7] The voluntary standards also specify that the owner's manual should provide instructions about handling and operating the gun safely, selecting safe and proper targets, caring for and maintaining the gun properly, storing of the gun in an unloaded state and in a safe and proper manner, and always confirming that the gun is unloaded when removed from storage or received from another person.[7] However, these standards do not include specifications regarding other important injury prevention measures pertinent to minors (e.g., limits on maximum velocity and impact force of BBs and pellets or design modifications to clearly indicate when a gun is loaded).[8]

In the United States, 14 states have enacted laws to regulate the sale or possession of nonpowder guns. Although most of these states restrict the purchase, possession, or use of these guns by minors aged less than 16 years or aged less than 18 years, such age restrictions on the purchase of these guns are void in most of these states when a minor has obtained permission from a parent or guardian.

Analysis of the NEISS data indicate that BB and pellet GSWs treated in hospital EDs typically result from an unintentional shooting of a young or adolescent male who either shot himself or was shot by a friend, acquaintance, or relative. Many of these shootings occur when using or playing with a gun in or around the home. These findings suggest that ready access to a BB or pellet gun and ammunition stored in the home and/or the lack of supervision during use of the gun may contribute substantially to the risk for injury among children and adolescents, especially for boys aged 10-14 years. Although most BB and pellet gun injuries are unintentional, the findings from this analysis and from a statewide ED-based surveillance system in Massachusetts[9] also indicate that BB and pellet guns sometimes have been used to purposefully inflict harm.

Unintentional BB and pellet gun-related injuries that occur during unsupervised activities are preventable. Parents considering the purchase of a BB or pellet gun for their children should be aware of the potential hazards of these guns, and should help to ensure the safety of their children in the presence of a BB or pellet gun. Children and teenage users should recognize that these guns are not toys but are designed and intended specifically for recreational and competitive sport use. Parents or other adults should provide direct supervision at all times for each child who is using or observing the use of these guns. Each user should be educated about the potential danger of these guns, the importance of gun safety practices, and how to safely handle and fire the gun. The use of protective eyewear should be enforced during shooting activities. When not in use, all guns in the home should be kept locked up and unloaded. Subsequent efforts to reduce the severity and frequency of injuries associated with BB and pellet guns should include determination of the effectiveness of a variety of interventions (e.g., technological, regulatory, environmental, and behavioral).

References

1. McNeill AM, Annest JL. The ongoing hazard of BB and pellet gun-related injuries in the United States. *Ann Emerg Med* 1995;26:187-94.

2. Annest JL, Mercy JA, Gibson DR, Ryan GW. National estimates of nonfatal firearm-related injuries: beyond the tip of the iceberg. *JAMA* 1995;273:1749-54.

3. Harris W, Luterman A, Curreri PW. BB and pellet guns: toys or deadly weapons? *J Trauma* 1983;23:566-9.

4. Wascher RA, Gwinn BC. Air rifle injury to the heart with retrograde caval migration. *J Trauma* 1995;38:379-81.

5. Schein OD, Enger C, Tielsch JM. The context and consequences of ocular injuries from air guns. *Am J Ophthalmol* 1994;117: 501-6.

6. Parver LM. The National Eye Trauma System. *Int Ophthalmol Clin* 1988;28:203.

7. Committee on Standards, American Society for Testing and Materials. Standard consumer safety specification for non-powder guns. Conshohocken, Pennsylvania: American Society for Testing and Materials, 1992.

8. Greensher J, Aronow R, Bass JL, et al. Injuries related to "toy" firearms: Committee on Accident and Poison Prevention. *Pediatrics* 1987;79:473-4.

9. CDC. Emergency department surveillance for weapon-related injuries—Massachusetts, November 1993-April 1994. *MMWR* 1995;44:160-3,169.

*In this report, the terms BB gun and pellet gun refer to nonpowder guns that use compressed air or gas to propel lead pellets or steel BBs.

**Distance is dependent on the type of gun and muzzle velocity.

Chapter 33

Risks Associated with Home Trampolines

Trampoline-related injuries have almost tripled since 1991 (Table 33.1). In 1999, CPSC estimates that almost 100,000[1] people were treated in U.S. hospital emergency rooms for injuries associated with trampolines. In 1991, by comparison, an estimated 37,500[2] people were treated for these injuries. Since 1990, CPSC has received reports of 11 deaths relating to trampoline use.

Death and Injury Data

- Victims who died from trampoline use ranged in age from 3 to 43, with 6 victims being teenagers, ages 12 to 19. Falls from the trampoline were the most frequent cause of death, followed by landing on the neck while attempting somersaults.

- Most trampoline-related injuries occur to children. Children ages 6 to 14 comprise almost two-thirds of the hospital emergency room injuries. Children under 6 were treated for about 15% of trampoline injuries in hospital emergency rooms.

- Most trips to hospital emergency rooms are the result of jumpers colliding with one another, falling on the trampoline springs or frame, falling or jumping off the trampoline, or doing stunts.

"Trampolines," U.S. Consumer Product Safety Commission, September 2000; "Trampoline Safety Alert," Consumer Product Safety Commission CPSC Document #085; and "Trampoline Safety," SafeUSA™, updated March 25, 2002.

- In 1999, injuries to the leg/foot were reported most frequently, accounting for 40% of the total. Injuries to the arm/hand, head/face/neck, and shoulder/trunk were associated with 29%, 20%, and 10% of the total, respectively.

- About 4% of all trampoline emergency room-treated injuries result in hospitalization.

- There is no indication that deaths or neck injuries resulting in paraplegia or quadriplegia have increased.

Market Data

- According to the International Trampoline Industry Association, an estimated 640,000 backyard trampolines were sold in 1998, more than a 350% increase in sales from an estimated 140,000 sold in 1989.

- An estimated 3 million backyard trampolines are in use today.

- Backyard trampolines, 10 to 14 feet in diameter, sell for about $200 to $600.

Safety Actions

- To address some known hazards associated with trampolines, CPSC staff requested changes to the ASTM voluntary safety standard for trampolines. Four provisions, effective in 1999, were added to the standard. These included:

  1. Padding must cover the entire frame, hooks, and springs.

  2. Labels on trampoline boxes must state that trampolines over 20 inches tall are not recommended for children under six years of age.

  3. Ladders cannot be sold with trampolines (to prevent young children's access to these products).

  4. Warnings visible on trampoline beds must alert jumpers against somersaults and multiple jumpers, which can cause deaths, paralysis, and the largest number of injuries.

- Trampoline net enclosures can prevent injuries from falling off trampolines.

As sales of trampolines have increased over the past decade, so have the number of trampoline-related injuries. Trampoline gymnastics was scheduled as an event at the 2000 Summer Olympics for the first time, which is likely to encourage more individuals to use trampolines.

To prevent further injuries, consumers who choose to use trampolines should follow safety guidelines. These include allowing only one person at a time on the trampoline, not attempting somersaults, and always supervising children who use trampolines.

References

1. The confidence interval of this estimate at the 95% level of confidence is 82,300–115,400.

2. The confidence interval of this estimate at the 95% level of confidence is 23,000–52,100.

Trampoline Safety Alert

The U. S. Consumer Product Safety Commission (CPSC) wants you and your family to be safe when using trampolines. The CPSC estimates that in 1998 there were 95,000 hospital emergency room-treated injuries associated with trampolines. About 75 percent of the victims are under 15 years of age, and 10 percent are under 5 years of age. Since 1990, CPSC has received reports of 6 deaths involving trampolines. The hazards that result in injuries and deaths are:

- Colliding with another person on the trampoline.
- Landing improperly while jumping or doing stunts on the trampoline.
- Falling or jumping off the trampoline.
- Falling on the trampoline springs or frame.

Almost all of the trampolines associated with injuries were at private homes, usually in backyards. Most of the injuries occurred on full-size trampolines. Here are the steps you can take to help prevent serious trampoline injuries, especially sprains, fractures, scrapes, bruises, and cuts.

- Allow only one person on the trampoline at a time.
- Do not attempt or allow somersaults.
- Do not allow trampoline to be used without shock-absorbing pads that completely cover the springs, hooks, and the frame.

- Place the trampoline away from structures and other play areas. Use shock-absorbent material on the ground around the perimeter.

- Do not use a ladder with the trampoline because it provides unsupervised access by small children. No child under 6 years of age should use a regular-size trampoline. Secure the trampoline to prevent unauthorized and unattended use.

- Always supervise children who use a trampoline.

American Academy of Pediatrics Advice for Parents

More than 83,000 injuries related to trampolines were treated in hospital emergency rooms in 1996. Nearly all of these injuries occurred on home trampolines. Because injuries are common and can be severe, the American Academy of Pediatrics recommends that trampolines be used only in supervised training programs—never at home, in outdoor playgrounds, or in schools.

Preventing Trampoline Injuries

A trampoline is not a toy. The American Academy of Pediatrics offers this advice for parents:

- Never buy a trampoline for use at home.

- Never allow your child to use a trampoline at someone else's home.

Who Is Affected?

As many as 500,000 trampolines intended for backyard use are sold in the U.S. each year. In 1996, the latest year for which data exist, more than 83,000 people were injured badly enough while using trampolines to seek treatment in hospital emergency departments. Almost all of those injured were using home trampolines. More than 75 percent of those injured were under age 15, and 10 percent of the injuries were sustained by children under 5 years old. Forty percent of trampoline-related injuries are sprains and strains, most frequently affecting the leg or foot. Nearly one-third of injuries are fractures, many of which require surgery. Younger children appear to be at the greatest risk for fractures, while older children more often suffer sprains and strains. Head and neck injuries account for about 10 percent of injuries associated with the trampoline, and about 15 percent of head injuries involve fractures, concussions, and closed-head trauma. Deaths from trampoline use are rare (on average, less than one per year).

Because of the injury risks associated with the trampoline, the American Academy of Pediatrics has recommended that trampolines never be used at home, on playgrounds, in physical education classes, or for athletic competition. The U.S. Consumer Product Safety Commission has stated that children under six years old, because of their immature motor skills, should not use trampolines in any setting.

Table 33.1. Estimated Number of Emergency Room Treated Injuries Associated with Trampolines, by Year, 1991–1999.

Year	Number of E.R. Treated Injuries
1991	37,555
1992	41,897
1993	44,116
1994	50,189
1995	62,416
1996	78,663
1997	82,722
1998	95,239
1999	98,889

Safety Resources

American Academy of Pediatrics (AAP)
141 Northwest Point Boulevard
Elk Grove Village, IL 60007-1098
Tel: 847-434-4000
Fax: 847-434-8000
Website: www.aap.org
E-mail: kidsdocs@aap.org

U.S. Consumer Product Safety Commission
4330 East-West Highway
Bethesda, MD 20814-4408
Toll-Free: 800-638-2772
Tel: 301-504-0990
Fax: 301-504-0124 and 301-504-0025
Website: www.cpsc.gov
E-mail: info@cpsc.gov

References

American Academy of Orthopaedic Surgeons Seminar (Sullivan J, Grana W, editors). *The Pediatric Athlete*. Park Ridge, IL: The Academy, 1990:137-138.

American Academy of Pediatrics. Trampolines at home, school, and recreational centers. *Pediatrics* 1999;103(5):1053-1056.

Smith G. Injuries to children in the United States related to trampolines, 1990-1995: A national epidemic. *Pediatrics* 1998;101(3):406-412.

Part Four

Diagnosis, Treatment, and Rehabilitation of Sports Injuries

Chapter 34

On-Field Examination and Care: An Emergency Checklist for Athletic Events

The on-site physician at an athletic event must be able to recognize life-threatening conditions, provide initial care for all conditions, and direct transport if needed. Preparation is critical for avoiding catastrophe; it involves establishing communication and protocol beforehand, as well as developing a mental checklist for assessing injuries. After ensuring an adequate airway, breathing, and circulation, the examiner determines the patient's level of consciousness, mental status, symptoms, and assesses for neck injury. The physician may then need to prepare for emergency transport or for further evaluation on the sidelines.

Medical coverage of sporting events is an enjoyable and important contribution for many sports medicine professionals. These providers carry the responsibilities of emergency care, triage, and judgment concerning return to play. They know that their initial response to an injury on the playing field can make the difference between life and death. Education and preparation are critical for making informed decisions and giving proper treatment, and part of preparation involves establishing a mental checklist as outlined below.

"On-Field Examination and Care: An Emergency Checklist," by Michael J. Stuart, MD, *The Physician and Sportsmedicine*, Vol. 26, No. 11, November 1998, © McGraw-Hill, Inc., reprinted with permission; and "Seriously Injured? Get to the ER—Stat!" by Cary Zigman, M.S., EMT-D, © Sports Medicine Performance Center of St. Francis Hospital, Milwaukee, Wisconsin, reprinted with permission.

Planning Ahead

Serious, catastrophic, and life-threatening injuries are rarely encountered at athletic events, especially in young participants. Despite these favorable odds, the on-site physician must always anticipate the worst. A cardiac emergency is more likely to occur in a spectator, such as a parent or grandparent. Brain injury and spine trauma with spinal cord involvement do occur in sports. The best approach is to plan for resuscitation and emergency transport before the event:

- Introduce yourself to the ambulance crew (if available on site).

- Establish a means of communication with a hospital and/or ambulance company, which can mean having a cellular phone or locating on-site phones for dialing 911. Phone numbers for non-emergencies should also be on hand.

- Identify potential help in attendance (e.g., athletic trainers, other physicians, emergency medical technicians, nurses, students, coaches).

- Establish the availability and location of emergency equipment (e.g., spine board, neck support, bolt cutters, first aid kit, crutches).

- Determine the levels of care available at the local medical facility and where to refer injuries that require specialized evaluation and treatment.

Initial Response

Start with basic cardiopulmonary resuscitation (CPR) by establishing responsiveness and initiating treatment as necessary. All medical personnel and preferably each member of the coaching staff should complete a basic CPR course available through the American Heart Association or the American Red Cross. Hands-on practice is excellent preparation.

Talk with the athlete without moving his or her head or neck and determine the level of consciousness. Proceed with the ABCs: airway (make sure the athlete has an adequate airway), breathing (ensure an air exchange: chest rise, breath sounds, and speech), and circulation (make sure the athlete has a pulse).

Evaluation of the Unconscious Athlete

An unconscious athlete is, of course, unable to communicate symptoms, and the physical examination provides very limited information.

Assume that the athlete has a serious neck injury until you ascertain otherwise. The athlete must remain in position: Place a hand or have an assistant place a hand on either side of the head to stabilize the neck until the evaluation is complete. Observe basic precautions:

- Do not move the athlete.
- Do not remove the helmet.
- Do not use ammonia inhalants, which may cause the head to jerk from the noxious stimulus.
- Do not give liquids or food.
- Do not rush the evaluation.
- Do not worry about delaying the game.

If the athlete is unresponsive, alert other medical personnel and coaches, and call for an ambulance.

The medical staff should then proceed with CPR steps as necessary. If the athlete is not breathing, start rescue breathing. For a football or ice hockey player, rescue breathing or CPR can be done with the helmet and shoulder pads in place once the face mask has been removed. A football face mask can often be removed by unscrewing the plastic mounting clips or cutting them with heavy-duty shears or bolt cutters.

Use the log roll method to turn the patient supine onto a spine board. Open the airway with a jaw-thrust maneuver, not neck hyperextension. If breathing is absent after 3 to 5 seconds, give respirations.

Similarly, CPR must be started if the athlete has no carotid pulse. Circulation is maintained through chest compressions.

If the patient has profuse bleeding, apply direct pressure with a sterile or clean dressing if possible. The major artery supplying the area can also be compressed.

In transporting the patient to the emergency department or trauma center, protective equipment should be left on because spinal alignment is closest to normal when the helmet and shoulder pads are in place. The head and neck should be stabilized at all times, and a spine board should be used. *Remember*: Transport can cause displacement of unstable cervical spine injuries and even lead to permanent spinal cord sequelae.

Evaluation of the Conscious Athlete

The initial on-field evaluation of a conscious athlete determines the presence of a serious or life-threatening condition. Obtain a brief

345

history and perform a screening physical examination. The athlete should not be allowed to sit up or walk until neck injury has been excluded.

Mental status. Assess orientation to person, place, time, and situation (ask the athlete to describe the circumstance of the injury). Check for retrograde amnesia (loss of memory of events immediately before the injury).

Symptoms. Ask about pain, headache, dizziness, nausea, blurred or double vision, and numbness, tingling, or electric-shock sensations in the extremities.

Mechanism of injury. Serious neck injuries (cervical spine fractures and dislocations) are most commonly caused by an axial load to the head with the spine in a flexed position (impact to the top of the head with the chin down).

Rule out neck injury. The athlete should not sit up or walk unless he or she has:

- no neck pain or tenderness;

- no pain, feeling of numbness, or tingling sensations in the arms or legs;

- normal sensation to touch on the chest, arms, hands, legs, and feet; and

- normal motor function on both sides (can make a fist, bend the elbow, lift the arm, curl the toes, move the ankle up and down, bend the knee, and lift the leg).

Regional physical exam. Briefly examine the area of the athlete's complaint. Check for deformity, swelling, bleeding, tenderness, and active range of motion.

Postural symptoms. Have the athlete sit up, and reassess for dizziness, nausea, pain, or other symptoms. When an athlete sits up, he or she should always do so under his or her own power, rather than be pulled up by helpful bystanders. It is often at this point that the athlete decides not to get up, and the injury is shown to be more serious than previously suspected.

Move to sidelines. If there is no evidence of head, neck, or spine trauma, unstable fractures, or uncontrolled bleeding, the athlete can be helped carefully off the field. If these serious injuries remain a possibility, the athlete should be transported off the field on a spine board.

Helping the athlete to the sidelines may require splinting of an injured extremity and/or assistance with walking to avoid weight bearing. Obtain a more detailed history and physical examination on the sidelines or in the locker room or training room.

Injury Severity

The initial assessment of injury severity will guide further evaluation and treatment (Table 34.1). Mild injuries are treated on-site according to first-aid principles. Moderate injuries may preclude immediate return to play. Referral to a specialist is indicated for dental or eye trauma or if there is any question about the type or severity of an injury. Severe injuries require prompt transport to a medical facility for further assessment and care.

Life-threatening injuries demand relevant resuscitation efforts and emergency transportation to the most appropriate trauma care facility available. These conditions include respiratory arrest or irregular breathing, severe chest or abdominal pain, excessive bleeding from a major artery, suspected spinal injury, head injury with prolonged loss of consciousness, fractures or dislocations with no pulse, and any signs of shock or internal hemorrhage.

An Orderly, Logical Assessment

The first responder at the scene of an athletic injury needs to be able to recognize a life-threatening condition, provide emergency care, and facilitate transportation to a medical facility when indicated. An orderly, logical primary assessment on the field can help identify serious conditions promptly and guide further evaluation and treatment.

Suggested Readings

Allman FL, Crow RW: On-field evaluation of sports injuries, in Griffin LY (ed): *Orthopaedic Knowledge Update: Sports Medicine.* Rosemont, IL, American Academy of Orthopaedic Surgeons, 1994, pp 141-149

Fox K: Emergency procedures, in Anderson MK, Hall SJ (eds): *Sports Injury Management.* Baltimore, Williams & Wilkins, 1995, pp 57-101

Table 34.1. Classification of Injury Severity

Type of Injury	Degree of Injury			
	Mild	Moderate	Severe	Life-Threatening
Skin or penetrating	Abrasion; superficial laceration	Deep laceration without neurovascular or articular involvement	Deep laceration with neurovascular or articular involvement	Major artery laceration
Musculoskeletal	Sprain, strain, or contusion without swelling or loss of motion	Sprain, strain, or contusion with some swelling, pain, and limitation of motion	Sprain, strain, or contusion with marked swelling, pain, and limitation of motion; fracture or dislocation	
Brain or spinal cord	Head trauma with transient confusion (complete resolution in <15 min)	Concussion with symptoms >15 min but without loss of consciousness	Concussion with retrograde amnesia or loss of consciousness	Head injury with prolonged loss of consciousness; cervical spine injury with spinal cord involvement
Miscellaneous	Blister	Dental injury		Cardiac arrest; respiratory failure or airway obstruction

Hunter-Griffin LY: *Emergency assessment of the injured athlete, in Athletic Training and Sports Medicine*. Park Ridge, IL, American Academy of Orthopaedic Surgeons, 1991, pp 156-166

Magee DJ: Emergency sports assessment, in Magee DJ: *Orthopedic Physical Assessment*, ed 3. Philadelphia, WB Saunders, 1997, pp 727-757

—by Michael J. Stuart, MD

Dr. Stuart [author] is an associate professor of orthopedic surgery and the co-director of the Mayo Clinic Sports Medicine Center in Rochester, Minnesota.

Dr. Warren B. Howe [Emergencies Series Editor] is the team physician at Western Washington University in Bellingham and an editorial board member of *The Physician and Sportsmedicine*.

Seriously Injured? Get to the ER—STAT!

In all serious medical emergencies do not delay in getting to the emergency room. The faster that you can get an individual to the hospital, the faster they can receive the proper medical treatment. Many athletes who get injured are transported to the hospital in a car rather than in an ambulance. This is not always advisable since many injuries may cause serious problems that do not always present themselves at the time of the injury.

What is the problem with taking an athlete in your car to the hospital? The problem is that too many individuals want to go home first. Others will take the time to soak in a hot tub, which causes further swelling and bleeding. Some athletes want to get "something to eat" prior to reaching the hospital. Eating can delay surgery for six hours.

What you should do for an injured athlete is administer first aid and consider the following prior to transporting someone to the emergency room by car. Recognize an emergency when you see one. If the following occur, do not attempt to transport by yourself. Call 9-1-1 immediately.

- Someone who has fallen and can't get up
- Seriously deformed joint or bone
- Uncontrolled bleeding
- Difficulty breathing
- Seizures

- Diabetic emergencies
- Victims with altered level of consciousness following an injury
- Heat exhaustion
- Serious allergic reaction

When any of these occur, call 9-1-1 and be prepared to tell:

- Your name
- What has happened
- Where it happened
- The age and gender of the injured person
- Status of patient
- Any other pertinent information

Quick First Aid Tips

- Do not move the patient unless the patient's location is an immediate threat to their life (i.e., patient is in water or in harm's way).
- Protect the individual from the environment. Keep them covered if cold.
- If the person is bleeding, apply a sterile bandage. If bleeding continues, apply additional dressings over the existing bandage. If possible, elevate the injury and apply direct pressure to the wound.
- If the patient is not breathing or does not have a pulse, begin rescue breathing and/or CPR.
- When in doubt, always contact 9-1-1.

Chapter 35

Pre-Hospital Care of the Spine Injured Athlete

On-the-Field Management and Immediate Care

The ideal care of a specific athletic incident begins with observation of the event that leads to the possibility of a spinal injury. The certified athletic trainers and medical staff should make every attempt to closely observe all of the plays because knowledge of the mechanism of injury and degree of contact are often helpful in understanding the likelihood of significant injury.

Initial Assessment. The initial assessment of an injured player begins by forming a general impression of the athlete's condition, which includes the consideration of basic life support. If any concerns regarding basic life support are present at this time, the emergency medical services (EMS) system should be activated immediately. The athlete should not be moved unless it is absolutely essential to maintain the airway, breathing, or circulation.

Airway. The evaluation and maintenance of a functional airway are rapidly performed with full consideration for the potential of a

The information in this chapter is excerpted from, Kleiner DM, Almquist JL, Bailes J, Burruss P, Feuer H, Griffin LY, Herring S, McAdam C, Miller D, Thorson D, Watkins RG, Weinstein S. *Prehospital Care of the Spine-Injured Athlete: A Document from the Inter-Association Task Force for Appropriate Care of the Spine-Injured Athlete*. Dallas, Texas, National Athletic Trainers' Association, March 2001. Reprinted with permission.

spinal injury. Any athlete who is suspected of having a spinal injury should not be moved until the appropriate personnel are present, and he or she should be managed as though a spinal injury exists. If unconscious, the player is presumed to have an unstable fracture until it is proven otherwise. If it is necessary to move the athlete, he or she should be placed in a supine position while the spine is safeguarded. However, as in any instance of trauma response, whatever method necessary to achieve an adequate airway must be used. If a jaw thrust maneuver is unsuccessful, an oral airway or endotracheal intubation may be required. The team physician and/or EMS personnel should be available if such intervention is required.

Breathing. Next, the presence of sufficient ventilatory exchange is confirmed through either observation of the chest respiratory excursions or listening and feeling for air movement at the upper airway. Ineffective breathing patterns, the use of accessory breathing muscles, or even apnea can be caused by a cervical spinal cord injury. High cervical cord damage may inhibit the output of the phrenic nerve, which controls the diaphragm and arises from the third, fourth, and fifth cervical nerves.

Circulation. Circulation is evaluated. A circulation abnormality with inadequate peripheral perfusion is rare and unlikely to be present in the absence of a primary cardiac event.

Level of Consciousness. The athlete's level of consciousness is assessed. The athlete should be oriented to person, place, time, and incident. A fully conscious player is questioned regarding the presence of pain, particularly in the spinal region or a limb, altered sensation or strength of any body part, weakness, and visual and hearing function. In the unconscious player or one who exhibits any abnormal neurological function, the Glasgow Coma Scale may be helpful as a rapid, objective, and reproducible measure of cerebral function and should be used until a more formal neurological examination is carried out.

Neurological Screening. A screening examination is performed to assess motor and sensory function in the four extremities. In a cooperative player, an accurate initial neurological examination of the extremities can be achieved and is vital for a full evaluation of the injury. A cranial nerve assessment should be performed as completely as possible while the helmet is left in place.

Transportation. If the athlete is suspected of having a vertebral column or spinal cord injury, he or she should be transported to an emergency department, where a more formal neurological examination can be conducted and serial assessments can be completed. When it becomes necessary to move the athlete, the head and trunk must be moved as one unit, which can be accomplished by manually splinting the head to the trunk as the body is moved (see Immobilization and Transportation). Due to the difficulty in attaining a definitive exclusion regarding the possibility of spinal injury in an on-field setting, the Inter-Association Task Force recommends that any player suspected of such be evaluated in a controlled environment, and that any athlete with significant neck or spine pain, diminished level of consciousness, or significant neurological deficits be transported, in an appropriate manner, to a medical receiving facility with definitive diagnostic and medical resources.

To transport the athlete, he or she should be secured to a suitable backboard (specific steps for this vary from situation to situation and are discussed later in Immobilization and Transportation). Should the airway, breathing, or circulation be compromised, spinal immobilization must be maintained when removing the face mask.

Emergency Plan Activation. On-the-field management procedures might include the presence of the team physician and the initiation of additional medical assistance, such as activation of the EMS system. When other medical or allied healthcare personnel arrive on the scene, a briefing of the situation must be completed efficiently and effectively. History, signs, and symptoms obtained by the first responder must be shared with all those involved. However, it is imperative that only proper medical or allied health personnel be involved. Good Samaritans who come down from the stands and who are unfamiliar with the protocols should not be allowed to participate. A potential on-the-field disagreement on protocol can be detrimental to the health and welfare of the injured athlete and should be avoided. Administrative personnel and coaches can be helpful in restricting the access of individuals other than the previously established appropriate personnel on the field while care is being given by the first responders and follow-up personnel.

A defined delegation of duties is essential to maintain on-the-field management and crowd control during a medical emergency. The primary athletic healthcare provider must work quickly and efficiently with full focus on the athlete in distress. Coaches and administrative personnel should immediately step into action, instructing teammates and bystanders to move away from the injured athlete. If a spinal injury is suspected, athletes and onlookers should be directed to an area away from the injured athlete. It is recommended that athletic teams be educated on the dangers of moving an injured player (well in advance of the onset of contact practices or contests). It is a common response to offer assistance to an injured teammate or an opponent. However, all participants on the field must be cognizant of the dangers of moving a player with a suspected spinal injury and must refrain from moving any player who shows signs of a severe injury.

The National Football League has developed guidelines for its game officials to use during a serious on-field player injury, such as a spinal injury. These guidelines are the first of their kind and show the importance of on-the-field management. In August 1999, the *Inter-Association Task Force for Appropriate Care of the Spine-Injured Athlete* commended the National Football League for these guidelines. The Inter-Association Task Force recommends that teammates and coaches be reminded to not move an injured player. A coach or game official should keep concerned teammates and family away from the injured athlete.

Skilled and practiced medical care should be readily available at the athletic event. When this is not possible, such as in many rural areas, a plan to obtain this type of care at the scene when needed must be in place. Deviation from a standard and practiced protocol should be avoided.

Immobilization and Transportation

For initial stabilization of an injured athlete, see On-the-Field Management and Immediate Care. Manual stabilization of the head, neck, and shoulders should be performed as the patient is being assessed. In most cases, the football helmet and shoulder pads should not be removed during evaluation, immobilization, and transportation, but when the helmet must be removed, the shoulder pads should be removed as well.

When a determination is made that transportation to an emergency receiving facility is imminent, the athlete will have to be secured to an appropriate immobilization device. Controversy has arisen over whether the athlete whose spine is found in a less than anatomically correct position should be repositioned. In the past, when an athlete could actively reposition his or her head into a neutral position without encountering resistance or pain, they were encouraged to do so. Recently, a more cautious approach has been observed since it is assumed that an unstable spinal injury can be converted to an injury with more severe damage if the athlete is mishandled.

The Inter-Association Task Force recommends only that stabilization of the head and spine be maintained. In most cases, this means that the head and spine are repositioned into a neutral position so in-line stabilization can be accomplished with appropriate immobilization devices. However, in some instances, it may be best for the athlete's head and neck to be immobilized in the position in which they are found. The appropriateness of repositioning the head into a spine-neutral position should be assessed on an individual basis. Techniques for spinal immobilization and the determination of whether in-line stabilization is required for transportation should be left to local protocols or the clinical judgment, expertise, and training of the individuals on-site.

The Inter-Association Task Force recognize that it may not be possible to apply a rigid cervical collar when the helmet and shoulder pads are left in place or when spinal immobilization is being accomplished in a position other than neutral. Other methods of padding, such as towels or blanket rolls, must then be used to secure the head to the spine board. It has also been suggested that a cervical vacuum splint is an effective immobilizer in the athlete wearing protective equipment. If the athlete's spine is being immobilized in a neutral (in-line) position, every attempt should be made to apply a rigid cervical collar. When the athlete is anchored to the spine board, the body should be secured using standard techniques. The application of a spine board should always include straps to secure the pelvis, shoulders, legs, and, last, the head. After removal of the face mask, with the chin strap left in place, the helmeted head is secured to the board with adhesive tape or straps. At least two straps should be used to secure the torso, pelvis, and legs. The straps must be applied snugly so the athlete does not move if rolled onto his or her side due to vomiting. Any gaps must be filled in with towels or rigid foam. Once the athlete is completely stabilized, the person at the head relinquishes his or her control, and the athlete is transported to an emergency medical facility. The Inter-Association Task Force recommends some form of acceleration/deceleration, or "trauma strapping," to prevent axial loading in the ambulance during braking. It is also a common practice and a local protocol in some districts to load the stretcher in the ambulance with the athlete's head at the rear to avoid axial loading during ambulance braking.

Patients with spinal injuries often have a component of head injury that can lead to vomiting. Athletes who are vomiting or bleeding from the oral cavity must be kept prone or placed on their side to prevent aspiration of blood or vomitus into the airway. However, this can be performed after the athlete is immobilized. Furthermore, proper equipment, such as a suction apparatus, should be readily available. These procedures should be identified and practiced often to ensure a smooth transfer to a spine board when an emergency occurs.

Transfer of the Athlete

To transfer a supine athlete, the Inter-Association Task Force recommends using a six-plus–person lift along with a scoop stretcher to lift the athlete onto a rigid long spine board rather than a log roll technique. A six-plus–person lift is recommended due to the size of many athletes and the interference by protective equipment. To transfer a prone athlete, the Inter-Association Task Force recommends log rolling the athlete directly onto a rigid long spine board. Movement of the athlete from the prone to the supine position should be done with a minimum of four persons, with one designated to maintain stabilization of the head and neck. All movement should be carefully coordinated to avoid shifting the head, neck, and torso.

Log Roll of a Prone Athlete. Due to the urgency of establishing an airway in the athlete, assessment must be made very quickly and efficiently. If a prone athlete is not breathing, a log roll should be performed immediately. Unless the immobilization device is readily available, the athlete must be log rolled into a supine position on the playing surface and then moved (lifted) a second time onto the long back board. Obviously, with each movement the chances of a secondary injury increase. If the athlete is conscious and stable, the log roll should be delayed until the backboard is available.

To immobilize the prone athlete, the rescuer at the head (rescuer 1) should maintain the athlete's head/neck complex in the position in which it was found until it is completely splinted on the full body splint. When possible, the athlete should be treated with a rigid cervical collar to ensure the immobilization of all segmental levels. Next, position the immobilization device by the injured athlete on the side of rescuer 1's lower hand. When the athlete is wearing protective equipment, the athlete's arms should be maintained at his or her side (with palm inward). Rescuers 2 and 3 will then roll the athlete onto his or her arm, which should be kept to the side during the log roll maneuver. An injury that involves the arm calls for the athlete to be log rolled to the opposite side, which may be difficult in the presence of shoulder pads. Shoulder pads are not easy to remove, especially if worn with a neck collar; thus, they should be only removed in the most extenuating of circumstances.

Rescuer 1 is in charge and will give every command to move the athlete. Rescuer 1 must continue to maintain the position of the head/neck complex until the athlete is completely immobilized. Rescuers 2 and 3 position themselves adjacent to the athlete. On the opposite side of the athlete, rescuer 4 positions himself or herself and the splinting device. Rescuer 2 is positioned at the chest area, and rescuer 3 is positioned at thigh level. Rescuer 3 is expected to control both legs during the log roll maneuver. To roll the athlete, rescuer 1 gives the command "prepare to roll, roll." The other rescuers should then roll the athlete onto his or her side, toward the rescuers. By rolling the athlete onto his or her arm, the head, shoulders, and pelvis are kept in anatomical alignment. Rescuer 4 places the splinting device against the athlete's back at a 30 degree angle. While positions are maintained, rescuer 1 gives the command "prepare to lower, lower," and the athlete is lowered onto the splint.

Six-Plus–Person Lift. Heavy persons, including many athletes, can be handled more efficiently with a six-plus–person lift; this is also preferred for suspected spine injuries. The Inter-Association Task Force recommends that the six-plus–person lift be used along with a scoop stretcher whenever possible. In the athletic arena, there are usually a sufficient number of certified athletic trainers, physicians, and EMS personnel on hand to effectively administer the six-plus–person lift.

For the six-plus–person lift, rescuer 1 immobilizes the neck. The rescuer's hands are placed on the athlete's shoulders (under the shoulder pads) with the thumbs pointed away from the athlete's face. The athlete's head will then be resting between the rescuer's forearms.

The other six rescuers position themselves along the athlete's sides: one on each side of the chest, pelvis, and legs. The hands are slid under the athlete and equipment, if any, to provide a firm, coordinated lift. To lift, rescuer 1 gives the command "prepare to lift, lift." The assistants lift the athlete 4 to 6 inches off the ground. It is imperative to maintain a coordinated lift and to prevent any movement of the spine. One of the rescuers at the thigh level must control the legs with his or her arms toward the feet so the splint can be slid into place from the foot end. After the splint is in place, while positions are maintained, rescuer 1 gives the command "prepare to lower, lower," and the athlete is lowered onto the splint.

In the case of larger athletes, as many as 10 individuals should participate in the lift, with one on each side of the chest and pelvis, two at the legs, one at the head, and one with the splint. The Inter-Association Task Force does not recommend the use of fewer than four-plus–persons to lift athletes suspected of having a spinal injury, even smaller athletes and children, in part due to the weight of the athlete while wearing protective equipment.

Immobilization Equipment

Any injured athlete who may have a cervical spine injury should be immobilized on a suitable full-body splint. The equipment used for splinting athletes with head or neck injuries will depend on the appliances that are available, as well as the training and knowledge of EMS personnel.

Certified athletic trainers should know how to use the equipment that is available and should be familiar with the equipment EMS providers will bring to the scene. EMS providers should take the lead in the immobilization of an athlete for transportation because they are far more practiced in immobilization techniques and will be responsible for the athlete during transportation. However, team physicians and certified athletic trainers are more familiar with athletic protective equipment and should therefore direct and assist the EMS providers in the immobilization process of the athlete with protective equipment. Certified athletic trainers and team physicians should familiarize themselves and rehearse the handling of such equipment on a regular basis because of their infrequent use of such equipment.

Equipment for spinal immobilization includes the Miller full-body splint, the standard rigid spine board, the vacuum mattress, and the scoop stretcher.

Miller Full-Body Splint. To use the Miller full-body splint, move the splint next to the athlete. Open the harness, and fold all straps onto themselves to prevent entanglement of the Velcro. Lift or log roll the athlete onto the Miller full-body splint. Align the athlete's shoulders with the shoulder pins on the Miller full-body splint. Place the chest straps loosely over the athlete's chest. Place the shoulder strap onto the chest strap. Thread the chest strap through the pins on the Miller full-body splint. Adjust the chest strap, and then adjust the shoulder straps. Do not overtighten either of the straps. Adjust the torso and the leg and ankle straps to secure the athlete to the Miller full-body splint.

If the athlete is wearing a protective helmet, tape the helmet directly to the Miller full-body splint headpiece. Apply the chin strap snugly but loose enough to allow the mouth to open.

Rigid Spine Board. Once the athlete has been placed on the board (by six-plus–person lift or log roll), apply blankets, rolled towels, or commercial head immobilizers, and strap the athlete into position. At least two straps should be used to secure the torso, pelvis, and legs. The Inter-Association Task Force recommends some form of acceleration/deceleration, or "trauma strapping." With the helmet and shoulder pads in place, towels or other padding are usually sufficient to fill the voids. Finally, the helmet should be secured to the backboard with adhesive tape. When completed, the athlete with protective equipment is said to be immobilized.

Vacuum Mattress. The vacuum mattress is one of the newest methods of immobilization. Unlike the rigid spine board, the vacuum splints consist of Styrofoam beads encapsulated in a vacuum nylon covering. When air is released, the splint provides support to the axial spine or total body. The splint includes wooden slats posteriorly for head-to-toe stability.

To prepare the splint for use, remove from the case at the beginning of each practice or game. Create a semirigid splint through partial removal of air. In the event of an injury, the semirigid splint can be moved into place as needed. When an injury occurs that necessitates total body immobilization, those who are providing care must decide how to move the athlete onto the splint. Always protect the athlete with a suspected spinal injury. Athletes in awkward positions may be moved onto the rigid spine board or vacuum splint with a scoop stretcher. When the vacuum mattress is used, release the buckles on the mattress before moving the athlete onto the splint. The person at the head maintains firm support, or pressure, to the head. Pressure includes gentle, in-line traction. When preparing the athlete for the vacuum mattress, use standard commands of "prepare to lift, lift" or "prepare to roll, roll." Once the athlete is positioned onto the mattress, continue stabilization of the head and neck. Open the valves at the head and foot ends to allow air to enter the mattress. Bunch the beads around the head and into the body to mold the splint. At this point, screw the valve at the head to the locked position. Continue the application of pressure so the beads form around the head and helmet. The person at the head works with the second rescuer to accomplish this molding around the head/helmet. Reattach the straps by connecting color-coded buckles. Take care not to twist the straps, which could create uncomfortable pressure points for the athlete. Move the excess strap down the body from head to toe. As tightened, attach the pump to the foot end and release air from the splint. As the splint becomes rigid, recheck the straps in a head-to-toe direction to remove any excess slack from the belt. Apply adhesive tape across the head area to secure the helmet to the splint. Screw all valves to the locked position.

Scoop Stretcher. The scoop stretcher, or split litter, is adjusted to the correct length and then separated, inserted, and fastened according to its design. The patient is lifted 4 to 6 inches off the ground while a rigid long board is slid underneath. The split litter should not be picked up from the head and foot ends or used to carry the patient before it has been placed on a long board because it can sag without center support. The scoop stretcher can be left in place or removed before the athlete is secured to the long board, but keep in mind that these devices are usually made of aluminum and x-rays do not penetrate easily. The Inter-Association Task Force recommends using a scoop stretcher along with the six-plus–person lift to facilitate the transfer of the supine athlete onto a long spine board for definitive immobilization.

Advanced Transportation and Care

Team physicians, certified athletic trainers, and EMS personnel who are caring for an athlete with a potential spinal injury should be familiar with local trauma networks and protocols. If the patient is hemodynamically stable, transport should be directed to a designated hospital with special capabilities for spinal injury. Critical patients may need to be stabilized at the closest appropriate hospital before transfer to a more definitive care facility. In remote areas where the distance to a trauma center is very long, the physician may elect to accompany the athlete to the hospital and participate in the treatment.

Any athlete who is suspected of having a spinal injury is to be transported by trained professionals in an ambulance. Transportation in a private vehicle is never to be attempted. In certain settings, air transportation may be preferred to ground transportation. A trauma center should be the first-choice destination for spine-injured athletes. Trauma center designation levels and capabilities will vary by state, so it is important to be familiar with the facilities available in your area.

Methylprednisolone. Methylprednisolone is used in cases of spinal cord injury, but it must be administered as soon as possible and over 24 hours. The dosage of this medication is 30 mg/kg body weight administered over 1 hour. The subsequent dosage is 5.6mg/kg body weight, administered over the next 23 hours. The first dose of intravenous methylprednisolone should be administered within 4 hours of the injury to be most effective. Therefore, team physicians in rural areas or those who travel substantial distances may elect to carry methylprednisolone or to ensure that the emergency receiving facilities and/ or EMS providers have the medication on hand. Many local EMS providers are able to begin this treatment while transporting the patient.

Injuries and Possible Mechanisms

Injuries can be classified as direct or indirect. Direct injuries occur as a result of sports participation and include closed head injuries and cervical spine trauma as a result of contact/collision. Indirect injuries can include heart attack, heat illness, or other preexisting medical conditions. Direct injuries are more common in contact/collision sports such as football, hockey, and rugby.

All of the anatomic components of the cervical spine are subject to traumatic injury, including soft tissues, bone and joint structures, and neurological elements. Within each category, these tissues are variably susceptible to both compressive and tensile overload, which will result in specific injury patterns and clinical presentations. Not all spinal injuries are catastrophic, although many of the same signs and symptoms can appear in catastrophic and noncatastrophic injuries. Therefore, an understanding of all of the possible injuries to the spine is warranted.

Soft Tissue Injuries

Soft tissue injuries to the cervical spine, including muscle, ligament, and tendon injuries, probably occur most frequently. Muscle contusions can result from direct impact in the neck region or can occur indirectly via forces transmitted through protective equipment (i.e., the shoulder pads and helmet). Tensile overload to the musculotendinous unit occurs most commonly and is often associated with tackling in football. This is particularly true with a blind-side tackle when the player is not prepared for the collision, which can result in a forceful eccentric muscle contraction that places the musculotendinous unit at risk. This risk is often increased when muscle fatigue is present.

Acute muscular spasm often develops secondary to an underlying spinal injury, so a spinal injury should be considered whenever an initial assessment reveals spasm, tenderness, or loss of active range of motion.

Ligamentous injuries typically result from tensile overload with varying degrees of disruption. The innervation of the ligamentous structures in the cervical spine includes receptors that respond to slow tonic input, which is important in postural control, rather than ballistic movement. Thus, ligaments are susceptible to sudden loads. Ligament injury may lead to instability patterns specific for the segmental location of the particular ligament and may be associated with neurological impairment. Instability must be considered in any player with neurological symptoms, especially if the symptoms are persistent.

Skeletal Injuries

The spatial and geometric orientation of the cervical zygapophyseal joints (also known as facet joints, or z-joints) allows a high degree of mobility of the cervical spine, which places all anatomic structures at risk for injury. The z-joints are loaded when the head and neck are moved into the posterior and posterolateral quadrants. Acute compressive overload or chronic repetitive loading of these structures may result in synovitis of the z-joint and, depending on the force, may have an impact on injury and microfracture of the articular cartilage and subchondral bone of the facet processes. Tensile overload injuries lead to a spectrum of capsular damage, from strain to complete disruption. Greater degrees of capsular incompetence contribute to segmental hypermobilities and instabilities. Whether resulting in hypomobility or hypermobility, z-joint injury at one segmental level may lead to a cascading effect of segmental motion abnormalities elsewhere in the cervical spine.

Fractures of the cervical spine can occur when a player's head unexpectedly strikes another object and the force of impact exceeds the compressive or tensile limit of the bony structure. Both the anterior column (i.e., vertebral body) and the posterior column (i.e., pedicle, lamina, or facet) structures are at risk. Fractures can be associated with instability, which must always be considered if neurological sequelae develop, but can also exist without neurological symptoms or signs. It is important to note that some fractures, particularly in the posterior column, can be difficult, if not impossible, to identify on plain radiography and require some type of advanced imaging technique.

Acute cervical fracture-dislocations occur most commonly as the result of an axial load to the top of the helmet with the neck slightly flexed, the so-called segmented column. The straightened spine buckles in the center in an accordion-type mechanism, which produces a fracture dislocation or a transitory subluxation. It is for this reason that spearing is illegal in football. However, inadvertent contact with another player, or even the ground, also can produce this injury. Catastrophic injuries almost universally result from the axial load mechanism, of which an understanding is important for injury prevention. Other injuries that can occur from axial loading include the following:

- Flexion rotation fracture dislocation of the midcervical spine
- Jefferson fracture of the ring of C1
- An anterior subluxation injury that involves a rupture of the posterior longitudinal ligament and ligamentum flavum
- Bilateral and unilateral facet dislocation
- Cervical disc herniation
- Vertebral body fracture
- Intervertebral facet fracture
- A rupture of the atlantoaxial ligament

A variety of other mechanisms can also result in fracture-dislocation or in dislocation without fracture (i.e., unilateral or bilateral facet dislocation), including forceful rotation with flexion or extension. These types of injuries usually result in an intervertebral disc injury, as well as a disc rupture or herniation. Less severe disc injury also can occur, due to excessive torque to the cervical spine and excessive shear force across the annulus fibrosus, leading to annular tears and possibly disc herniations.

Predisposing Conditions. Numerous injuries can be acquired from head contact. Predisposing conditions can make certain players more vulnerable even though they are unaware of this predisposition. The most common abnormality is congenital stenosis, in which the spinal canal is too small for the spinal cord. Klippel-Feil syndrome is a congenital abnormality that involves the fusion of different segments of the neck to produce compensatory hypermobility in other areas. Most players and physicians are not aware of congenital abnormalities until some symptoms develop. These findings can be a major factor in determining potential risk and in decisions concerning continued play after an injury.

Spinal stenosis, whether congenital or acquired, means the player is more likely

- To have an episode of transient quadriplegia
- To have "stingers"
- To require surgery after a cervical disc herniation
- To run the risk of potential paralysis without a fracture-dislocation
- To develop paralysis and a greater degree of paralysis after a fracture-dislocation

Neurological Injuries

From a mechanical basis, the neurological contents of the spinal canal can be compromised by bone or disc fragment, malalignment, or instability. Vascular insult also may contribute to various neurological syndromes. The three main neurological elements at risk are the spinal cord, nerve root/spinal nerve complex, and brachial plexus. Catastrophic injury that results in transient or permanent quadriplegia is rare, with an incidence of approximately 0.6 to 1.5 per 100,000 participants in high school and college, respectively, during the 19-year period of 1977 to 1995.

As previously described, central spinal canal compromise is associated with fracture-dislocation and other instability patterns. The spinal cord is deformable and can accommodate some change in the length of the spinal canal without injury. However, the presence of spinal stenosis, developmental or acquired, decreases the chances for full neurological recovery if an athlete develops quadriplegia due to cervical spine trauma. Spinal cord injury may be neurapraxic (a reversible concussive event) with motor and sensory function returning within approximately 24 hours.

The most typical pattern of incomplete spinal cord injury is the central cord syndrome. Due to the lamination of the corticospinal tracts located toward the center of the spinal cord, the upper extremities are most susceptible to impairment with swelling or contusion to the cord. A variety of incomplete spinal cord injuries can develop due to a combination of mechanical and vascular effects on the spinal cord.

Burners and Stingers. The more common neurological injury is the stinger, or burner. The stinger is a peripheral nerve injury, not a spinal cord injury. It is characterized by burning dysesthesias that usually begin in the shoulder and radiate unilaterally into the arm and hand. Weakness, numbness, or both are occasionally associated in a C5-6 nerve root distribution. Recovery from an initial stinger usually occurs in minutes, but the symptoms and signs (most commonly numbness or weakness) can persist for several days to a few weeks, particularly if it is a recurrent condition.

Stingers typically result from one of two mechanisms of injury, which can vary depending on the skill and physical maturity of the athlete. A compressive mechanism develops when the head and neck are forcibly moved into a posterolateral direction toward the symptomatic upper limb. The other mechanism, a tensile mechanism, occurs when the involved arm and neck are forced in opposite directions. With either pathomechanism (tension or compression), the cervical spine nerve is probably at greater risk than the brachial plexus. Thus, stingers are more appropriately considered a cervical radiculopathy than a brachial plexopathy, although a brachial plexopathy can occur from a direct blow to the upper thorax or from tension. Cervical radiculopathy also can occur due to a cervical disc herniation, cervical foraminal stenosis, and instability.

Burners and stingers typically produce loss of function and pain only for a limited period of time. Often the player will flex and laterally bend his or her head and neck away from the involved arm. As the pain decreases, the player will gradually demonstrate improved range of motion. There can be a great deal of posterior cervical tenderness with the stinger because the posterior primary ramus of the nerve innervates the skin in that area and comes directly off the dorsal ganglion.

The symptoms of a stinger should be distinguished from those of a spinal cord injury to initiate an appropriate treatment relative to the severity of the injury. The key clinical distinction between spinal cord injury and a stinger is that the spinal cord injury results in multiple limb involvement (i.e., two to four), whereas the stinger always results in unilateral upper extremity impairment. The determination of whether an injury is related to the spinal cord or is a stinger should be made with great caution due to the importance of initial management of the injury. Unlike the consequences of a spinal cord injury, players with burners and stingers often are headed off the field when their symptoms are discovered.

Transient quadriplegia is a temporary paralysis that is characterized by a loss of motor or sensory function, or both. It is current neurosurgical thinking that a common mechanism of transient quadriplegia is a contusion of the spinal cord that produces a temporary restriction of blood flow to a portion of the cervical spinal cord. The extent of neurological deficit and how long it lasts are critical and determine prognosis. The mechanism of injury may be varied and complex. The most significant factor is the initial head first contact. If subsequent neck flexion follows, the spinal cord becomes taut and is stretched over the floor of the spinal canal, producing a transitory plastic deformation of the cord. This produces a collapse of blood vessels and an interruption of blood supply to the cord. Neck extension after head contact produces the opposite effect, or slackening of the cord. Further extension narrows the central spinal canal, and the posterior disc, osteophytes, and ligamentum flavum protrude into the spinal canal and compress the spinal cord. In addition, the intervertebral foramen diameter narrows and becomes smaller in extension as the two articular facets slide into a small relative subluxation. Conversely, flexion produces a larger central canal diameter through removal of the relative infolding of ligamentum flavum and posterior disc bulging from the canal. Extension and flexion can produce a pincer effect between the posterior edge of one vertebral body and the lamina of another. This is a relative subluxation between two vertebral segments that squeezes the spinal cord producing a contusion and localized deformation of the cord. Transient quadriplegia is, by definition, a temporary condition, a neurapraxia, but the player initially presents with paralysis and must be managed accordingly.

Summary and Conclusions

Injuries to the spine are relatively rare in athletics. However, when they occur, they must be treated promptly and correctly. Certified athletic trainers and other providers of pre-hospital care must know which procedures to use in these situations. They must have the necessary equipment readily available and be proficient in its use. The regular practice of immobilization of athletes with potential cervical spine injuries is a must for individuals who expect to perform these important tasks in an actual emergency.

Care of the injured athlete should follow a carefully designed protocol. The athlete's airway, breathing, and circulation; neurological status; and level of consciousness should be assessed, and the EMS system should be activated.

Because unconscious individuals are unable to speak, they are unable to tell the rescuer whether they have a spinal injury. Therefore, all unconscious athletes in a situation that may have included a collision or a fall and conscious athletes with any sign or symptoms that suggest cervical spine trauma must be treated as if they have a cervical spine injury.

Any athlete suspected of having a head or spinal injury should not be moved unless absolutely essential to maintain airway, breathing, and circulation. If the athlete must be moved to maintain airway, breathing, and circulation, the athlete should be placed in a supine position while spinal immobilization is maintained.

In the conscious athlete, a possible cervical spine injury must be identified early. Athletes who display spasm, tenderness, or loss of active range of motion should be suspected of having significant cervical spine trauma and should be treated accordingly. Cervical spine injuries are usually orthopedic in nature and may or may not have immediately observable neurological sequelae.

Athletes with no neurological signs or symptoms and no findings that suggest trauma to the cervical spine can be safely moved to a more suitable site for further evaluation. However, if there is any question as to medical status, it is best to err on the side of safety and to treat the injury as if it were a significant cervical spine injury.

When it becomes necessary to transport the athlete, the head and trunk should be moved as a unit. It takes many people to correctly move an injured athlete, with one rescuer responsible for stabilizing the athlete's head and cervical spine; as a general rule, this should be the most qualified and experienced person on the scene. It is imperative that this rescuer maintains cervical stabilization throughout the procedure. The rescuer who is stabilizing the head must continue to keep it stabilized until the athlete is completely immobilized with an appropriate device.

Injuries to the head and neck are difficult to evaluate and treat in the athletic environment. To adequately prepare for these and other critical injuries to athletes, an emergency plan should be developed. Providers of emergency care must make sure to have the proper equipment readily available and that it is in good working order.

The sports medicine team must be prepared for any emergency; preparation includes education and training, maintenance of appropriate emergency equipment and supplies, utilization of appropriate person-nel (including certified athletic trainers), and the formation and imple-mentation of an emergency plan.

Emergency plans should be comprehensive and practical, yet flex-ible enough to adapt to any emergency situation. The emergency plan must be established, approved, revised, and rehearsed on a regular basis. Each emergency plan may vary but should include information on education, emergency equipment, personnel, communication, and a rehearsal schedule. The emergency plan should also address equip-ment issues, which are particularly important in managing and pack-aging persons with suspected head or cervical spine injuries. Each member of the emergency team should be knowledgeable and prac-ticed in the function and operation of emergency equipment. It would be helpful for each member of the sports medicine team to be multi-skilled and cross-trained in the use of all emergency equipment. For example, it has been suggested that practice with tools required for face mask removal of the catastrophically injured football player is essential.

Emergency medical personnel must take extreme caution when evaluating and treating an athlete with a suspected head or spinal injury. The proper management of head and neck injuries can prevent further damage from occurring.

Guidelines for Appropriate Care of the Spine-Injured Athlete

General Guidelines

- Any athlete suspected of having a spinal injury should not be moved and should be managed as though a spinal injury exists.

- The athlete's airway, breathing, circulation, neurological status, and level of consciousness should be assessed.

- The athlete should not be moved unless absolutely essential to maintain airway, breathing, and circulation.

- If the athlete must be moved to maintain airway, breathing, and circulation, the athlete should be placed in a supine position while maintaining spinal immobilization.

- When moving a suspected spine-injured athlete, the head and trunk should be moved as a unit. One accepted technique is to manually splint the head to the trunk.

- The Emergency Medical Services system should be activated.

Face Mask Removal

- The face mask should be removed prior to transportation, regardless of current respiratory status.
- Those involved in the pre-hospital care of injured football players should have the tools for face mask removal readily available.

Football Helmet Removal

The athletic helmet and chin strap should only be removed:

- If the helmet and chin strap do not hold the head securely, such that immobilization of the helmet does not also immobilize the head;
- If the design of the helmet and chin strap is such that, even after removal of the face mask, the airway cannot be controlled nor ventilation provided;
- If the face mask cannot be removed after a reasonable period of time;
- If the helmet prevents immobilization for transportation in an appropriate position.

Helmet Removal

Spinal immobilization must be maintained while removing the helmet.

- Helmet removal should be frequently practiced under proper supervision.
- Specific guidelines for helmet removal need to be developed.
- In most circumstances, it may be helpful to remove cheek padding and/or deflate air padding prior to helmet removal.

Equipment

Appropriate spinal alignment must be maintained.

- There needs to be a realization that the helmet and shoulder pads elevate an athlete's trunk when in the supine position.

- Should either the helmet or shoulder pads be removed—or if only one of these is present—appropriate spinal alignment must be maintained.

- The front of the shoulder pads can be opened to allow access for CPR and defibrillation.

Additional Guidelines

- This task force encourages the development of a local emergency care plan regarding the pre-hospital care of an athlete with a suspected spinal injury. This plan should include communication with the institution's administration and those directly involved with the assessment and transportation of the injured athlete.

- All providers of pre-hospital care should practice and be competent in all of the skills identified in these guidelines before they are needed in an emergency situation.

Recommendations for Appropriate Care of the Spine-Injured Athlete

- The Inter-Association Task Force for Appropriate Care of the Spine-Injured Athlete commends the current and ongoing commitment of helmet and face guard manufacturers for integrating safety in the development of their products.

- The Inter-Association Task Force for Appropriate Care of the Spine-Injured Athlete encourages manufacturers to continue to support research promoting helmet and face guard safety.

- The Inter-Association Task Force for Appropriate Care of the Spine-Injured Athlete recommends that manufacturers provide information to purchasers on the best methods for the emergency removal of the face guard.

- The Inter-Association Task Force for Appropriate Care of the Spine-Injured Athlete recommends that NOCSAE develop equipment standards that would allow for the emergency removal of helmets and face guards.

- The Inter-Association Task Force for Appropriate Care of the Spine-Injured Athlete recommends that helmets and face guards that meet current NOCSAE standards be worn by all football, lacrosse, baseball, and softball players.

• The Inter-Association Task Force for Appropriate Care of the Spine-Injured Athlete recommends that football helmet face guards be attached by loop straps and not bolted on, in order to facilitate appropriate emergency management by medical personnel (from the May 1998 meeting in Indianapolis, Indiana).

• The Inter-Association Task Force for Appropriate Care of the Spine-Injured Athlete recommends that loop straps be made of material that is easily cut, and that the producers of loop straps provide appropriate tools to cut/remove the loop straps that they manufacture (from the May 1998 meeting in Indianapolis, Indiana).

These guidelines were developed as a consensus statement by the Inter-Association Task Force of Appropriate Care of the Spine-Injured Athlete.

Chapter 36

Diagnostic Procedures and Treatments for Sports Injuries

Athletes who suffer a moderate to severe injury should see an orthopaedist to receive a professional diagnosis and the necessary proper medical care. Prompt medical care following a sports-related injury can limit the extent of damage and significantly reduce the recovery period.

Invasive Diagnostic Procedures

Arthrography involves injecting a contrast dye into a joint and taking an x-ray to determine the exact site and extent of an injury within the joint. It is typically used when there is a suspicion of a ruptured ligament or torn cartilage in the knee or a torn rotator cuff in the shoulder. It may be performed on other joints as well.

Arthroscopy involves inserting a fiber optic device connected to a camera through a small incision to examine the interior of a joint. Arthroscopy is frequently used to confirm the surgeon's clinical diagnosis and then to perform surgical procedures if they are indicated in the joint.

Non-Invasive Diagnostic Procedures

Clinical Examination is done to assess the history of an injury, as well as the structure and function of the injured area. Orthopaedists conduct an exam to determine how the injury occurred, the degree of pain and swelling, the stability of the joint, and the range of motion. This information helps the physician determine the site, extent, and nature of an injury.

Computerized Tomography (CT) is a computerized diagnostic imaging tool used to obtain information about the body. The information is presented as an image generated by a computer that synthesizes x-rays obtained from many different directions. CT is particularly useful for detecting hidden bone injuries or soft tissue masses that may not be detected by simple x-ray.

Magnetic Resonance Imaging (MRI) is another computerized procedure in which the patient's body is placed in a magnetic field. The effects of the field on the tissue can then be measured. This technique does not involved radiation like conventional x-rays or CT scans and can provide a very accurate and detailed image of an injured area.

Ultrasound Imaging uses sound waves to produce images that aid physicians in the diagnosis of injuries. This does not involve the use of radiation, but generally is not as specific as the MRI. Ultrasound is frequently used to assess rotator cuff injuries.

X-ray Machines use electromagnetic radiation x-rays to create an image of an injury. X-rays are helpful in determining the extent of injuries primarily to the bone and, to some extent, the soft tissue.

Surgical Treatment

Arthroplasty is a surgical procedure used to help stabilize or improve the function of a joint. In some cases, arthroplasty refers to procedures used to repair torn ligaments or the capsule around a joint, as in the shoulder to tighten the capsule for a shoulder that dislocates. It also may refer to the use of artificial materials such as metal alloys or plastics to create a new or artificial joint to help restore the range of motion and functional strength to the joint.

Arthroscopy is a common procedure used both for diagnostic and surgical procedures. It can be used to repair or remove torn cartilage or remove bone or cartilage fragments from the joint and assist in repairing certain ligament injuries. Arthroscopy is the least invasive form of surgery and is often performed on an outpatient basis.

Open Repair Reconstructive Surgery is a procedure that requires a larger incision than arthroscopy so that the orthopaedist can assess and repair a serious injury. Open surgery is commonly used to repair ligament injuries around the joint and bone fractures that require the insertion of screws and metal plates.

Immobilization

Immobilization is a common treatment for sports-related injuries. Immobilization helps an injury settle and allows the healing process to begin. Immobilization helps control the blood supply to the injury which reduces pain and swelling. Methods of immobilization include the use of hard casts, soft casts, splints, slings and leg immobilizers.

Hard casts are made of plaster or plastic and are used to immobilize serious injuries, including broken bones and severe sprains.

Soft casts (bandage wraps) are used to provide compression to an injury which helps control and reduce swelling.

Splints and slings are often used to immobilize injuries to the upper body including the arms and shoulders. Splints and slings hold an injury stationary until the range of motion returns to the joint.

Leg immobilizers are devices that immobilize the leg after a knee injury. As with other immobilization techniques, the leg immobilizers help an injury settle and speed healing.

Chapter 37

Understanding Nuclear Medicine Imaging

What Is Nuclear Medicine?

Nuclear medicine is a medical specialty that uses safe, painless, and cost-effective techniques both to image the body and treat disease. Nuclear medicine imaging is unique in that it documents organ function and structure, in contrast to diagnostic radiology, which is based upon anatomy. It is a way to gather medical information that may otherwise be unavailable, require surgery, or necessitate more expensive diagnostic tests.

As an integral part of patient care, nuclear medicine is used in the diagnosis, management, treatment, and prevention of serious disease. Nuclear medicine imaging procedures often identify abnormalities very early in the progression of a disease—long before some medical problems are apparent with other diagnostic tests. This early detection allows a disease to be treated early in its course when there may be a more successful prognosis.

Nuclear medicine uses very small amounts of radioactive materials or radiopharmaceuticals to diagnose and treat disease. Radiopharmaceuticals are substances that are attracted to specific organs, bones, or tissues. The radiopharmaceuticals used in nuclear medicine emit gamma rays that can be detected externally by special types of cameras:

This chapter includes the following copyrighted documents reprinted by permission of the Society of Nuclear Medicine: "What Is Nuclear Medicine," "Fast Facts about Nuclear Medicine," "Nuclear Medicine, X-rays, CT, and MRI," "Bone Imaging," "Brain Imaging," and "Frequently Asked Questions."

gamma or PET cameras. These cameras work in conjunction with computers used to form images that provide data and information about the area of body being imaged. The amount of radiation from a nuclear medicine procedure is comparable to that received during a diagnostic x-ray.

Today, nuclear medicine offers procedures that are helpful to a broad span of medical specialties, from pediatrics to cardiology to psychiatry. There are nearly one hundred different nuclear medicine imaging procedures available and not a major organ system which is not imaged by nuclear medicine.

Fast Facts about Nuclear Medicine

- An estimated 10 to 12 million nuclear medicine imaging and therapeutic procedures are performed each year in the United States.

- Nuclear medicine procedures are unique, safe, and cost-effective.

- There are nearly 100 different nuclear medicine imaging procedures available today.

- Nuclear medicine uniquely provides information about both the function and structure of virtually every major organ system within the body.

- Nuclear medicine procedures are among the safest diagnostic imaging tests available.

- The amount of radiation in a nuclear medicine procedure is comparable to that received during a diagnostic x-ray.

- Nuclear medicine procedures are painless and do not require anesthesia.

- Children commonly undergo nuclear medicine procedures to evaluate bone pain, injuries, infection, or kidney and bladder function. Common nuclear medicine applications include diagnosis and treatment of hyperthyroidism (Grave's Disease), cardiac stress tests to analyze heart function, bone scans for orthopedic injuries, lung scans for blood clots, and liver and gall bladder procedures to diagnose abnormal function or blockages.

- There are approximately 2,700 full-time equivalent nuclear medicine physicians and 14,000 certified nuclear medicine technologists nationwide.

Nuclear Medicine, X-Rays, CT, and MRI

Nuclear medicine began approximately 50 years ago and has evolved into a major medical specialty for both diagnosis and therapy of serious disease. More than 3,900 hospital-based nuclear medicine departments in the United States perform over 10 million nuclear medicine imaging and therapeutic procedures each year. Despite its integral role in patient care, nuclear medicine is still often confused with other imaging procedures, including general radiology, CT, and MRI.

Nuclear medicine studies document organ and function and structure, in contrast to conventional radiology, which creates images based upon anatomy. Many of the nuclear medicine studies can measure the degree of function present in an organ, often times eliminating the need for surgery. Moreover, nuclear medicine procedures often provide important information that allows the physician to detect and treat a disease early in its course when there may be more success. It is nuclear medicine that can best be used to study the function of a damaged heart or restriction of blood flow to parts of the brain. The liver, kidneys, thyroid gland, and many other organs are similarly imaged.

General Radiology

The image, or a x-ray film, is produced when a small amount of radiation passes through the body to expose sensitive film on the other side. The ability of x-rays to penetrate tissues and bones depends on the tissue's composition and mass. The difference between these two elements creates the images. The chest x-ray is the most common radiologic examination. Contrast agents, such as barium, can be swallowed to highlight the esophagus, stomach, and intestine and are used to help visualize an organ or film.

Computed Tomography (CT)

Computed tomography or CT, shows organs of interest at selected levels of the body. They are visual equivalent of bloodless slices of anatomy, with each scan being a single slice. CT examinations produce detailed organ studies by stacking individual image slices. CT can image the internal portion of organs and separate overlapping structures precisely. The scans are produced by having the source of the x-ray beam encircle or rotate around the patient. X-rays passing through the body are detected by an array of sensors. Information from the sensors is computer processed and then displayed as an image on a video screen.

MRI

Like CT, MRI produces images, which are the visual equivalent of a slice of anatomy. MRI, however, is also capable of producing those images in an infinite number of projections through the body. MRI uses a large magnet that surrounds the patient, radio frequencies, and a computer to produce its images. As the patient enters a MRI scanner, his body is surrounded by a magnetic field up to 8,000 times stronger than that of the earth. The scanner subjects nuclei of the body's atoms to a radio signal, temporarily knocking select ones out of alignment. When the signal stops, the nuclei return to the aligned position, releasing their own faint radio frequencies from which the scanner and computer produce detailed images of the human anatomy. Patients who cannot undergo a MRI examination include those people dependent upon cardiac pacemakers and those with metallic foreign bodies in the brain or around the eye.

Bone Imaging

Bone scans are used to detect arthritis, osteoporosis, fractures, sports injuries, tumors, and even cases of child abuse. Bone scans may also be used to evaluate unexplained bone pain, malignancies in the breast, prostate or thyroid, and certain types of heart or brain damage.

Test Preparation

For most bone studies, you will be asked to drink as many fluids as possible, both before and after the procedure.

Exam Procedure

During the first part of the test, the tracer is injected. It generally takes about two hours for the tracer to be absorbed by the bones. The technologist will let you know if it is okay to eat during this waiting period. During the waiting period, you should try to urinate as often as possible because it will help eliminate the tracer from your body that is not going to the bones.

Depending on the study, the technologist may take pictures of your bones as the tracer is moving through your bloodstream before it reaches your bones. It takes about 30 minutes to complete the images. In most bone studies, however, the imaging portion takes much longer, from two to four hours. For most bone scans, you will lie on the imaging table with the camera positioned above or below you. Several images may be taken or the camera may move slowly, imaging the entire length of your body. Although the imaging session takes a long time, it is extremely important that you remain as still as possible so that the scan results are accurate.

For children, the procedure is the same as for adults, except that after the tracer injection, the child may be given a sedative. If the child is given a sedative, he or she will have to remain in the nuclear medicine department until they are fully awake. After the test, the child should be able to resume daily activities, and there are no restrictions to eating, drinking, or contact with others. If the child has been sedated, you may wish to let him or her rest for a day before resuming normal play activity.

Brain Imaging

A brain scan may be necessary to investigate problems within the brain itself or in blood circulation to and from the brain (perfusion imaging).

Test Preparation

Generally, no special preparation is needed. If special preparation is required, your doctor will let you know.

Exam Procedure

Perfusion Imaging: After relaxing in a dimly lit room, the tracer is injected in the arm. Thirty to 60 minutes after the injection, you will lie on your back under the camera and pictures of your brain will be taken for 30 to 60 minutes. You will be asked not to move, touch your head or cough while the pictures are being taken.

Stress/Rest Test: Most brain scans are taken while the patient is resting, but some medical conditions require evaluation of different activity levels of the brain during active and rest periods. This test is performed using a special drug or while doing certain tasks which activate brain function. The test is performed in two parts: first, a rest image is obtained, and the next day, the necessary stress test is performed.

Cisternography: This test determines if there is abnormal flow of cerebral spinal fluid around or in the brain. The tracer is injected into the lower back region by a doctor. After the injection, you will lie still for a few hours. It usually takes two to three days to complete the images.

Frequently Asked Questions about Nuclear Medicine

Why May Several Different Tests Be Needed?

Sometimes a variety of diagnostic tests are performed to determine the nature of a medical problem and the most appropriate treatment. Although a diagnosis is usually made with one nuclear medicine test, it may be necessary to confirm the test results with another test or studies.

Are Nuclear Medicine Procedures Safe?

Nuclear medicine procedures are very safe. A patient only receives an extremely small amount of tracer, just enough to provide accurate diagnostic information. The amount of radiation in a nuclear medicine test is no more than that received during an x-ray.

Who Performs Nuclear Medicine Tests?

- A nuclear medicine technologist, a health care professional trained and experienced in the theory and practice of nuclear medicine procedures, performs the test by administering the tracer, positioning the patient under the camera, and operating the equipment used in the test.

- A nuclear medicine physician, who is specially trained in physics and chemistry and is licensed to use tracers, interprets the images.

How Should I Prepare for the Test?

Generally, no special preparation is required, but if preparation is needed, you will be notified before the test. Certain tests may require some slight preparation. For example, if you are having a cardiac stress-rest test, you may be asked not to eat three to four hours before the test because the pictures of your heart will be easier to interpret if the stomach is empty. Or, if you are having a prostate, ovarian, or colorectal cancer scan, it is important to let the technologist know if you have had a nuclear medicine test recently, have had previous surgery, or are allergic or sensitive to any substances or drugs.

You need not worry about stopping your regular, daily activities or stop taking previously prescribed medications. Although you should check with your doctor, most medications generally do not affect the accuracy of the test results.

The key to having a successful nuclear medicine test is to remain as still as possible. Any movement may distort the image results, making them difficult to interpret and increasing the possibility of redoing the test. Be sure to dress comfortably so that you are relaxed during the test. You should also dress warmly since some imaging rooms may be cold. Also, if lying on your back for long periods of time causes discomfort, you may take a pain reliever before the test is performed.

What Should I Tell My Doctor before the Test Is Scheduled?

You should tell your doctor if you are pregnant or think that you are pregnant. You should also tell your doctor if you are breastfeeding.

Why Do Nuclear Medicine Tests Take a Long Time to Perform?

The amount of time needed for a procedure depends on the type of test. Nuclear medicine tests are performed in three parts: tracer administration, taking the pictures, and analyzing the images. For many tests, a certain amount of time is needed (from a few hours to a few days) for the tracer to accumulate in the part of the body being studied before the pictures can be taken. During the imaging session, the time needed to obtain the pictures (from minutes to hours) will vary depending on the test.

Does the Tracer Cause Side Effects?

Adverse reactions, or side effects, are rare, but do let the technologist know if you experience any symptoms during or after the tracer injection.

What Happens after the Test?

When the exam is completed, the nuclear medicine physician reviews your images, prepares a report, and discusses the results with your doctor. Your doctor will explain the test results to you and discuss what further procedures, if any are needed.

After the test, should I avoid physical contact with others? No. If you have had radioiodine treatment, however, there are guidelines that your doctor may recommend that you follow to reduce the chance of radiation exposure to others. In general, the tracer you are given will remain in your body for a short period of time and is cleared from the body through natural bodily functions. Drinking fluids will help eliminate the tracer more quickly.

Can I Resume My Daily Activities after the Test?

You should be able to resume your daily activities after a nuclear medicine test. If you were temporarily asked to stop taking any medication prior to the test or if your doctor changed your usual dosage because of the test, be sure to ask when and if you should resume taking your medication(s).

Are Nuclear Medicine Tests Performed on Children?

Yes, scans are performed on children. The tests are usually done to evaluate bone pain, injuries, infection, or kidney or bladder functions. The amount of tracer is carefully adjusted based on the child's size. Sedation is sometimes required, depending on the child and type of test being given.

What You Should Know

- Remember to remain still while the pictures are being taken. Movement may distort the images and make the test results difficult to interpret.

- Do now worry about the amount of radiation you will receive during the test. It is no more than what you would receive from similar x-ray procedures.

- Be sure to tell your doctor if you are pregnant, think you are pregnant, or are a nursing mother.

- Let the technologist know if you experience any symptoms during or after the tracer is administered.

- The radioactive tracer remains in your body for a short time and it is cleared from the body through natural bodily functions. Drinking plenty of fluids will help the tracer clear through your body more quickly.

- Ask the technologist to explain any part of the procedure that you do not understand.

Nuclear Medicine Procedures

Scans may be used to diagnose a host of medical problems. Some of the more frequently performed tests include:

- Bone scans to examine orthopedic injuries, fractures, tumors, or unexplained bone pain.

- Heart scans to identify normal or abnormal blood flow to the heart muscle, measure heart function, or determine the existence or extent of damage to the heart muscle after a heart attack.

- Breast scans which are used in conjunction with mammograms to more accurately detect and locate cancerous tissue in the breasts.

- Liver and gallbladder scans to evaluate liver and gallbladder function.

- Ovarian and colorectal cancer imaging to detect tumors and determine the severity (staging) of various types of cancer.

- Prostate cancer imaging to detect tumors and to determine the extent and spread of various types of cancers.

- Brain imaging to investigate problems within the brain itself or in blood circulation to the brain.

- Renal imaging in children to examine kidney function.

Other commonly performed procedures include thyroid uptake scans to analyze the overall function of the thyroid and show the structure of the gland; lung scans to evaluate the flow of blood and movement of air into and out of the lung as well as determine the presence of blood clots; gallium scans to evaluate infection and certain types of tumors; and gastrointestinal bleeding scans.

Nuclear medicine can also be used for treatment (therapy). Radioiodine treatment for the thyroid is a common therapeutic procedure.

The material presented here is for informational purposes only and is not intended as a substitute for discussion between you and your physician. Be sure to consult with your physician or the nuclear medicine department where the test will be performed if you require more information about specific nuclear medicine procedures.

Chapter 38

Treatment and Management of Concussion in Sports

One of the most challenging problems faced by medical personnel responsible for the health care of athletes is the recognition and management of concussions.[8,11] Concussions can be defined as any alteration in cerebral function caused by a direct or indirect (rotation) force transmitted to the head resulting in one or more of the following acute signs or symptoms: a brief loss of consciousness, light-headedness, vertigo, cognitive and memory dysfunction, tinnitus, blurred vision, difficulty concentrating, amnesia, headache, nausea, vomiting, photophobia, or a balance disturbance. Delayed signs and symptoms may also include sleep irregularities, fatigue, personality changes, an inability to perform usual daily activities, depression, or lethargy. Although many concussions are mild, the range of injury is wide. Nevertheless, concussions are a form of traumatic brain injury.

In recent years, these injuries have captured many news headlines as several professional football and hockey players have retired because of the effects of concussions. Interestingly, depending on the nature of the sport and the type (for example, rotation) and degree of contact expected, these injuries are many times viewed as just part of the game. While many of these injuries are minor, some can be quite serious, with long-term consequences. Therefore, early detection through a thorough knowledge of the signs and symptoms and specific documentation of the injury is critical to the management of concussion and the monitoring of the natural history of the injury.[7,8] Unfortunately, attempts to characterize and classify the spectrum of concussions by stratifying the signs and symptoms as indicators of relative severity have been difficult.[1,2] Yet the need to accurately diagnose the severity of these injuries is obvious, especially at the time of injury when the triage decision could be critical to the patient's future. Returning an injured athlete to competition when the brain needs time to recover is an obvious concern. One of the reasons for concern is the second-impact syndrome,[5,6,10,13] a rare but ominous consequence of an untimely blow to a vulnerable central nervous system. While recent reviews cast a shadow of doubt on the occurrence and frequency,[9] the catastrophic nature of these events requires its consideration in the evaluation and treatment of concussions. Also, the cumulative effects of repeated injuries, even mild injuries, over time remains a serious concern to those involved in sports medicine.[3] The fact that some athletes do not recover as expected from concussions and are hampered by persistent symptoms for weeks or months is troublesome. In 1999, a complete understanding of the pathobiology of cerebral concussion is still lacking,[14] as is an explanation as to why the brain of some athletes may become so vulnerable to secondary injury after a seemingly mild insult.

Because of these lingering concerns, an American Orthopaedic Society for Sports Medicine-sponsored Concussion Workshop was held in December 1997 to assemble representatives from the medical community who routinely diagnose and treat these injuries in athletes. Invited participants included healthcare professionals who perform research on brain injuries, a variety of clinicians responsible for the care of the athlete, and representatives of organized contact sports (NFL, NHL, NCAA). These representatives met with the hope of defining areas of agreement and disagreement in the detection and management of concussion in sports.

Realizing that differences do exist among clinicians regarding the safety of return-to-play at various time points after concussion, defining areas of disagreement was also a goal of the concussion workshop so that these differences could be subjected to discussion and investigation. Lastly, participants focused on the key elements of the initial evaluation of concussion so that data collection, future studies, and follow-up reports could benefit from the use of common terminology and evaluation tools.

Initial Evaluation—Anticipation, Awareness, Preparation

The goal of this section on initial evaluation was to define and prioritize the steps that should be taken by medical personnel responding to an athlete who has sustained a potential concussion. The evaluation process has been subdivided into those measures that should be addressed on the playing field, when an athlete is down, and those that can be performed on the sideline after the player has either been removed from the playing surface or has come off the field independently.

On-the-Field Evaluation

The most important objective of on-the-field evaluation is to make an accurate and complete diagnosis of the level of consciousness and to rule out the presence of significant associated injuries, especially to the cervical spine. Those responsible for the care of athletic teams must have a plan formulated in advance that should include a routine protocol for assessing athletes with head injuries. This should include the presence of adequately trained personnel, appropriate equipment, and an emergency back-up plan to evacuate a critically injured player safely and promptly, should it become necessary. Medical personnel must review these procedures before the season and be assured that all responsible persons understand the routine.

Medical personnel must understand the mechanisms of head injury, realizing that concussions may occur either by direct contact of the head against a hard surface or from sudden rotational or shear forces transmitted to the brain. Rapid acceleration or deceleration of the head and neck from a whiplash type of force can be as harmful as direct contact with a hard surface. Whereas a brief attempt to determine the mechanism of injury is advisable, prolonged questioning about the mechanism should not delay the initial assessment on the field. When approaching a player who is injured, observing the posture of the athlete and noting any spontaneous motion or verbalization from the player is the first step. Total lack of motion in the extremities should always alert those at the scene to the potential for a cervical spine injury. Incoherent speech would suggest a significant concussion. The player's helmet should not be removed initially unless a cervical spine injury can be ruled out. The face guard may require removal in emergent situations.

The ABCs of Evaluation. The respondents' initial obligation is to determine whether the injured player is breathing spontaneously, has an unobstructed airway, and has a pulse. Second, medical personnel should quickly determine whether further evaluation on the sidelines is appropriate or whether emergent transport to a hospital is needed.

For the cardiovascular assessment, the carotid and radial pulses are usually the most accessible. If the patient has an adequate airway, respiration, and pulse, the initial assessment of the level of consciousness should be performed in the position in which the athlete lies. If the player is unconscious, one must assume that the athlete has an associated cervical spine injury until proven otherwise.

In the absence of a pulse and adequate respiration, the neck should be stabilized by an experienced person. With the assistance of two or three trained personnel, the athlete may then be log-rolled into a supine position so that cardiopulmonary resuscitation can be initiated effectively.

Athletes with closed head injuries frequently have a blank expression, may appear confused, exhibit delayed verbal responses, and seem emotionally labile. The standard method of assessing the level of consciousness is by establishing a Glasgow Coma Scale[57] rating.

By observing the patient's eyes and motor and verbal responses, one can quantify the level of consciousness. A Glasgow Coma Scale of 11 or higher is usually associated with an excellent prognosis for recovery. On the other hand, a Glasgow Coma Scale of 7 or less is considered very serious.

The athlete's orientation to time, place, and person should be determined by asking the date, month, day of the week, the score, the period of the game, or the play in which he or she was injured. It is also important to establish the presence of retrograde amnesia, which is associated with a more significant injury. This can be done by asking about events earlier in the day, such as what was consumed for breakfast, how the athlete traveled to the game, or the location of the locker room. The presence of symptoms such as dizziness, blurring of vision, and head or neck pain should be noted before moving the patient.

When an associated cervical spine injury has been ruled out and the level of confusion and orientation has improved to the point where the athlete can understand and follow commands, the patient may be assisted into a sitting position. This position will often decrease intracranial pressure and help to relieve the patient's confusion and apprehension. Keep the patient in the sitting position until you are satisfied that the symptoms are improving and that the athlete has adequate strength, coordination, and orientation to follow instructions. At this point, the athlete may be assisted into the standing position with people on either side for support. If the athlete is unsteady in the upright position, it is safer to remove him or her from the field seated in a motorized cart or on a stretcher. However, if the athlete does have adequate strength and coordination, he or she can be assisted from the field, being sure there are people on either side for assistance, if necessary.

On-the-Bench Evaluation

When a player with a head injury is brought to the sidelines, he or she should be thoroughly evaluated in a routine manner to further

Table 38.1. Glasgow Coma Scale [a]

Response	Point/s	Action
Eye opening		
Spontaneously	4	Reticular activity system is intact; patient may not be aware
To verbal command	3	Opens eyes when told to do so
To pain	2	Opens eyes in response to pain
None	1	Does not open eyes to any stimuli
Verbal		
Oriented, converses	5	Relatively intact CNS; aware of self and environment
Disoriented, converses	4	Well articulated, organized, but disoriented
Inappropriate words	3	Random, exclamatory words
Incomprehensible	2	Moaning, no recognizable words
No response	1	No response or intubated
Motor		
Obeys verbal commands	6	Readily moves limbs when told to
Localizes to painful stimuli	5	Moves limb in an effort to avoid pain
Flexion withdrawal	4	Pulls away from pain in flexion
Abnormal flexion	3	Decorticate rigidity
Extension	2	Decerebrate rigidity
No response	1	Hypotonic, flaccid: suggests loss of medullary function or concomitant cord injury

[a]Normal, 15

define the level of injury. This should include a review of symptoms, a careful neurologic examination, and neuropsychologic testing. Players with concussion are frequently confused, irritable, and, at times, even combative. They frequently ask to be left alone. It is preferable to take the player to a quiet spot on the sidelines near the end of the bench or into the locker room. The player should be questioned about the symptoms of dizziness, light-headedness, vertigo, blurring or double vision, photophobia, ringing in the ears, headache, nausea, and vomiting. Many of these symptoms may be present initially after an acute head injury, while headache, nausea, and vomiting may not become evident for several minutes after the precipitating trauma. Vomiting is not very common after athletic injuries, but when it is present, it suggests a significant injury with elevated intracranial pressure and should be cause for concern.

The initial clinical examination should also include careful inspection and palpation of the head and neck followed by a careful neurologic evaluation. A baseline evaluation is important to accurately appreciate any changing clinical signs and symptoms in a deteriorating situation. In all contact injuries to the head or facial region, particularly those in which a helmet is not worn, the scalp, skull, and facial bones should be palpated, in search of lacerations and tenderness. If there is a laceration, it should be cleansed and then inspected carefully with a sterile glove for crepitus, which is indicative of an underlying skull fracture. The periorbital, mandibular, and maxillary areas should be carefully palpated after blunt trauma. Having an athlete open and close the mouth and clench the teeth will often lead to detection of a malocclusion or pain secondary to a mandibular fracture. The nose should also be observed for deformity and palpated for crepitus and tenderness in facial injuries. The presence of clear fluid around the nose (rhinorrhea) is indicative of a skull fracture in the cribriform plate region.

The neurologic examination should include a careful eye examination. About 3% of the population has one pupil larger than the other (anisocoria). This should have been detected on a pre-participation physical examination and the information should be available in the athlete's record. A direct blow to the face can result in a unilateral dilation of the pupil due to sympathetic nerve response. Serious head injuries, such as a skull fracture or subdural hematoma, may damage the third cranial nerve (oculomotor), but this is generally evident later in the clinical course. It is, therefore, essential to have a baseline evaluation of the size and symmetry of the pupils to appreciate subsequent changes that may result from increasing intracranial pressure.

Visual acuity (ability to read small print), visual fields, extraocular motion, the level of the eyes (asymmetric with infraorbital blow-out fracture), and the presence of nystagmus should be part of the initial assessment. Nystagmus may be seen after a sudden rotational or shearing injury to the brain stem. It may be transient and is most frequently detected by the initial observer. A baseline evaluation of the 7th cranial nerve (facial) is also essential because paralysis of the 7th nerve may be the result of a basilar skull fracture, resulting in increasing intracranial pressure. The tympanic membrane should be visualized while looking for a spinal fluid leak (otorrhea) from a fracture in the petrous region of the temporal bone. Bleeding behind the tympanic membrane may be seen with skull fractures. Ecchymosis posterior to the ear over the mastoid region (Battle's sign) is a subsequent finding indicative of skull fractures in the posterior region of the head.

The cervical spinous processes and the brachial plexus in the supraclavicular region should be palpated. Pain with movement or tenderness warrants further assessment. Even though neck pain is common after head injuries, radiographic examination of the cervical spine is indicated in the presence of pain and tenderness.

Upper extremity strength should be thoroughly assessed, including the rotator cuff muscles, biceps, triceps, deltoid, wrist extensors and flexors, and the intrinsic muscles. Sensation in the arms and legs should be tested, and a baseline Hoffman test performed. Functional lower extremity strength and coordination can be evaluated by observing the athlete while standing, toe and heel walking, and squatting. Coordination can be evaluated by the finger-nose test, tandem walking, and the Romberg test.

On the sidelines, neuropsychologic testing can be performed to document defects in orientation, concentration, and memory. Orientation and retrograde amnesia are usually evaluated on the field. If the player has come off the field under his or her own power and was not examined on the field, these functions should be assessed immediately. Memory can be tested by asking the player to recall three words or three objects at 0 and 5 minutes. Detailed concentration can be evaluated by asking the player to repeat three, four, and five digits backward, to recite the months of the year in reverse order, or to do serial 7s. Knowledge of the player's capabilities through pre-season testing is usually necessary in evaluating cognitive performance.

A player should be initially observed for a minimum of 15 minutes on the sidelines and reevaluated as needed. If any symptoms develop, the athlete should not return to competition that day. If the player has not lost consciousness, is oriented, and is asymptomatic, provocative testing should be performed next to determine whether symptoms will occur with physical stress. A 40-yard dash, five sit-ups, five push-ups, or five deep knee bends are usually adequate to increase intracranial pressure. Having the patient recline supine with the feet elevated for several seconds may also increase intracranial pressure sufficiently to cause symptoms. If there are any symptoms after these maneuvers, the player should not be allowed to return to play.

If a player is asymptomatic and returns to the game, it is essential that the athlete be reevaluated repeatedly during the contest to detect any change in clinical course. These subsequent evaluations are preferably performed by the same person who performed the initial examination. It is also helpful to communicate to the player the importance of being extremely honest about symptoms, realizing that many players will deny symptoms to be able to return to competition. The seriousness of the second-impact syndrome and post-concussion syndrome should be explained to the player before he or she is allowed to return to competition. A conservative approach would be to not allow the athlete who has had a head injury back into the game because of the potential risk.

Recommendations for Concussion Work-Up and Return to Play

In general, if an athlete has any symptoms on the field that are related to a concussion, the athlete should not be allowed to continue to play. Additionally, athletes with concussions should always be evaluated by a physician before return to athletic play. Parameters for return to activity in the asymptomatic athlete should be the same for all sports, regardless of the degree of contact or use of protective equipment such as helmets. A small number of symptomatic athletes may require subsequent evaluation by a neurosurgeon or a neurologist because of persistent symptoms. Caution should always be exercised by the medical staff responsible for making return-to-play decisions because the athlete's motivation as well as peer or coaching pressure may be significant factors.

Most importantly, any athlete who is symptomatic after a concussion requires serial neurologic evaluations. These examinations should be performed, as needed, for as long as symptoms persist to determine if the athlete's condition is deteriorating. If a neurologic evaluation at any time reveals any deterioration in mental status or a loss of consciousness after a concussion, immediate transport to an appropriate emergency facility is indicated where a neurosurgeon or neurologist and diagnostic neuroimaging are available. No other abnormalities on the neurologic examination would be needed to warrant such emergent treatment.

When a concussion occurs, the athlete should be observed and evaluated for a minimum of 15 minutes. The medical personnel at the competition may allow the athlete to return to play if there was no loss of consciousness and all signs and symptoms are normal. If the athlete's symptoms do not abate during the initial 15 to 20 minutes of observation, the athlete should be disqualified from that day's competition. Only when the athlete is totally asymptomatic, passes memory and concentration tests, and has no symptoms after provocative testing, may the athlete be returned to play. Once the athlete has returned to competition, medical personnel should continue to observe and reexamine the athlete carefully for any signs that the athlete is not 100% recovered. The increased stress of competition may produce signs and symptoms that are not produced by the provocative maneuvers off the field. If the athlete is not 100% recovered, the athlete should be disqualified. This is especially important in sports where breaks in the action are infrequent and frequent reevaluations off the field are not possible.

Several clinical rules are important to keep in mind when evaluating athletes with concussion. Any observed period of unconsciousness is significant and should always preclude return to play. Even brief episodes of loss of consciousness are usually associated with other symptoms that will preclude play. While a brief loss of consciousness is only one factor to consider in the clinical evaluation, it should be evaluated in context with other signs and symptoms. As with any other injury, careful serial follow-up examinations are always recommended.

Return-to-Play Classifications

Return to Play (Same Day)

1. Signs and symptoms cleared within 15 minutes or less both at rest and exertion.

2. Normal neurologic evaluation

3. No documented loss of consciousness

Delayed Return to Play (Not the Same Day)

1. Signs and symptoms did not clear in 15 minutes at rest or with exertion

2. Documented loss of consciousness

Any new headache in the first 48 to 72 hours after a concussion or an unusual headache should be considered a significant symptom and should preclude play; either is also an indication that further medical evaluation is needed. Caution should always be exercised in the younger athlete with headache, particularly a unilateral headache.

The other symptoms that should preclude play at any time are dizziness, slowness in responding to questions, evidence of difficulty concentrating, physical sluggishness, and memory loss, especially if there is a loss of memory of events before the injury (retrograde amnesia). Athletes who experience retrograde amnesia do not usually recover during the athletic contest. If the player has had any symptoms or difficulty with concentration tests, that player should not return to play. While a loss of consciousness usually receives a lot of attention by those attending an injured athlete, a brief loss of consciousness, such as a matter of a couple of seconds during the time it takes medical personnel to reach the athlete on the playing surface, may not be as significant as other symptoms that do not clear in the first 15 minutes.

While some concussion scenarios present challenges to the clinician, there is no question about a symptomatic athlete's status: the athlete should not return to play. However, the clinical decisions become more difficult when symptoms clear after 20 to 30 minutes, after the game, or the next day. All of these situations should be classified as prolonged symptoms and are cause for concern. Unfortunately, at the present time, it is not known if neurocognitive function returns to normal when symptoms subside in humans. Therefore, it cannot be assumed that an athlete is normal when he or she feels fine. The return to play for a young (for example, high school) athlete who experienced symptoms for longer than 15 minutes continues to be a difficult decision and represents a gray zone in the medical literature. Current medical knowledge does not adequately address this situation. While some athletes may benefit from 5 to 7 days of rest after experiencing initial symptoms in excess of 15 minutes,[13] others may be able to safely return to play much sooner.

Until neuropsychologic testing can be done on enough asymptomatic athletes in the first 48 hours after symptoms resolve, correlation between the absence of symptoms and neurocognitive function in humans cannot be drawn, and even if it could, it may still not mean the player is safe to return to play. Presently, the NHL is performing neuropsychologic testing on all players after concussion. The relationship between neurofunction and symptoms in this group of athletes may soon be known. However, these same correlative studies, between symptoms and cognitive function, will have to be repeated in all age ranges and athletic groups to determine the safety of a return to play. It is very important not to generalize the results of these correlative studies. What is medically acceptable in adults may not be safe in teenagers or adolescents. Further studies in the various age groups and sports will be needed to answer these clinical problems safely. Unfortunately, as far as we know, there are no ongoing studies in child or adolescent athletes such as those being conducted by the NHL and the NFL.

Recommendations

1. Every athlete with concussion should be evaluated by a physician.

2. Loss of consciousness precludes return to play that day.

3. Persistence of (longer than 15 minutes) or delayed onset of any symptoms such as headache, dizziness, malaise, slowness to respond mentally or physically at rest, or with provocation (supine with legs elevated), or with exercise precludes return to play that day.

4. Any deterioration in physical or mental status after the initial trauma, such as increasing headache, dizziness, or nausea, warrants immediate transport to an emergency facility where neurologic or neurosurgical consultation and neuroimaging are available.

5. When prolonged symptoms (greater than 15 minutes) are experienced after a concussion, great care must be exercised in returning an asymptomatic athlete to practice or competition. Without at least 5 to 7 days of rest, neurofunction may not yet be normal. Further research is needed to demonstrate the association, or lack of association, between symptoms, neurocognitive function, and injury susceptibility. Until this age-specific information is available, such decisions must be approached with great concern. Repeated examinations of the athlete are needed during a gradual increase in physical exertion to determine if these stresses trigger symptoms. If symptoms recur, the athlete is not ready to return to play. Current neuroscience knowledge in humans does not give a safe, firm

timetable for return to play after concussion in most circumstances. Therefore, each athlete with prolonged symptoms (more than 15 minutes) must be evaluated individually. Repeated and thorough evaluations, preferably by the same clinician, are most helpful in determining readiness to play.

6. Newer tools, such as balance testing,[4] cannot be recommended for clinical decision-making after concussion at this time. However, their use for further data collection is encouraged. The balance test may prove to be a useful tool for identifying impairment associated with concussion.

7. We recommend further study of the SAC48-50 as part of the initial evaluation of an athlete with concussion to gain experience with its use. Furthermore, wide-scale examination of this instrument is needed at all levels of competition and in different athletic groups. While recognizing its clinical potential, we believe it is premature to recommend its generalized use as the sole determinant of clinical decisions after concussion. We do recommend continued wide-scale clinical testing of this instrument.

8. We recognize the need for continued clinical and basic science research of sports-induced concussions. The clinical use of neuropsychologic assessments in the study of athletes has been limited by a current lack of research studies that have specifically investigated the use of these assessments in sports. We recommend the establishment of cooperative studies across athletic organizations at the junior, high school, college, and professional levels that would promote the longitudinal study of large groups of athletes.

9. We specifically promote the establishment of databases on all athletes with concussions. If similar neuropsychologic instruments are used at all levels, longitudinal analysis of test results for specific athletes will be possible as the athlete progresses from one level to the next. This type of information would be particularly useful to athletes, their families, and physicians to assess the risk of future injury and further difficulties.

References

1. Cantu RC: Guidelines for return to contact sports after cerebral concussion. *Physician Sportsmed* 14: 75-83, 1986

2. Clifton GL, Hayes RL, Levin HS, et al: Outcome measures for clinical trials involving traumatically brain-injured patients: Report of a conference. *Neurosurgery* 31: 975-978, 1992

3. Evans RW: The postconcussion syndrome: 130 years of controversy. *Semin Neurol* 14: 32-39, 1994

4. Guskiewicz KM, Riemann BL, Perrin DH, et al: Alternative approaches to the assessment of mild head injury in athletes. *Med Sci Sports Exerc* 29 (7 Suppl): S213-S221, 1997

5. Hovda DA, Badie H, Karimi S, et al: Concussive brain injury produces a state of vulnerability for intracranial pressure perturbation in the absence of morphological damage, in Avezaat CJJ, Van Eijndhoven JHM, Maas AIR, et al (eds): *Intracranial Pressure VIII*. New York, Springer-Verlag, 1993, pp 469-472

6. Jenkins LW, Marmarou A, Lewelt W, et al: Increased vulnerability of the traumatized brain to early ischemia, in Baethmann A, Go GK, Unterberg A (eds): *Mechanisms of Secondary Brain Damage*. Wien, Springer, 1996, pp 273-282

7. Kelly JP, Rosenberg J: Practice parameter: The management of concussion in sport: Report of the Quality Standards Subcommittee. *Neurology* 48: 581-585, 1997

8. Landry G: Mild brain injury in athletes, in National Athletic Trainers Association Research and Education Foundation: Proceedings from Mild Brain Injury Summit. Washington, DC, April 16-18, 1994

9. McCrory PR, Berkovic SF: Second impact syndrome. *Neurology* 50: 677-683, 1998

10. McQuillen JB, McQuillen EN, Morrow P: Trauma, sports, and malignant cerebral edema. *Am J Forensic Med Pathol* 9: 12-15, 1988

11. Muizelaar JP: Cerebral blood flow, cerebral blood volume, and cerebral metabolism after severe head injury, in Becker DP, Gudeman SK (eds): *Textbook of Head Injury*. Philadelphia, WB Saunders, 1989, pp 221-240

12. Rosen P, Barkin RM: *Emergency Medicine: Concepts of Clinical Practice*. Fourth edition. St. Louis, Mosby Year Book, 1998

13. Saunders RL, Harbaugh RE: The second impact in catastrophic contact sports head trauma. *JAMA* 252: 538-539, 1984

14. Walker AE: The physiological basis of concussion: 50 years later [Commemorative Article]. *J Neurosurg* 81: 493-494, 1994

Chapter 39

Traumatic Brain Injury (TBI) Rehabilitation

Models of Comprehensive Rehabilitation for Traumatic Brain Injury

Howard A. Rusk is generally credited with being the pioneer of comprehensive, general rehabilitation in the United States; he was an early advocate for multidisciplinary, rehabilitative care. However, specialized models of brain injury rehabilitation were not initiated until the 1970s with the advent of the Glasgow Coma Scale (Teasdale, Jennett, 1974) and the Glasgow Outcome Scale (Jennett, Bond, 1975). Indeed, Rosenthal (1996) has described the period from 1975 to 1979 as the era of enlightenment for the field of rehabilitation following traumatic brain injury (TBI). During this period, improvements occurred in emergency medical services and acute care, and individuals began to be transferred to comprehensive TBI rehabilitation programs rather than to facilities for purely custodial care. According to Rosenthal (1996), the years from 1980 to 1984 can be described as the era of proliferation for TBI programs. In just a few years, the number of TBI rehabilitation programs swelled to approximately 500 (Rosenthal, 1996), and the continuum of care expanded substantially (Cope, 1985). Rosenthal (1996) has described the years from 1985 to 1989 as the era of refinement. During these years, skepticism about the efficacy of TBI rehabilitation arose, and the scientific literature began to expand

"Report of the Consensus on Rehabilitation of Persons with Traumatic Brain Injury," National Institute of Child Health and Human Development (NICHD), October 26–28, 1998.

401

rapidly. New professional journals dedicated to TBI emerged, training programs for TBI professionals expanded, and major governmental funding became available. Rosenthal (1996) has described the years from 1990 to 1994 as the era of accountability. During those years, allegations of provider abuse and fraud were published (Kerr, 1992), and a congressional subcommittee was charged to investigate consumer complaints. As a result, ethical guidelines and rehabilitation standards were assimilated by TBI professionals. Finally, Rosenthal (1996) has noted that the field of TBI rehabilitation has now entered the era of consolidation; this era mirrors the nationwide changes that are occurring in the health care industry. Specifically, there is an increasing shift toward outpatient care, reduction of costs, and earlier discharge from inpatient rehabilitation programs. After nearly 25 years of rapid evolution, the field of TBI rehabilitation is in need of an in-depth, scientific review.

A review of the TBI rehabilitation literature presents many difficulties, as has been noted by several authors. First, studies vary widely with regard to the definition of TBI, which complicates comparisons across studies. Second, most rehabilitation programs are heterogeneous in terms of treatments; that is, many rehabilitation strategies are used simultaneously so there is difficulty ascertaining which of the multiple components are actually effective. Third, studies vary widely in terms of the adequacy of outcome measures; the consistent use of standardized and ecologically valid measures is needed. Fourth, definitive outcome research requires a no-treatment control group, but a deliberate decision not to provide rehabilitative care for persons with TBI may be considered unethical. Therefore, randomized no-treatment studies generally have not been considered as an option. Fifth, many studies have relied on convenience samples rather than representative, national cohorts. For these reasons, the existing literature on TBI rehabilitation must be viewed with caution and with a recognition that definitive conclusions are difficult to draw.

A Conceptual Model of TBI Rehabilitation

The articulation of a model of TBI rehabilitation is challenging in its own right. The literature is replete with imprecise terms and labels that have been used by different authors in different ways. For example, terms such as acute, post-acute, and sub-acute have been applied inconsistently. However, Malec and Basford (1996) have presented a conceptual framework that serves as a good starting point for a discussion of a comprehensive model of TBI rehabilitation. In

Malec and Basford's model, the acute phase of care following TBI includes emergency medical treatment, emergency room care, intensive care unit/acute hospital care, acute rehabilitation, and sub-acute rehabilitation (e.g., coma management). Accordingly, everything that follows acute-phase treatment is described as post-acute care. In Malec and Basford's model, the post-acute phase includes interdisciplinary rehabilitation assessment, outpatient community reentry programs, comprehensive day treatment programs, residential community reintegration programs, neurobehavioral programs, and community-based services. Although not specifically mentioned in the Malec and Basford model, post-acute programs also include home-based rehabilitation, independent living programs, and, more recently, clubhouse programs. Jacobs (1997) described the concept of a clubhouse as a member-directed residential/rehabilitation setting designed to facilitate community reentry and return to employment. To establish a firm basis for the consistent use of terminology, the Malec and Basford model has been adopted here as a framework for organizing this literature review.

Overview of the Literature

A literature review by Cope (1995) examined the efficacy of key components of a comprehensive model of TBI rehabilitation. Cope reviewed the literature from the standpoint of several rehabilitation settings as follows: (1) ICU/acute neurosurgical care, (2) acute inpatient hospital rehabilitation, (3) outpatient/day treatment rehabilitation, (4) residential post-acute rehabilitation, and (5) neurobehavioral programs. Cope selected studies with quasi-experimental designs that included significant elements of experimental methodology, validity, and functional and/or economic outcome measures. This review updates (and expands) the Cope review; the studies selected for discussion include observational reports and uncontrolled trials that were viewed by the Consensus Panel as representative studies in the TBI rehabilitation literature. However, this review is by no means all inclusive. Studies of TBI rehabilitation vary on many important parameters such as nature of injury, severity of impairment, sampling methodology, treatment setting, and experimental design, among many others. A full description of these relevant parameters is beyond the scope of this review. However, the evidence tables from the *Evidence Report on Rehabilitation of Persons with Traumatic Brain Injury* (Chesnut et al., 1998) contain this relevant information in a concise, well-organized format.

ICU/Acute Neurosurgical Care

In the Cope (1995) review, two studies of the ICU/acute neurosurgical care setting were described. ICU/acute neurosurgical care refers to the practice of including physiatrists and other rehabilitation specialists at the earliest possible point following TBI. Morgan and colleagues (1988) found that persons with TBI given early rehabilitation had significantly shortened lengths of stays and better functional outcomes at discharge. Mackey and colleagues (1992) found that persons with TBI who received early rehabilitation had shorter coma lengths and shorter rehabilitation stays in comparison with a matched control group who did not receive acute rehabilitation. However, a cautionary note about the Mackey study is that the shorter coma length for the rehabilitation group may be construed as a potential methodological shortcoming.

Acute Inpatient Hospital Rehabilitation

Cope (1995) reviewed several studies on TBI in the category of acute inpatient hospital rehabilitation, which refers to the use of an interdisciplinary approach to in-hospital rehabilitative care; this typically includes medical stabilization, physical rehabilitation, and cognitive/behavioral rehabilitation. Heinemann and colleagues (1990) conducted a descriptive study of persons with TBI discharged from an inpatient rehabilitation program and found demonstrative improvements in functional status and ADL capacity at 3 months after discharge. Blackerby (1990) found that increasing the intensity of rehabilitation activities led to a reduced length of stay. Cope and Hall (1982) found that individuals referred for early comprehensive rehabilitation had a greater than 50 percent reduction in hospital treatment days compared with individuals who were referred for late rehabilitation. However, the groups in the Cope and Hall study did not differ in terms of functional recovery or functional status at 2 years post-injury. Spivack and colleagues (1992) found that both length of stay and intensity of treatment were associated with improved outcomes as measured by both physical and cognitive skills. Aronow (1987) found that individuals who received inpatient TBI rehabilitation had better outcomes than those who received only acute neurotrauma care on such measures as living arrangements, functional status, daily care requirements, and vocational status.

In addition to the studies reviewed by Cope in 1995, Davis and Acton (1988) examined the outcomes following acute inpatient rehabilitation for a group of persons with TBI who were elderly and found that 85 percent eventually returned to a home setting; more than half the sample achieved independence in activities of daily living. Keyser and colleagues (1995) examined persons with TBI immediately following acute inpatient rehabilitation and found generally low mean factor scores on the Neurobehavioral Rating Scale. Whitlock and Hamilton (1995) examined functional outcome following acute inpatient rehabilitation and found that even the most severely disabled persons with TBI can show a large degree of measurable functional improvement following acute inpatient rehabilitation. Heinemann and colleagues (1995) studied a cohort of persons with TBI following acute inpatient rehabilitation and found that the intensity of the rehabilitative therapies was not related to functional status gains. Tobis and colleagues (1992) examined outcomes following acute inpatient rehabilitation and found improvements in self-care and ambulation but limited benefits in terms of social and vocational functioning.

Outpatient/Day Treatment Rehabilitation

The Cope (1995) review included nine studies in the category of outpatient/day treatment rehabilitation, which refers to post-acute rehabilitative strategies that deliver integrated, interdisciplinary rehabilitation services on an outpatient basis. Ben-Yishay and associates (1987) treated individuals in an outpatient cognitive rehabilitation program and found statistically significant improvement in employment at discharge and at 3-year follow-up. Prigatano and colleagues (1984) examined a post-acute rehabilitation group, compared with a matched control group, on measures of neuropsychological functioning, emotional distress, and productivity; the treated group showed little improvement on neuropsychological measures but demonstrated improved productivity and decreased emotional distress. Ruff and Niemann (1990) compared outpatient day treatment with formal cognitive rehabilitation and found essentially equal outcomes on measures of depression. Scherzer (1986) followed a cohort of individuals who participated in a multidisciplinary day treatment program; he found improvements in neuropsychological status. Malec and associates (1993) found improvements in independent living and work outcome in two subgroups of persons with TBI (i.e., those treated within 1 year and those treated later than 1 year following injury). Fryer and Haffey (1987) found that a group of individuals with TBI who received an outpatient cognitive retraining program showed better outcomes on ratings of disability and psychosocial status in comparison with a matched control group. Haffey and Abrams (1991) found that persons with TBI who participated in a work reentry program, as contrasted with comparison groups, showed an improved employment rate. Wehman and colleagues (1990) used a vocational rehabilitation program (i.e., supported employment model) as an intervention and found increased employment rates at follow-up. Mills and colleagues (1992) reported on the treatment of persons with TBI in an outpatient rehabilitation program and found improvement in five-point level but not on cognitive measures.

In addition to the studies reviewed by Cope (1995), Lyons and Morse (1998) evaluated a community-based therapeutic work program and found that 79 percent of the participants returned to meaningful occupational activities. Buffington and Malec (1997) demonstrated that early vocational intervention (closely integrated with medical rehabilitative treatment) resulted in the placement of 40 percent of program participants within a 3-month period. Namerow (1987) followed a group of persons with TBI before and after an outpatient rehabilitation program and found modest improvements on both neuropsychological measures and functional scores. Switzer and Hinebaugh (1991) reported functional, vocational, or academic improvements in approximately 78 percent of participants with TBI in an intensive day treatment program. Rattok and associates (1992) studied three types of rehabilitation programs: (1) a balanced program emphasizing cognitive remediation and interpersonal therapies, (2) a program emphasizing primarily cognitive remediation, and (3) a program emphasizing primarily interpersonal therapies. All three rehabilitation programs were equally effective with regard to capacity to return to work and level of vocational achievement. Stern and associates (1985) studied a cohort of individuals with TBI who completed a daily treatment rehabilitation program and found cognitive improvements in 37 percent of the sample and improvement in family life/occupational status in approximately one-third of the sample. Prigatano and colleagues (1994) found that persons with TBI who underwent a neuropsychological rehabilitation program were more productive (as students or workers) than a matched historical group who did not participate in the rehabilitation program.

Residential Post-Acute Rehabilitation

Cope (1995) identified two studies in the category of residential post-acute rehabilitation, which refers to residential rehabilitative programs that provide integrated cognitive, behavioral, physical, and vocational rehabilitation services to persons who are unable to participate in outpatient programs. Johnston and Lewis (1991) reported results from nine post-acute rehabilitation programs and found a decreased need for supervision and/or care following the intervention. Cope and colleagues (1991) reported that comprehensive post-acute rehabilitation resulted in improvements on measures of residential status, productivity, and dependency.

In addition to the studies reviewed by Cope (1995), Jones and Evans (1992) conducted a follow-up of persons with TBI who received services in a residential post-acute rehabilitation program; they found that there was a significant increase in the percentage of clients living at home and a subsequent reduction in the need for inpatient care. Harrick and colleagues (1994) found improvements in productive activity, place of residence, and level of supervision for persons with TBI who participated in a transitional living program. McLaughlin and Peters (1993) reported that individuals with TBI participating in an innovative transitional living program were more independent in activities of daily living than those who engaged in only inpatient rehabilitation.

Neurobehavioral Programs

In the Cope (1995) review, three studies were identified within the category of neurobehavioral rehabilitation programs, which refers to residential programs that provide intensive behavioral treatments for persons with TBI who manifest severe behavioral disturbances. Eames and Wood (1985) reported that an intensive inpatient neurobehavioral intervention for persons with severe TBI (late-stage post-injury) resulted in improvements in residential options after treatment and better scores on behavioral and daily living scales. Ashley and associates (1990) found that individuals assessed at admission and discharge from an inpatient post-acute rehabilitation program showed improvements on ratings of disability and living status. Sundance and colleagues (1992) found that individuals treated in a residential neurobehavioral program showed improvements in Rancho Los Amigos levels and disability ratings; 84 percent of the sample of persons with brain injuries were discharged home.

In addition to the outcomes reviewed by Cope in 1995, Eames and associates (1995) found that an intensive rehabilitation program for persons with TBI resulted in improvements in functional skills and social behavior. Ashley and colleagues (1997) found a pattern of positive long-term outcome stability following post-acute TBI rehabilitation, except that vocational status decreased over the follow-up interval. Burke and colleagues (1988) followed the outcomes for persons with TBI discharged from a rehabilitation center and reported that nearly 70 percent of adults were placed in a less restrictive setting; approximately two-thirds were successfully placed in employment situations.

Outcomes Following Unspecified Rehabilitation or No Treatment

An evaluation of the TBI rehabilitation literature requires an examination of outcomes following unspecified rehabilitation or no treatment at all. Studies in this category examine outcomes for persons with TBI following unspecified rehabilitation, minimal rehabilitative programming, or no apparent rehabilitation. Kraft and associates (1993) surveyed occupational and educational achievements of Vietnam veterans with TBI 15 years post-injury and found that 56 percent were gainfully employed and that the occupational distribution was little different from uninjured controls. Dombovy and Olek (1996) conducted a telephone follow-up of persons with TBI (most of whom were discharged without rehabilitation) and found that physical disability was minimal but that approximately one-third remained cognitively impaired at 6 months; approximately two-thirds of persons with TBI remained unemployed. Brooks and colleagues (1987) conducted a follow-up of persons with TBI for the first 7 years after severe head injury and found that the employment rate had dropped from a pre-injury level of 86 percent to a post-injury level of 29 percent. Stambrook and colleagues (1990) conducted a follow-up on a group of individuals with severe impairments following TBI; whereas all had been employed full-time before their injury, only 55 percent were employed full-time following their injury. Schalen and colleagues (1994) described a nonspecific management protocol for persons with TBI; the authors found that the number of individuals who returned to work was significantly higher after the introduction of the management protocol. Ruff and associates (1993) conducted a follow-up of a cohort of persons with severe TBI; after 6 months, only 18 percent of former workers had returned to gainful employment and only 62 percent of former students had returned to school. Dikmen and colleagues (1993) found that many persons who were moderately to severely impaired following TBI were unable to support themselves and work independently at 2 years post-injury.

Home-Based Rehabilitation, Independent Living Programs, and Clubhouse Programs

The post-acute phase of TBI rehabilitation has been extended into home-based situations, independent living programs, and clubhouse programs. However, outcome data on the effectiveness of these new post-acute rehabilitation approaches are mostly nonexistent. Lockhart and colleagues (1994) described a home-based rehabilitation approach for persons with TBI, although outcome data were not provided. In the home-based approach, visiting providers from home health agencies deliver rehabilitation services in the client's home environment. In addition, rehabilitation services are increasingly available in the context of independent living programs and clubhouse programs. In general, there is an increasing emphasis on rehabilitation services in the "natural" setting (Carnevale, 1996); this emphasis typically includes training caregivers to implement and sustain behavioral management programs or other appropriate rehabilitation strategies (Fujii et al., 1996; Ragnarsson et al., 1993). These new post-acute TBI rehabilitation programs appear to have promise, but there are limited data to support their efficacy at this time.

TBI Model Systems

The National Institute on Disability and Rehabilitation Research (NIDRR) funded the Traumatic Brain Injury Model Systems of Care. Until 1998, the TBI Model Systems encompassed five sites: (1) Rehabilitation Institute of Michigan/Wayne State University, (2) Santa Clara Valley Medical Center in San Jose, California, (3) Institute for Rehabilitation and Research in Houston, (4) Ohio State University, and (5) Moss Rehabilitation Research Institute in Philadelphia, but recently other such centers have been funded. These original five centers were involved in a prospective, longitudinal study examining the recovery and outcomes of a coordinated system of acute neurotrauma and rehabilitation. This multi-site trial incorporates measures of impairment, disability, and handicap, according to the definitions of the World Health Organization. The TBI Model Systems are of particular interest because the continuum of care includes the following: (1) emergency medical services, (2) acute neurosurgical care, (3) comprehensive rehabilitation services, and (4) long-term interdisciplinary follow-up and rehabilitation services (Ragnarsson et al., 1993); this prospective, multi-site trial has already generated valuable epidemiologic information regarding the causes and course of TBI. However, there appear to be distinct limitations to the Model Systems trial. First, there is no control group (or even a comparison group) to permit an examination of the effectiveness of the Model Systems approach in comparison with a no-treatment group. Second, there is an inevitable selection bias in a sample restricted to only five sites. Third, the treatments provided at the various Model Systems sites are not uniform, which complicates outcome analyses. Fourth, attrition during the first year has been found to be high (39 percent). Last, there are methodological limitations in the ability to track post-acute service utilization. In spite of these limitations, data collection by the TBI Model Systems trial may provide considerable information on demographics, course, and outcome following comprehensive, multidisciplinary rehabilitation in the future.

Institute of Medicine Rehabilitation Model

In 1997, an important report titled *Enabling America: Assessing the Role of Rehabilitation Science and Engineering* was published by the Institute of Medicine (IOM), National Academy of Sciences (Brandt, Pope, 1997). The IOM report is particularly instructive because conventional models of rehabilitation are strongly challenged. Traditionally, rehabilitation has been conceptualized as the process of restoring a person's functionality to permit him or her to live optimally in the environment. In short, the focus of rehabilitation has typically been on the individual and the restoration of his or her functional capacity. The IOM model depicts the disabling process as the situation in which a person's needs are large in relation to the existing environment.

In contrast with traditional rehabilitation, the IOM model depicts the enabling process as containing two strategic possibilities. First, a program of functional restoration (i.e., rehabilitation) might be pursued to permit a person to regain the capacity to function within the existing environment. Or second, a systematic effort could be made to enlarge the existing environment to make everyday functioning easier for a person with TBI. In this latter approach, the focus is more on changing the environment than on changing the individual. From this new IOM perspective, the manifestation of a disability occurs at the interaction of the person with his or her environment. A person brings to his or her environment a certain potential for pathology, impairment, or functional limitation. In turn, environments vary dramatically in terms of the physical and social factors that make them either more or less supportive. Therefore, for a given individual, disability becomes a function of the interaction between himself or herself and a specific environment. If the environment is sufficiently supportive for a given person, disability is minimized (or possibly nonexistent). If the environment is not sufficiently supportive for that person, then potential disability becomes manifest. The IOM model is highly instructive because it shifts the focus away from rehabilitation in the traditional sense to enablement in the broader sense of permitting a person to function within his or her environment. In the field of TBI, there will be a need to explore the utility of the new IOM model for its ability to generate new approaches to the minimization of disability.

Perspective of Persons with Brain Injuries and Their Families

In 1994, the Office of Special Education and Rehabilitation Services sponsored a national TBI conference titled *Life After Brain Injury: Finding Answers I Can Live With*. The advocacy statement of the conference attendees was that services for persons with TBI must be consumer driven and focused on consumer preferences to be effective. In short, consumer involvement and choice throughout the entire TBI rehabilitation and enablement process are the clear expectation of the majority of persons with TBI and their families. However, the literature on TBI models is surprisingly lacking in the area of consumer involvement. Therefore, the entire literature on comprehensive, multidisciplinary rehabilitation models for TBI can be questioned from the standpoint of its applicability to the real life needs of persons with TBI. Clearly, future research on TBI rehabilitation and enablement will need to be much more attentive to the expressed needs of consumers.

One development viewed as positive from a consumer standpoint is the requirement of projects funded by the National Institute on Disability and Rehabilitation Research that participatory action research (PAR) (Whyte, 1991) be incorporated into the study methodology. With the PAR approach, consumers are included as participants in the research process at all levels. Specifically, consumers help define relevant research questions, conceptualize clinically meaningful methodologies, and participate in the interpretation of findings. In the PAR process, there is a commitment to a partnership between experts who possess scientific skills and consumers who can enhance clinical relevance. To date, the field of TBI outcomes research appears to be lacking in studies describing the area of appropriate consumer involvement.

411

References

Aronow HU. Rehabilitation effectiveness with severe brain injury: translating research into policy. *J Head Trauma Rehabil* 1987;2:24-36.

Ashley MJ, Krych DK, Lehr RP. Cost/benefit analysis for post-acute rehabilitation of the traumatically brain-injured patient. *J Ins Med* 1990;22:156-61.

Ashley MJ, Persel CS, Clark MC, Krych DK. Long-term follow-up of post-acute traumatic brain injury rehabilitation: a statistical analysis to test for stability and predictability of outcome. *Brain Inj* 1997; 11:677-90.

Ben-Yishay Y, Silver SM, Piasetsky E, et al. Relationship between employability and vocational outcome after intensive holistic cognitive rehabilitation. *J Head Trauma Rehabil* 1987;2:35-8.

Blackerby WF. Intensity of rehabilitation and length of stay. *Brain Inj* 1990;4:167-73.

Brandt EN Jr, Pope AM. *Enabling America: assessing the role of rehabilitation science and engineering.* Washington (DC): National Academy Press; 1997.

Brooks N, McKinlay W, Symington C, Beattie A, Campsie L. Return to work within the first seven years of severe head injury. *Brain Inj* 1987;1:5-19.

Buffington ALH, Malec JF. The vocational rehabilitation continuum: maximizing outcomes through bridging the gap from hospital to community-based services. *J Head Trauma Rehabil* 1997;12:1-13.

Burke WH, Wesolowski MD, Guth ML. Comprehensive head injury rehabilitation: an outcome evaluation. *Brain Inj* 1988;2:313-22.

Carnevale GJ. Natural-setting behavior management for individuals with traumatic brain injury: results of a three-year caregiver training program. *J Head Trauma Rehabil* 1996;11(1):27-38.

Chesnut RM, Carney N, Maynard H, Patterson P, Mann NC, Helfand M. *Evidence report on rehabilitation of persons with traumatic brain injury,* 1998. Contract No.: AHCPR 290-97-0018.

Cope DN. The effectiveness of traumatic brain injury rehabilitation: a review. *Brain Inj* 1995;9:649-70.

Cope DN. Traumatic closed head injuries: status of rehabilitation treatment. *Semin Neurol* 1985;5:212-20.

Cope DN, Cole JR, Hall KM, et al. Brain injury: analysis of outcomes in a post-acute rehabilitation system. Part 1: general analysis. *Brain Inj* 1991;5:111-25.

Cope DN, Hall K. Head injury rehabilitation: benefit of early intervention. *Arch Phys Med Rehabil* 1982;63:433-7.

Davis CS, Acton P. Treatment of the elderly brain-injured patient: experience in a traumatic brain injury unit. *J Am Geriatr Soc* 1988;36:225-9.

Dikmen S, Machamer J, Temkin N. Psychosocial outcome in patients with moderate to severe head injury: 2-year follow-up. *Brain Inj* 1993; 7:113-24.

Dombovy ML, Olek AC. Recovery and rehabilitation following traumatic brain injury. *Brain Inj* 1996;11:305-18.

Eames P, Cotterill G, Kneale TA, Storrar AL, Yeomans P. Outcome of intensive rehabilitation after severe brain injury: a long-term follow-up study. *Brain Inj* 1995;10:631-50.

Eames P, Wood R. Rehabilitation after severe brain injury: a special unit approach to behavior disorder. *Int Rehabil Med* 1985;7:130-3.

Fryer LJ, Haffey WJ. Cognitive rehabilitation and community readaptation: outcomes from two model programs. *J Head Trauma Rehabil* 1987;2:51-63.

Fujii D, Hanes S, Kokuni Y. Family intervention in the rehabilitation and community reintegration of individuals with brain injury. *Cog Rehabil* 1996;14(2):6-17.

Haffey WJ, Abrams DL. Employment outcomes for participants in a brain injury work reentry program: preliminary findings. *J Head Trauma Rehabil* 1991;6:24-34.

Harrick L, Krefting L, Johnston J, Carlson P, Minnes P. Stability of functional outcomes following transitional living programme participation: 3-year follow-up. *Brain Inj* 1994;8:439-47.

Heinemann AW, Hamilton B, Linacre JM, Wright BD, Granger C. Functional status and therapeutic intensity during inpatient rehabilitation. *Am J Phys Med Rehabil* 1995;74:315-26.

Heinemann AW, Saghal V, Cichowski K, et al. Functional outcome following traumatic brain injury rehabilitation. *J Neurol Rehabil* 1990; 4:27-37.

Jacobs HE. The clubhouse: addressing work-related behavioral challenges through a supportive social community. *J Head Trauma Rehabil* 1997;12:14-27.

Jennett B, Bond MR. Assessment of outcome after severe brain damage. *Lancet* 1975;1:480.

Johnston MV, Lewis FD. Outcomes of community re-entry programmes for brain injury survivors. Part 1: independent living and productive activities. *Brain Inj* 1991;5:141-54.

Jones ML, Evans RW. Outcome validation in post-acute rehabilitation: trends and correlates in treatment and outcome. *J Ins Med* 1992; 24:186-92.

Kerr P. Centers for head injury accused of earning millions for neglect. *New York Times* 1992 March 16;1.

Keyser L, Witol AD, Kreutzer JS, Rosenthal M. A multi-center investigation of neurobehavioral outcome after traumatic brain injury. *J Neurol Rehabil* 1995;5:255-67.

Kraft JF, Schwab KA, Salazar AM, Brown HR. Occupational and educational achievements of head injured Vietnam veterans at 15-year follow-up. *Arch Phys Med Rehabil* 1993;74:596-601.

Lockhart C, Mandel J, Grossett D, Green D. The paradigm shift: behavioral home care. *Caring magazine* 1994;13:10-11,74-6.

Lyons JL, Morse AR. A therapeutic work program for head-injured adults. *Am J Occup Ther* 1988;42:364-70.

Mackey LE, Bernstein BA, Chapman PE, et al. Early intervention in severe head injury: long-term benefits of a formalized program. *Arch Phys Med Rehabil* 1992;73:635-41.

Malec JF, Basford JS. Postacute brain injury rehabilitation. *Arch Phys Med Rehabil* 1996;77:198-207.

Malec JF, Smigielski JS, DePompolo RW, et al. Outcome evaluation and prediction in a comprehensive-integrated post-acute outpatient brain injury rehabilitation programme. *Brain Inj* 1993;7:15-29.

McLaughlin AM, Peters S. Evaluation of an innovative cost-effective programme for brain injury patients: response to a need for flexible treatment planning. *Brain Inj* 1993;7:71-5.

Mills VM, Nesbeda T, Katz DI, et al. Outcomes for traumatically brain-injured patients following post-acute rehabilitation programmes. *Brain Inj* 1992;6:219-28.

Morgan AS, Chapman P, Tokarski L. *Improved care of the traumatically brain injured.* Proceedings of the Eastern Association for Surgery of Trauma—First Annual Conference; Longboat Key (FL); 1998.

Namerow NS. Cognitive and behavioral aspects of brain-injury rehabilitation. *Neuro Clin* 1987;5:569-83.

Prigatano GP, Fordyce DJ, Zeiner HK, et al. Neuropsychological rehabilitation after closed head injury in young adults. *J Neurol Neurosurg Psychiatry* 1984;47:505-13.

Prigatano GP, Klonoff PS, O'Brien KP, Altman IM, Amin K, Chiapello D, et al. Productivity after neuropsychologically oriented milieu rehabilitation. *J Head Trauma Rehabil* 1994;9:91-102.

Ragnarsson KT, Thomas JP, Zasler ND. Model systems of care for individuals with traumatic brain injury. *J Head Trauma Rehabil* 1993; 8:1-11.

Rattok J, Ben-Yishay Y, Ezrachi O, Lakin P, Piasetsky E, Ross B, et al. Outcome of different treatment mixes in a multidimensional neuropsychological rehabilitation program. *Neuropsychology* 1992;6:395-415.

Rosenthal M. 1995 Sheldon Berrol MD senior lectureship: the ethics and efficacy of traumatic brain injury rehabilitation—myths, measurements, and meaning. *J Head Trauma Rehabil* 1996;11:88-95.

Ruff RM, Marshall LF, Crouch J, Klauber MR, Levin HS, Barth J, et al. Predictors of outcome following severe head trauma: follow-up data from the traumatic coma data bank. *Brain Inj* 1993;7:101-11.

Ruff RM, Neimann H. Cognitive rehabilitation versus day treatment in head-injured adults: is there an impact on emotional and psychosocial adjustment? *Brain Inj* 1990;4:339-47.

Schalen W, Nordstrom G, Nordstrom C. Economic aspects of capacity for work after severe traumatic brain lesions. *Brain Inj* 1994;8:37-47.

Scherzer BP. Rehabilitation following severe head trauma: results of a three-year program. *Arch Phys Med Rehabil* 1986;67:366-74.

Spivack G, Spettle CM, Ellis DW, et al. Effects of intensity of treatment and lengths of stay on rehabilitation outcomes. *Brain Inj* 1992; 6:419-34.

Stambrook M, Moore AD, Peters LC, Deviaene C, Hawryluk GA. Effects of mild, moderate, and severe closed head injury on long-term vocational status. *Brain Inj* 1990;4:183-90.

Stern JM, Groswasser Z, Alis R, Geva N, Hochberg J, Stern B, et al. Day center experience in rehabilitation of craniocerebral injured patients. *Scand J Rehabil Med Suppl* 1985;12:53-8.

Sundance PL, Jolander DK, Bryant ET, et al. *Short-term neurobehavioral program for achievement of stable community placement*. Paper presented at the 10th AAPM&R annual meeting; San Francisco (CA); 1992.

Switzer SF, Hinebaugh FL. Outcome results of post-acute rehabilitation after head injury: five conservative studies of 198 individuals over a five-year period. *J Ins Med* 1991;23:239-44.

Teasdale G, Jennett B. Assessment of coma and impaired consciousness. *Lancet* 1974;2:81.

Tobis JS, Puri KB, Sheridan J. Rehabilitation of the severely brain-injured patient. *Scand J Rehabil Med* 1992;14:83-8.

Wehman PH, Kreutzer JS, West MD, et al. Return to work for persons with traumatic brain injury: a supported employment approach. *Arch Phys Med Rehabil* 1990;71:1047-52.

Whitlock JA Jr, Hamilton BB. Functional outcome after rehabilitation for severe traumatic brain injury. *Arch Phys Med Rehabil* 1995; 76:1103-12.

Whyte WF. *Participatory action research*. Newbury Park (CA): Sage Publications; 1991.

Chapter 40

Rehabilitation Speeds Return to Play

Rehabilitation is the restoration of the ability to function in a normal or near-normal manner following an illness or injury. In sports medicine, rehabilitation usually involves reducing pain and swelling, restoring range of motion, and increasing strength. Rehabilitation for sports-related injuries is usually performed on an outpatient basis. Rehabilitation programs reduce recovery time and speed the return to work and sports activity.

Rehabilitation Methods

Rehabilitation methods differ among patients based on the type and severity of their injuries and the level of physical wellness prior to injury.

Electrostimulation provides pain relief by preventing nerve cells from transmitting pain impulses to the brain. Electrostimulation also is used to make a muscle contract, which helps prevent muscle atrophy and maintain or increase muscle strength.

Heat is applied to soft tissue injuries and causes the blood vessels to dilate, increasing the blood flow to the injury site. Increased blood flow aids the healing process by removing dead tissues and substances that cause swelling and pain. Heat is generally used 48 hours after the injury occurs.

Ice is generally used within the first 48 hours after an injury. Icing an injury causes blood vessels to constrict and limits blood flow to the injury. Ice is primarily used to reduce swelling but it also reduces pain by numbing injured tissue.

Nonsteroidal anti-inflammatory drugs (NSAIDS) such as aspirin, ibuprofen, and naproxen sodium can help reduce inflammation, swelling, and pain.

Physical therapy is used to increase the range of motion and strength after an injury. Physical therapy includes various exercise and physical fitness programs that can be customized to meet each patient's needs.

Rest is the cessation of physical activity. Limiting activity can help stabilize an injury, which allows the body to heal itself more rapidly.

Ultrasound uses the vibrations from sound waves to stimulate blood flow to soft tissue such as muscles and ligaments. Stimulation of blood flow helps reduce swelling and aids healing.

Whirlpools operate similarly to heat and ultrasound. Whirlpools can increase circulation and blood flow to an injury to facilitate healing.

What Does Return to Play Mean?

Return to play refers to the point in recovery from an injury when a person is able to go back to playing their sport or participating in an activity at a level close to that which they participated at before.

No one likes to be sidelined with an injury. One of the goals of sports medicine is to try to get an athlete back into action as soon as possible. Returning too soon, before adequate healing or recovery, can put you at risk for re-injury and possibly an even longer down time. With the right game plan for sports injuries, from early diagnosis and treatment to full functional rehabilitation, you can often safely accelerate your return to play.

A Lesson from the Pros

Why does it seem that professional athletes return to play so much faster? Professional athletes are usually in tremendous physical condition at the time of their injury. This fitness level helps them in many ways because studies have shown that good conditioning can not only prevent injuries, but can also lessen the severity of an injury and speed recovery.

Professional athletes also get prompt treatment when an injury occurs and this lessens the acute phase of the injury. Early treatment means that there is less swelling, stiffness, and loss of muscle tone. In addition, they work extremely hard with a physical therapist and/or certified athletic trainer during their recovery.

In addition, they bring to their recovery what they bring to their sport—a positive attitude. While you may not have access to many things professional athletes have, you can harness the power of a positive attitude for your own benefit during recovery.

Tips from the Pros to Speed Your Recovery

- Maintain year round balanced physical conditioning.
- Make sure that injuries are recognized early and treated promptly.
- Participate in a full functional rehabilitation program.
- Stay fit while injured.
- Keep a positive, upbeat attitude.

Your Recovery Plan

Recovery from an injury involves a series of logical steps from the time of the injury until you are able to be back on the field or court. Each step should be outlined and monitored by your physician and physical therapist.

During the acute phase, the focus should be on minimizing swelling. This involves the RICE formula: Rest, Ice, Compression and Elevation, along with a limitation of activities. Depending on the type and severity of your injury, treatment may also involve surgery, bracing, or even casting.

During this period, it is very important to maintain overall conditioning while the injury heals. Creative techniques can be used to

419

safely work around the injury. For example, a runner with a leg injury can often run in water or use a stationary bicycle to maintain conditioning. Even if one leg is in a cast, the rest of the body can be exercised by performing strength training exercises. Do not wait until your injury is healed to get back into shape.

In the next phase of recovery, you should work on regaining full motion and strength of the injured limb or joint. An exact plan should be outlined by your physician, therapist, or certified athletic trainer. For most injuries, gentle protective range of motion exercises can be started almost immediately. Muscle tone can be maintained with the use of electrical stimulation or simple strengthening exercises.

When strength returns to normal, functional drills can be started. This may include brisk walking, jumping rope, hopping, or light jogging for lower extremity injuries and light throwing or easy ground strokes for upper extremity injuries. Specific balance and agility exercises can bring back coordination that may have been lost in the injury.

Once you have progressed with motion, strength, endurance, and agility, and are tolerating functional drills, you can try higher levels of functional tests and drills that incorporate sport specific movement patterns on the field or court. This is monitored by your physical therapist or certified athletic trainer. You may find that tape, braces, or supports help during this transition time.

Only when you are practicing hard without significant difficulty and the healing has progressed to the point where the likelihood of injury or harm is low, are you ready to return to play. During these final phases of recovery, you should be closely monitored and special attention should be given to adequate warm-up before and icing after activity.

A Word of Caution

Following the rational progression of recovery not only lessens the chance of re-injury but assures that you will be able to perform at your best when you return to play. All too often, athletes think they are ready to return as soon as the limp or the swelling subsides. They may feel good, but they are probably only 70 to 75% recovered. This invites re-injury.

Sports medicine experts are working on ways to help athletes get as close to 100% recovery from injuries as possible, as quickly as safety allows. There is often tremendous pressure to get the athlete back as soon as possible, but the athlete's health and safety must be placed above all other concerns.

A systematic recovery plan is successfully used every day, at all levels of play, from the recreational athlete to the elite professional or Olympic athlete.

Additional Information

The American Orthopaedic Society for Sports Medicine
6300 N. River Road, Suite 200
Rosemont, Illinois 60018
Tel: 847-292-4900
Fax: 847-292-4905
Website: www.sportsmed.org

Part Five

Conditioning and Training

Chapter 41

How to Begin Weight Training

What Is Weight Training?

Weight training means adding resistance to the body's natural movements in order to make those movements more difficult, and encourage the muscles to become stronger.

Why Weight Train?

Weight training increases fitness by:

- Increasing muscle strength and endurance
- Enhancing the cardiovascular system
- Increasing flexibility
- Maintaining the body's fat within acceptable limits

Weight training can be an important component of your fitness program, regardless of your age or gender.

What Equipment Is Needed to Weight Train?

Weight training programs can be done with free weights or with weight machines. Free weights are less expensive than weight machines and are more easily adapted to smaller and larger body types.

"How to Begin a Weight Training Program," © 2000 The American Orthopaedic Society for Sports Medicine, reprinted with permission.

Machines are safer than most free weights because the weight is more controlled.

With multiple purpose machines, like the Universal™ gym, several individuals can exercise simultaneously on the same piece of equipment within a small space. If you use free weights, select a set of barbells or dumbbells and a weight bench for the upper extremities and barbells for the lower extremities.

For all lifting, use a weight belt. Some people feel that weight gloves give them better grip strength, but they are not necessary. Good athletic shoes that provide firm floor traction are a must.

How Do I Start a Weight Training Program?

First, you should establish goals for your program. Decide if you want to exercise to obtain good muscular tone and cardiovascular endurance, to build muscle strength in a particular muscle group, to improve sports performance, or to rehabilitate an injured muscle.

If you want to improve muscle tone and cardiovascular performance, design your program along the lines of a circuit program. In such a program, exercises are done at least four times a week for approximately 20 to 30 minutes a session, and very short rest periods (30 seconds or less) are allowed between exercises. This program would generally consist of 15 to 20 repetitions of an exercise for each major muscle group.

If you want to build strength, you should exercise the muscle group you are strengthening to fatigue. This program incorporates fewer repetitions than circuit training. For example, you would do three sets of repetitions, but only 8 to 10 repetitions per set, with a longer rest period of 60 to 90 seconds between each exercise. This may be done every other day, but not as frequently as a circuit program because the fatigued muscles need longer to recover.

If you want to rehabilitate an injured muscle, your program would be similar to the circuit training program of higher repetitions and lower weights. However, a rehabilitation program, unlike a circuit training program, focuses on working the injured muscle group.

An exercise professional, like a certified athletic trainer, a sports physical therapist, an exercise physiologist, or a strength and conditioning coach, can help you design a program that's suitable for your needs.

Limitations

It is extremely important to check with your doctor before beginning a weight training program, particularly if you are over 30 or have any physical limitations. If you have musculoskeletal problems, check with an orthopaedist to make sure that the program will not aggravate those problems.

Precautions

To avoid injury when weight training, you should:

- Wear appropriate clothing.
- Keep the weight training area clean and free of debris.
- Stay well hydrated while lifting.
- Get adequate rest.
- Eat sensibly.
- Stretch after warming up but before lifting.
- Always use a spotter when doing when doing bench presses and squats.
- Lift with a buddy, whenever possible.

Chapter 42

Sports Nutrition

What Is the Best Diet for an Athlete?

It's important that an athlete's diet provides the right amount of energy, the 50-plus nutrients the body needs and adequate water. No single food or supplement can do this. A variety of foods are needed every day. But, just as there is more than one way to achieve a goal, there is more than one way to follow a nutritious diet.

Do the Nutritional Needs of Athletes Differ from Non-Athletes?

Competitive athletes, sedentary individuals, and people who exercise for health and fitness all need the same nutrients. However, because of the intensity of their sport or training program, some athletes have higher calorie and fluid requirements. Eating a variety of foods to meet increased calorie needs helps to ensure that the athletes diet contains appropriate amounts of carbohydrate, protein, vitamins, and minerals.

Are There Certain Dietary Guidelines Athletes Should Follow?

Health and nutrition professionals recommend that 55-60% of the calories in our diet come from carbohydrate, no more than 30% from

"Questions Most Frequently Asked about Sports Nutrition," The President's Council on Physical Fitness and Sports. Produced as a public service by The Sugar Association Inc.

fat, and the remaining 10-15% from protein. While the exact percentages may vary slightly for some athletes based on their sport or training program, these guidelines will promote health and serve as the basis for a diet that will maximize performance.

How Many Calories Do I Need a Day?

This depends on your age, body size, sport, and training program. For example, a 250-pound weight lifter needs more calories than a 98-pound gymnast. Exercise or training may increase calorie needs by as much as 1,000 to 1,500 calories a day.

The best way to determine if you're getting too few or too many calories is to monitor your weight. Keeping within your ideal competitive weight range means that you are getting the right amount of calories.

Which Is Better for Replacing Fluids—Water or Sports Drinks?

Depending on how muscular you are, 55-70% of your body weight is water. Being hydrated means maintaining your body's fluid level. When you sweat, you lose water which must be replaced if you want to perform your best. You need to drink fluids before, during, and after all workouts and events.

Whether you drink water or a sports drink is a matter of choice. However, if your workout or event lasts for more than 90 minutes, you may benefit from the carbohydrates provided by sports drinks. A sports drink that contains 15-18 grams of carbohydrate in every 8 ounces of fluid should be used. Drinks with a higher carbohydrate content will delay the absorption of water and may cause dehydration, cramps, nausea, or diarrhea. There are a variety of sports drinks on the market. Be sure to experiment with sports drinks during practice instead of trying them for the first time the day of an event.

What Are Electrolytes?

Electrolytes are nutrients that affect fluid balance in the body and are necessary for our nerves and muscles to function. Sodium and potassium are the two electrolytes most often added to sports drinks. Generally, electrolyte replacement is not needed during short bursts of exercise since sweat is approximately 99% water and less than 1% electrolytes. Water, in combination with a well-balanced diet, will restore normal fluid and electrolyte levels in the body. However, replacing electrolytes may be beneficial during continuous activity of longer than 2 hours, especially in a hot environment.

What Do Muscles Use for Energy During Exercise?

Most activities use a combination of fat and carbohydrate as energy sources. How hard and how long you work out, your level of fitness, and your diet will affect the type of fuel your body uses. For short-term high intensity activities like sprinting, athletes rely mostly on carbohydrate for energy. During low-intensity exercises like walking, the body uses more fat for energy.

What Are Carbohydrates?

Carbohydrates are sugar and starches found in foods like breads, cereals, fruits, vegetables, pasta, milk, honey, syrups, and table sugar. Carbohydrates are the preferred source of energy for your body. Regardless of origin, your body breaks down carbohydrates into glucose that your blood carries to cells to be used for energy. Carbohydrates provide 4 calories per gram, while fat provides 9 calories per gram. Your body cannot differentiate between glucose that comes from starches or sugars. Glucose from either source provides energy for working muscles.

Is It True That Athletes Should Eat a Lot of Carbohydrates?

When you are training or competing, your muscles need energy to perform. One source of energy for working muscles is glycogen which is made from carbohydrates and stored in your muscles. Every time you work out, you use some of your glycogen. If you don't consume enough carbohydrates, your glycogen stores become depleted, which can result in fatigue. Both sugars and starches are effective in replenishing glycogen stores.

When and What Should I Eat Before I Compete?

Performance depends largely on the foods consumed during the days and weeks leading up to an event. If you regularly eat a varied, carbohydrate-rich diet you are in good standing and probably have ample glycogen stores to fuel activity. The purpose of the pre-competition meal is to prevent hunger and to provide the water and additional energy the athlete will need during competition. Most athletes eat 2 to 4 hours before their event. However, some athletes perform their best if they eat a small amount 30 minutes before competing, while others eat nothing for 6 hours beforehand.

For many athletes, carbohydrate-rich foods serve as the basis of the meal. However, there is no magic pre-event diet. Simply choose foods and beverages that you enjoy and that don't bother your stomach. Experiment during the weeks before an event to see which foods work best for you.

Will Eating Sugary Foods Before an Event Hurt My Performance?

In the past, athletes were warned that eating sugary foods before exercise could hurt performance by causing a drop in blood glucose levels. Recent studies, however, have shown that consuming sugar up to 30 minutes before an event does not diminish performance. In fact, evidence suggests that a sugar-containing pre-competition beverage or snack may improve performance during endurance workouts and events.

What Is Carbohydrate Loading?

Carbohydrate loading is a technique used to increase the amount of glycogen in muscles. For five to seven days before an event, the athlete eats 10-12 grams of carbohydrate per kilogram body weight and gradually reduces the intensity of the workouts. (To find out how much you weigh in kilograms, simply divide your weight in pounds by 2.2.) The day before the event, the athlete rests and eats the same high-carbohydrate diet. Although carbohydrate loading may be beneficial for athletes participating in endurance sports which require 90 minutes or more of non-stop effort, most athletes needn't worry about carbohydrate loading. Simply eating a diet that derives more than half of its calories from carbohydrates will do.

As an Athlete, Don't I Need to Take Extra Vitamins and Minerals?

Athletes need to eat about 1,800 calories a day to get the vitamins and minerals they need for good health and optimal performance. Since most athletes eat more than this amount, vitamin and mineral supplements are needed only in special situations. Athletes who follow vegetarian diets or who avoid an entire group of foods (for example,

Table 42.1. Nutrient Content of Selected Foods Rich in Carbohydrates (CHO), Protein, Iron, and/or Calcium.

Food	Serving Size	Energy (kcal)	Protein (g)	CHO (g)	Fat (g)	Calcium (mg)	Iron (mg)
Lean Beef	3 ounces	189	27	0	8	4	2.9
Hamburger	3 ounces	246	20	0	18	9	2.1
Lean Pork, Broiled	3 ounces	196	27	0	9	4	.8
Chicken, Breast	3 ounces	167	25	0	7	12	.9
Egg, Hard-Boiled	1 whole	77	6	1	5	25	.6
Peanut Butter	2 Tbsp	190	8	7	16	11	.5
Roasted Peanuts	1 ounce	164	7	5	14	24	.5
Navy Beans, Cooked	1/2 cup	129	8	24	0	64	2.2
Salmon, Broiled/Baked	3 ounces	183	23	0	9	6	.5
Salmon, Canned with Bones	3 ounces	118	17	0	5	182	.7
Milk, Whole	1 cup	150	8	11	8	291	.1
Milk, 2% Low-Fat	1 cup	121	8	12	5	297	.1
Milk, 1% Low-Fat	1 cup	102	8	12	3	300	.1
Milk, Skim	1 cup	86	8	12	0	302	.1
Yogurt, Low-Fat	1 cup	193	11	31	3	388	.2
Cheddar Cheese	1.5 ounces	171	11	0	14	305	.3
Cottage Cheese, 2%	1/2 cup	102	16	4	2	78	.2
Ice Cream, Vanilla	1/2 cup	134	2	16	7	88	.1
Bread, White/Wheat	1 slice	72	3	13	1	35	1.0
Bran Flakes, Fortified	1 ounce	91	4	25	0	14	8.1
Muffin, Bran	1 whole	125	3	19	6	60	1.4
Cookie, Choc. Chip	3 whole	139	2	19	8	8	.8
Baked Potato	1 whole	220	5	51	0	20	2.8
Spaghetti	1/2 cup	98	3	20	0	5	1.0
Green Peas	1/2 cup	63	4	11	0	19	1.2
Broccoli, Cooked	1/2 cup	22	2	4	0	36	.7
Banana	1 whole	105	1	28	0	7	.1
Orange	1 whole	60	1	15	0	52	.1
Butter	1 Tbsp	102	0	0	12	3	0
Margarine	1 Tbsp	102	0	0	11	4	0
Table Sugar	1 tsp	16	0	4	0	0	0
Jelly	1 tsp	16	0	4	0	1	0

The nutrient analysis for each food was obtained using The Food Processor II computer program.

never drink milk) may need a supplement to make up for the vitamins and minerals not being supplied by food. A multivitamin-mineral pill that supplies 100% of the Recommended Dietary Allowance (RDA) will provide the nutrients needed. An athlete who frequently cuts back on calories, especially below the 1,800 calorie level, is not only at risk for inadequate vitamin and mineral intake, but also may not be getting enough carbohydrates. Since vitamins and minerals do not provide energy, they cannot replace the energy provided by carbohydrates.

Will Extra Protein Help Build Muscle Mass?

Many athletes, especially those on strength-training programs or who participate in power sports, are told that eating a ton of protein or taking protein supplements will help them gain muscle weight. However, the true secret to building muscle is training hard and consuming enough calories. While some extra protein is needed to build muscle, most American diets provide more than enough protein. Between 1.0 and 1.5 grams of protein per kilogram body weight per day is sufficient if your calorie intake is adequate and you're eating a variety of foods. For a 150-pound athlete, that represents 68-102 grams of protein a day.

Why Is Iron so Important?

Hemoglobin, which contains iron, is the part of red blood cells that carries oxygen from the lungs to all parts of the body, including muscles. Since your muscles need oxygen to produce energy, if you have low iron levels in your blood, you may tire quickly. Symptoms of iron deficiency include fatigue, irritability, dizziness, headaches, and lack of appetite. Many times, however, there are no symptoms at all. A blood test is the best way to find out if your iron level is low. It is recommended that athletes have their hemoglobin level checked once a year.

The RDA for iron is 15 milligrams a day for women and 10 milligrams a day for men. Red meat is the richest source of iron, but fish and poultry also are good sources. Fortified breakfast cereals, beans, and green leafy vegetables also contain iron. Our bodies absorb the iron found in animal products best.

Should I Take an Iron Supplement?

Taking iron supplements will not improve performance unless an athlete is truly iron deficient. Too much iron can cause constipation, diarrhea, nausea, and may interfere with the absorption of other nutrients such as cooper and zinc. Therefore, iron supplements should not be taken without proper medical supervision.

Why Is Calcium so Important?

Calcium is needed for strong bones and proper muscle function. Dairy foods are the best source of calcium. However, studies show that many female athletes who are trying to lose weight cut back on dairy products. Female athletes who don't get enough calcium may be at risk for stress fractures and, when they're older, osteoporosis. Young women between the ages of 9 and 18 need about 1,300 milligrams of calcium a day. Adults aged 19 through 50 need 1,000 milligrams daily, while those 51 and older should aim for 1,200 milligrams. Low-fat dairy products are a rich source of calcium and also are low in fat and calories.

Additional Information

The Sugar Association Inc.
1101 15ᵗʰ Street, N.W., Suite 600
Washington, DC 20005
Tel: 202-785-1122
Fax: 202-785-5019
Website: www.sugar.org
E-mail: sugar@sugar.org

Chapter 43

Youth Fitness Reduces Injuries

Fit Plan for Youth

In our sedentary society, it is difficult to achieve physical fitness through our daily lifestyle. Even children spend much of their time sitting in schoolrooms, living rooms, and automobiles. In fact, you may want to note how many hours your child spends sitting during a typical day. Be sure to include time on the school bus, in the classroom, in music lessons, watching television, utilizing computers, playing table games, and reading.

Assessing Fitness in Youth

Before beginning a fitness program, it is advisable to assess your child's present abilities in the areas of cardiovascular endurance, joint flexibility, and muscular strength/endurance. This allows for periodic reassessment to identify improvement and enhance motivation. Any child who has a pre-existing medical condition should see a physician before starting an exercise program.

The following fitness evaluation protocols are taken from the American Alliance of Health, "Physical Education, Recreation, and Dance's Physical Best" booklet. These tests are easy to administer and score.

"The Fit Plan for Youth," by Wayne L. Westcott, Ph.D, © Massachusetts Governor's Committee on Physical Fitness and Sports. This material is reprinted with permission of the Massachusetts Governor's Committee on Physical Fitness and Sports, Youth Fitness Subcommittee.

Table 43.1 and Table 43.2 present the health/fitness standards for boys and girls between 5 and 18 years of age. However, it should be emphasized that individual improvement is more important than attaining a specific test score. The key to better fitness and a physically active lifestyle is personal satisfaction with both the process and the product of regular exercise.

Contrast this to the number of hours your child spends performing vigorous physical activity. Include physical education classes and sports participation, but remember that few schools offer daily physical education and few athletic events provide comprehensive physical conditioning.

The general lack of vigorous physical activity among youth, necessitates a "Fit Plan" to foster the development of cardiovascular endurance, joint flexibility, and muscular strength/endurance. While the specific activities may vary according to personal preferences, the same basic conditioning principles should be applied to all exercise programs.

Physical Best Fitness Evaluation Techniques

Cardiovascular Endurance

Test Item: One Mile Walk/Run

Test Objective: To walk or run one mile in the fastest time possible.

Instructions: Students are instructed to run one mile in the fastest possible time. Emphasis should be placed on the development of the fastest pace that can be sustained for the mile distance. Participants should always warm-up, and should be encouraged to practice walking or running the required distance prior to the official day of the test.

As the students cross the finish line, elapsed time should be called to the participants (or their partners). Walking is permitted, but since the objective is to cover the distance in the shortest possible time, students should be encouraged to run as much as possible for the one mile distance.

Test Area: The one mile run can be conducted on a track or on any other flat, measured area.

Equipment: Stopwatch, scorecards and pencils.

Record: Distance___ Time___

Joint Flexibility

Test Item: Sit and Reach

Test Objective: To evaluate the flexibility of the lower back and hamstring muscles.

Instructions: Students should stretch the low back and hamstrings prior to testing. The warm-up should include slow, sustained, steady (no bobbing) stretching of the low back and hamstring muscles.

Have students remove shoes and be seated at the test apparatus with their knees straight in front of them; the heels should be approximately shoulder-width apart and the feet flat against the end board. Have the students lean forward extending the fingertips, palms down and hands together, as far forward along the ruler as possible. Each student is allowed four tries.

Equipment: Sit and Reach Box, a specially constructed box with a measuring scale where 23 cm is at the level of the feet. (You may substitute a milk crate and a yard stick to measure the cm.)

Scoring: The score is the most distant point reached on the fourth trial by both hands and held for one second. Measure to the nearest centimeter. The trial should be considered invalid and readministered if the knees fail to remain straight, or if the hands reach unevenly.

Record Score:_____

Muscular Strength/Endurance

Test Item: Modified Sit-Ups

Test Objective: To evaluate abdominal muscular strength/endurance.

Instructions: Students are instructed to lie on their back with knees bent, feet on floor, and heels between 12 and 18 inches from the buttocks. The arms are crossed on the chest with the hands on the opposite shoulders. The feet are held on the floor by a partner. On the command "ready-go," the student curls to a sitting position until the elbows touch the thighs. The arms maintain contact with the chest throughout the motion. The student then returns to the starting position with the midback making contact with the floor. Students are encouraged to repeat a correctly performed sit-up as many times as possible in the one-minute time limit. Rest between sit-ups is allowed in either the up or down position.

Test Area: Mats or other comfortable surfaces are recommended although any area with sufficiency may be used.

Equipment: Stopwatch and mats.

Scoring: Record the number of correctly executed sit-ups that are complete in 60 seconds. Number of sit-ups: _____

Guidelines for Youth Fitness Development

Now that you have determined your child's fitness levels, you can work together to provide a safe and effective means for improvement. The following guidelines for developing higher levels of muscular strength, cardiovascular endurance, and joint flexibility are well-suited to boys and girls between 8 and 15 years of age.

Guidelines for Youth Strength Development *

Muscular strength is very important for boys and girls. To begin, our muscles function as the engines of our bodies, producing movement

Table 43.1. Health Fitness Standards for Boys

Age	One Mile Walk/Run (minutes)	Sit & Reach Modified (cm)	Sit-Ups
5	13:00	25	20
6	12:00	25	20
7	11:00	25	24
8	10:00	25	26
9	10:00	25	30
10	9:30	25	34
11	9:00	25	36
12	9:00	25	38
13	8:00	25	40
14	7:45	25	40
15	7:30	25	42
16	7:30	25	44
17	7:30	25	44
18	7:30	25	44

and power for athletic activities. Our muscles also serve as the shock absorbers of our bodies, thereby playing a major role in injury prevention. Also, strong muscles are closely related to strong tendons, ligaments, and bones.

It should never be assumed that children will increase muscle strength through their sports participation. Rather, coaches should ensure that each player develops sufficient muscle strength prior to the competitive season. This may be safely accomplished through the use calisthenics, rubber tubing, free weights, or resistance machines, as long at the training stimulus is increased gradually and progressively.

Calisthenics, such as push-ups, pull-ups, sit-ups, and bench dips are the easiest form of muscle conditioning. Although exercises performed with bodyweight permit additional repetitions, they do not allow for systematic increases in resistance which is the key to strength development.

Free weights (barbells, dumbbells) and resistance machines (Universal Gym, Heartline, Nautilus) provide adjustable weight loads and a wide variety of exercise movements. However this equipment

Table 43.2. Health Fitness Standards for Girls

Age	One Mile Walk/Run (minutes)	Sit & Reach Modified (cm)	Sit-Ups
5	14:00	25	20
6	13:00	25	20
7	12:00	25	24
8	11:30	25	26
9	11:00	25	28
10	11:00	25	30
11	11:00	25	33
12	11:00	25	33
13	8:00	25	33
14	7:45	25	35
15	7:30	25	35
16	7:30	25	35
17	7:30	25	35
18	7:30	25	35

should be used only under the direction of trained (certified) strength instructors in accordance with the following guidelines established by the American Orthopaedic Society for Sports Medicine (1985).

1. A pre-participation physical exam is mandatory.

2. The child must have the emotional maturity to accept coaching and instruction.

3. There must be adequate supervision by coaches who are knowledgeable about strength training and the special problems of prepubescents.

4. Strength training should be a part of an overall program designed to increase physical fitness.

5. Strength training should be preceded by warm-up exercises and followed by cool-down exercise.

6. Emphasis should be on controlled lifting and lowering movements through a full range of joint motion, but avoiding a lockout position in pressing movements.

7. Competition is prohibited.

8. No maximum lift should ever be attempted.

The following recommendations for a safe, effective, and efficient youth strength training program are taken from the college textbook, *Strength Fitness: Physiological Principles and Training Techniques* (1991).

1. Warm-Up and Cool-Down: Begin and end each session with some moderate activity such as stationary cycling, bodyweight exercises, and stretching to serve as a transition to and from the strength exercise.

2. Exercise Selection: Perform exercises that involve the front thighs, rear thighs, lower back, abdominals, chest, upper back, shoulders, front arms, rear arms, front neck, rear neck, lower legs, and forearms.

3. Exercise Sequence: Generally perform the exercises for the lower body prior to the exercises for the upper body, moving from larger to smaller muscles groups.

4. Exercise Speed: Execute all strength training movements in a slow and controlled manner, with strict adherence to proper exercise technique.

5. Exercise Sets: Complete 1 properly performed set of each strength training exercise.

6. Exercise Repetitions: Each exercise set should consist of no less than 8 and no more than 12 repetitions.

7. Exercise Resistance: The resistance should be sufficient to produce muscle fatigue within 8-12 repetitions.

8. Exercise Range: Each exercise movement should encompass a comfortable range of joint movement.

9. Exercise Progression: The training resistance should be increased by no more than 5 percent (1-5 pounds) whenever 12 strict repetitions can be completed.

10. Exercise Frequency: Strength training should be performed 2 or 3 equally spaced days per week for approximately 15-20 minutes per session.

Guidelines for Youth Endurance Development*

Cardiovascular endurance is a critical factor in health and fitness for persons of all ages, and should be included in youth sports programs. Our cardiorespiratory system includes the cardiovascular system (heart and blood vessels), and respiratory system (lungs), and functions as the fuel pump of our bodies. That is, the cardiovascular system is responsible for delivering oxygen and energy to all areas of the body. Our ability to perform prolonged physical activity is directly related to the fitness level of our cardiovascular system.

Cardiovascular conditioning is obviously important for participation in aerobic activities such as soccer, basketball, and swimming, and should be an integral part of each practice session. Although not essential for performing well in football, baseball, and other stop-and-go sports, some endurance training should be included in these practice sessions as well.

In addition to training consistency, there are two key requisites for endurance development. First, the exercise must be vigorous enough to raise the heart rate above 50 percent of maximum. For most young people this corresponds to about 120-160 heartbeats per minute. Second, the exercise must be performed long enough to stimulate beneficial cardio-vascular adaptations. Fifteen to twenty minutes of endurance exercise is usually considered the minimum training duration for boys and girls.

Consider the following guidelines for developing cardiovascular endurance in a safe and sensible manner:

1. Warm-Up: Precede each endurance exercise session with a few minutes of warm-up activity such as brisk walking, bodyweight exercises, and stretching.

2. Activity Selection: Try to incorporate a variety of large muscle activities such as jogging, interval running, cycling, short-rest relays, rope jumping, and games that involve continuous movement.

3. Initial Conditioning Phase: Begin endurance workouts with a relatively slow pace for a short period of time (5 minutes).

4. Progression Principle: Gradually increase the training duration as the young participants' endurance fitness improves.

5. Maintenance Phase: Perform 15-20 minutes of endurance exercise at least twice a week, working at about three-quarters effort (70-80 percent of maximum heart rate).

6. Cool-Down: Follow each endurance exercise session with a few minutes of cool-down activities such as walking and stretching.

7. Positive Attitude: Be sure to present a positive and supportive attitude towards endurance training as it is important for youth to establish cardiovascular conditioning habits.

Guidelines for Youth Flexibility Development*

Flexibility refers to the range of movement in our joints. Flexibility frequently varies from joint to joint. Lack of flexibility is most often attributed to tight muscles, and can be a contributing factor to many sports injuries.

Although children are typically more flexible than adolescents and adults, there is usually some room for improvement. Stretching may be perceived as monotonous and unnecessary by some youth sports participants. However, it is particularly important in growing adolescents, because they experience decreases in flexibility during rapid growth periods.

Flexibility is specific to each joint movement, making it advisable to address the major muscle groups in a sequence of stretching exercises. A basic flexibility session should include stretches for the muscles of the neck, shoulder, upper torso, midsection and low back, front thigh, rear thigh, inner thigh, and lower leg.

Flexibility exercises are designed to increase the range of joint movements by gently and progressively stretching the surrounding muscles. In order to reduce muscle tension and relax the muscle fibers it is necessary to perform each stretch slowly, without bouncing or ballistic movements that actually cause the muscles to contract in a protective manner. Whenever possible, the fully stretched position should be held for about 60 seconds, thereby allowing the muscle fibers time to adapt to their stretched position.

For example, an excellent exercise to stretch the muscles of the calves, rear thighs, and low back is known as the Figure Four Stretch. This exercise is performed by sitting with the right leg extended and the left leg bent so that the left foot touches the right inner thigh. Reach the right hand towards the right foot, grasping either the ankle or the toes. Hold this stretched position for 30 seconds, relax momentarily and repeat. The second time, it should be possible to reach a little further as the calf, rear thigh, and low back muscles become more relaxed. Switch leg positions and perform the same stretching sequence with the left leg and hand.

Although some stretches, such as rotational exercises, may involve continuous movement they should be performed very slowly for maximum safety and effectiveness. Fast stretching movements are counter productive and dangerous, and should be avoided at all costs. Research indicates that stretching exercises may be performed before practice or after practice with equal benefit. It may be a good ideal to include a few stretching exercises during both the before practice warm-up and the after practice cool-down.

Recommendation

Physical fitness contributes to physical and mental well-being and is important for everyone. The benefits of good physical fitness allow children and adolescents to enjoy an active lifestyle. We encourage you to emphasize regular exercise in your family and to encourage and assist your children in achieving a high level of physical conditioning. You will all enjoy the process and be pleased with the results.

* The sections on Youth Strength Development, Youth Endurance Development, and Youth Flexibility Development have been reprinted by permission of the National Youth Sports Foundation for the Prevention of Athletic Injuries.

Additional Information

Massachusetts Governor's Committee on Physical Fitness and Sports
The Children's Hospital
Department of Orthopaedics
300 Longwood Avenue
Boston, MA 02215
Tel: 617-735-6934

The National Youth Sports Safety Foundation, Inc.
One Beacon Street, Suite 3333
Boston, MA 02108
Tel: 617-277-1171
Fax: 617-722-9999
Website: www.nyssf.org
E-mail: NYSSF@aol.com

Chapter 44

Steroids and Sports: A Losing Combination

Since the 1950s, some athletes have been taking anabolic steroids to build muscle and boost their athletic performance. Increasingly, other segments of the population also have been taking these compounds. The *Monitoring the Future* study, which is an annual survey of drug abuse among adolescents across the country, showed a significant increase from 1998 to 1999 in steroid abuse among middle school students. During the same year, the percentage of 12th-graders who believed that taking these drugs causes great risk to health, declined from 68 percent to 62 percent.

Studies show that, over time, anabolic steroids can indeed take a heavy toll on a person's health. The abuse of oral or injectable steroids is associated with higher risks for heart attacks and strokes, and the abuse of most oral steroids is associated with increased risk for liver problems. Steroid abusers who share needles or do not use sterile techniques when they inject steroids are at risk for contracting dangerous infections, such as HIV/AIDS, hepatitis B and C, and bacterial endocarditis.

Anabolic steroid abuse can also cause undesirable body changes. These include breast development and genital shrinking in men, masculinization of the body in women, and acne and hair loss in both sexes.

"Steroid Abuse and Addiction," NIDA Research Report, National Institute on Drug Abuse, NIH Publication No. 00-3721, printed 1991, reprinted 1994, 1996; revised April, 2000.

What Are Anabolic Steroids?

Anabolic steroids is the familiar name for synthetic substances related to the male sex hormones (androgens). They promote the growth of skeletal muscle (anabolic effects) and the development of male sexual characteristics (androgenic effects), and also have some other effects. The term *anabolic steroids* will be used throughout this report because of its familiarity, although the proper term for these compounds is *anabolic-androgenic steroids*.

Anabolic steroids were developed in the late 1930s primarily to treat hypogonadism, a condition in which the testes do not produce sufficient testosterone for normal growth, development, and sexual functioning. The primary medical uses of these compounds are to treat delayed puberty, some types of impotence, and wasting of the body caused by HIV infection or other diseases.

During the 1930s, scientists discovered that anabolic steroids could facilitate the growth of skeletal muscle in laboratory animals, which led to use of the compounds first by bodybuilders and weightlifters and then by athletes in other sports. Steroid abuse has become so widespread in athletics that it affects the outcome of sports contests.

More than 100 different anabolic steroids have been developed, but they require a prescription to be used legally in the United States. Most steroids that are used illegally are smuggled in from other countries, illegally diverted from U.S. pharmacies, or synthesized in clandestine laboratories

Commonly Abused Steroids

Oral Steroids

- Anadrol (oxymetholone)
- Oxandrin (oxandrolone)
- Dianabol (methandrostenolone)
- Winstrol (stanozolol)

Injectable Steroids

- Deca-Durabolin (nandrolone decanoate)
- Durabolin (nandrolone phenpropionate)
- Depo-Testosterone (testosterone cypionate)
- Equipoise (boldenone undecylenate)

What Are Steroidal Supplements?

In the United States, supplements such as dehydroepiandrosterone (DHEA) and androstenedione (street name Andro) can be purchased legally without a prescription through many commercial sources including health food stores. They are often referred to as dietary supplements, although they are not food products. They are often taken because the user believes they have anabolic effects.

Steroidal supplements can be converted into testosterone (an important male sex hormone) or a similar compound in the body. Whether such conversion produces sufficient quantities of testosterone to promote muscle growth or whether the supplements themselves promote muscle growth is unknown. Little is known about the side effects of steroidal supplements, but if large quantities of these compounds substantially increase testosterone levels in the body, they also are likely to produce the same side effects as anabolic steroids.

What Is the Scope of Steroid Abuse in the United States?

From 1998 to 1999, the *Monitoring the Future Survey* reported an increase in lifetime use of steroids among 10th graders and a decrease in perceived risk of harm among seniors.

Recent evidence suggests that steroid abuse among adolescents is on the rise. The 1999 *Monitoring the Future* study, a NIDA-funded survey of drug abuse among adolescents in middle and high schools across the United States, estimated that 2.7 percent of 8th and 10th graders and 2.9 percent of 12th graders had taken anabolic steroids at least once in their lives. For 10th graders, that is a significant increase from 1998, when 2.0 percent of 10th graders said they had taken anabolic steroids at least once. For all three grades, the 1999 levels represent a significant increase from 1991, the first year that data on steroid abuse were collected from the younger students. In that year, 1.9 percent of 8th graders, 1.8 percent of 10th graders, and 2.1 percent of 12th graders reported that they had taken anabolic steroids at least once.

Few data exist on the extent of steroid abuse by adults. It has been estimated that hundreds of thousands of people aged 18 and older abuse anabolic steroids at least once a year.

Among both adolescents and adults, steroid abuse is higher among males than females. However, steroid abuse is growing most rapidly among young women.

Why Do People Abuse Anabolic Steroids?

One of the main reasons people give for abusing steroids is to improve their performance in sports. Among competitive bodybuilders, steroid abuse has been estimated to be very high. Among other athletes, the incidence of abuse probably varies depending on the specific sport.

Another reason people give for taking steroids is to increase their muscle size and/or reduce their body fat. This group includes some people who have a behavioral syndrome (muscle dysmorphia) in which a person has a distorted image of his or her body. Men with this condition think that they look small and weak, even if they are large and muscular. Similarly, women with the syndrome think that they look fat and flabby, even though they are actually lean and muscular.

Some people who abuse steroids to boost muscle size have experienced physical or sexual abuse. They are trying to increase their muscle size to protect themselves. In one series of interviews with male weightlifters, 25 percent who abused steroids reported memories of childhood physical or sexual abuse, compared with none who did not abuse steroids. In a study of women weightlifters, twice as many of those who had been raped reported using anabolic steroids and/or another purported muscle building drug, compared to those who had not been raped. Moreover, almost all of those who had been raped reported that they markedly increased their bodybuilding activities after the attack. They believed that being bigger and stronger would discourage further attacks because men would find them either intimidating or unattractive.

Finally, some adolescents abuse steroids as part of a pattern of high-risk behaviors. These adolescents also take risks such as drinking and driving, carrying a gun, not wearing a helmet on a motorcycle, and abusing other illicit drugs.

While conditions such as muscle dysmorphia, a history of physical or sexual abuse, or a history of engaging in high-risk behaviors may increase the risk of initiating or continuing steroid abuse, researchers agree that most steroid abusers are psychologically normal when they start abusing the drugs.

How Are Anabolic Steroids Used?

Some anabolic steroids are taken orally, others are injected intramuscularly, and still others are provided in gels or creams that are rubbed on the skin. Doses taken by abusers can be 10 to 100 times higher than the doses used for medical conditions.

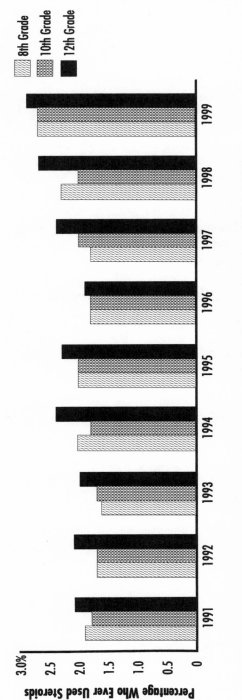

Figure 44.1. Lifetime Use of Steroids: 8th Graders, 10th Graders, and Seniors (1991-1999)

Steroid abusers typically *stack* the drugs, meaning that they take two or more different anabolic steroids, mixing oral and/or injectable types and sometimes even including compounds that are designed for veterinary use. Abusers think that the different steroids interact to produce an effect on muscle size that is greater than the effects of each drug individually, a theory that has not been tested scientifically.

Often, steroid abusers also *pyramid* their doses in cycles of 6 to 12 weeks. At the beginning of a cycle, the person starts with low doses of the drugs being stacked and then slowly increases the doses. In the second half of the cycle, the doses are slowly decreased to zero. This is sometimes followed by a second cycle in which the person continues to train but without drugs. Abusers believe that pyramiding allows the body time to adjust to the high doses and the drug-free cycle allows the body's hormonal system time to recuperate. As with stacking, the perceived benefits of pyramiding and cycling have not been substantiated scientifically.

What Are the Health Consequences of Steroid Abuse?

Possible Health Consequences of Anabolic Steroid Abuse

Hormonal system

- men
  - infertility
  - breast development
  - shrinking of the testicles
- women
  - enlargement of the clitoris
  - excessive growth of body hair
- both sexes
  - male-pattern baldness

Musculoskeletal system

- short stature
- tendon rupture

Cardiovascular system

- heart attacks
- enlargement of the heart's left ventricle

Liver

- cancer
- peliosis hepatis

Skin

- acne and cysts
- oily scalp

Infection

- HIV/AIDS
- hepatitis

Psychiatric effects

- homicidal rage
- mania
- delusions

Anabolic steroid abuse has been associated with a wide range of adverse side effects ranging from some that are physically unattractive, such as acne and breast development in men, to others that are life threatening, such as heart attacks and liver cancer. Most are reversible if the abuser stops taking the drugs, but some are permanent.

Most data on the long-term effects of anabolic steroids on humans come from case reports rather than formal epidemiological studies. From the case reports, the incidence of life-threatening effects appears to be low, but serious adverse effects may be under-recognized or under-reported. Data from animal studies seem to support this possibility. One study found that exposing male mice for one-fifth of their life span to steroid doses comparable to those taken by human athletes caused a high percentage of premature deaths.

Hormonal System

Steroid abuse disrupts the normal production of hormones in the body, causing both reversible and irreversible changes. Changes that can be reversed include reduced sperm production and shrinking of the testicles (testicular atrophy). Irreversible changes include male-pattern baldness and breast development (gynecomastia). In one study of male bodybuilders, more than half had testicular atrophy, and more than half had gynecomastia. Gynecomastia is thought to occur due to the disruption of normal hormone balance.

In the female body, anabolic steroids cause masculinization. Breast size and body fat decrease, the skin becomes coarse, the clitoris enlarges, and the voice deepens. Women may experience excessive growth of body hair but lose scalp hair. With continued administration of steroids, some of these effects are irreversible.

Musculoskeletal System

Rising levels of testosterone and other sex hormones normally trigger the growth spurt that occurs during puberty and adolescence. Subsequently, when these hormones reach certain levels, they signal the bones to stop growing, locking a person into his or her maximum height.

When a child or adolescent takes anabolic steroids, the resulting artificially high sex hormone levels can signal the bones to stop growing sooner than they normally would have done.

Cardiovascular System

Steroid abuse has been associated with cardiovascular diseases (CVD), including heart attacks and strokes, even in athletes younger than 30. Steroids contribute to the development of CVD, partly by changing the levels of lipoproteins that carry cholesterol in the blood. Steroids, particularly the oral types, increase the level of low-density lipoprotein (LDL) and decrease the level of high-density lipoprotein (HDL). High LDL and low HDL levels increase the risk of atherosclerosis, a condition in which fatty substances are deposited inside arteries and disrupt blood flow. If blood is prevented from reaching the heart, the result can be a heart attack. If blood is prevented from reaching the brain, the result can be a stroke.

Steroids also increase the risk that blood clots will form in blood vessels, potentially disrupting blood flow and damaging the heart muscle so that it does not pump blood effectively.

Liver

Steroid abuse has been associated with liver tumors and a rare condition called peliosis hepatis, in which blood-filled cysts form in the liver. Both the tumors and the cysts sometimes rupture, causing internal bleeding.

Skin

Steroid abuse can cause acne, cysts, and oily hair and skin.

Infection

Many abusers who inject anabolic steroids do not use sterile injection techniques or share contaminated needles with other abusers. In addition, some steroid preparations are manufactured illegally under non-sterile conditions. These factors put abusers at risk for acquiring life-threatening viral infections, such as HIV and hepatitis B and C. Abusers also can develop infective endocarditis, a bacterial illness that causes a potentially fatal inflammation of the inner lining of the heart. Bacterial infections also can cause pain and abscess formation at injection sites.

What Effects Do Anabolic Steroids Have on Behavior?

Case reports and small studies indicate that anabolic steroids, particularly in high doses, increase irritability and aggression. Some steroid abusers report that they have committed aggressive acts, such as physical fighting, committing armed robbery, or using force to obtain something. Some abusers also report that they have committed property crimes, such as stealing from a store, damaging or destroying others' property, or breaking into a house or a building. Abusers who have committed aggressive acts or property crimes generally report that they engage in these behaviors more often when they take steroids than when they are drug-free.

Some researchers have suggested that steroid abusers may commit aggressive acts and property crimes not because of steroids' direct effects on the brain but because the abusers have been affected by extensive media attention to the link between steroids and aggression. According to this theory, the abusers are using this possible link as an excuse to commit aggressive acts and property crimes.

One way to distinguish between these two possibilities is to administer either high steroid doses or placebo for days or weeks to human volunteers and then ask the people to report on their behavioral symptoms. To date, four such studies have been conducted. In three, high steroid doses did produce greater feelings of irritability and aggression than did placebo; but in one study, the drugs did not have that effect. One possible explanation, according to researchers, is that some but not all anabolic steroids increase irritability and aggression.

Anabolic steroids have been reported also to cause other behavioral effects, including euphoria, increased energy, sexual arousal, mood swings, distractibility, forgetfulness, and confusion. In the studies in which researchers administered high steroid doses to volunteers, a minority of the volunteers developed behavioral symptoms that were so extreme as to disrupt their ability to function in their jobs or in society. In a few cases, the volunteers' behavior presented a threat to themselves and others.

In summary, the extent to which steroid abuse contributes to violence and behavioral disorders is unknown. As with the health complications of steroid abuse, the prevalence of extreme cases of violence and behavioral disorders seems to be low, but it may be underreported or not recognized.

Are Anabolic Steroids Addictive?

An undetermined percentage of steroid abusers become addicted to the drugs, as evidenced by their continuing to take steroids in spite of physical problems, negative effects on social relations, nervousness, and irritability. Also, they spend large amounts of time and money obtaining the drugs and experience withdrawal symptoms such as mood swings, fatigue, restlessness, loss of appetite, insomnia, reduced sex drive, and the desire to take more steroids. The most dangerous of the withdrawal symptoms is depression, because it sometimes leads to suicide attempts. Untreated, some depressive symptoms associated with anabolic steroid withdrawal have been known to persist for a year or more after the abuser stops taking the drugs.

What Can Be Done to Prevent Steroid Abuse?

Early attempts to prevent steroid abuse concentrated on drug testing and on educating students about the drugs' adverse effects. A few school districts test for abuse of illicit drugs, including steroids, and studies are currently under way to determine whether such testing reduces drug abuse.

Research on steroid educational programs has shown that simply teaching students about steroids' adverse effects does not convince adolescents that they personally can be adversely affected. Nor does such instruction discourage young people from taking steroids in the future. Presenting both the risks and benefits of anabolic steroid use is more effective in convincing adolescents about steroids' negative effects, apparently because the students find a balanced approach more credible and less biased, according to the researchers. However, the balanced approach still does not discourage adolescents from abusing steroids.

A more sophisticated approach has shown promise for preventing steroid abuse among players on high school sports teams. In the ATLAS program, developed for male football players, coaches and team leaders discuss the potential effects of anabolic steroids and other illicit drugs on immediate sports performance, and they teach how to refuse offers of drugs. They also discuss how strength training and proper nutrition can help adolescents build their bodies without the use of steroids. Later, special trainers teach the players proper weightlifting techniques. An ongoing series of studies has shown that this multicomponent, team-centered approach reduces new steroid abuse by 50 percent. A program designed for adolescent girls on sports teams, patterned after the program designed for boys, is currently being tested.

What Treatments Are Effective for Steroid Abuse?

Few studies of treatments for anabolic steroid abuse have been conducted. Current knowledge is based largely on the experiences of a small number of physicians who have worked with patients undergoing steroid withdrawal. The physicians have found that supportive therapy is sufficient in some cases. Patients are educated about what they may experience during withdrawal and are evaluated for suicidal thoughts. If symptoms are severe or prolonged, medications or hospitalization may be needed.

Some medications that have been used for treating steroid withdrawal restore the hormonal system after its disruption by steroid abuse. Other medications target specific withdrawal symptoms—for example, antidepressants to treat depression, and analgesics for headaches and muscle and joint pains.

Some patients require assistance beyond simple treatment of withdrawal symptoms and are treated with behavioral therapies.

Glossary

Addiction: A chronic, relapsing disease, characterized by compulsive drug-seeking and use and by neurochemical and molecular changes in the brain.

Anabolic effects: Drug-induced growth or thickening of the body's nonreproductive tract tissues—including skeletal muscle, bones, the larynx, and vocal cords—and decrease in body fat.

Analgesics: A group of medications that reduce pain.

Androgenic effects: A drug's effects upon the growth of the male reproductive tract and the development of male secondary sexual characteristics.

Antidepressants: A group of drugs used in treating depressive disorders.

Cardiovascular system: The heart and blood vessels.

Hormone: A chemical substance formed in glands in the body and carried in the blood to organs and tissues, where it influences function, structure, and behavior.

Musculoskeletal system: The muscles, bones, tendons, and ligaments.

Placebo: An inactive substance, used in experiments to distinguish between actual drug effects and effects that are expected by the volunteers in the experiments.

Sex hormones: Hormones that are found in higher quantities in one sex than in the other. Male sex hormones are the androgens, which include testosterone; and the female sex hormones are the estrogens and progesterone.

Withdrawal: Symptoms that occur after chronic use of a drug is reduced or stopped.

References

Bahrke, M.S., Yesalis, C.E., and Wright, J.E. Psychological and behavioral effects of endogenous testosterone and anabolic-androgenic steroids: an update. *Sports Medicine* 22(6): 367-390, 1996.

Blue, J.G., and Lombardo, J.A. Steroids and steroid-like compounds. *Clinics in Sports Medicine* 18(3): 667-689, 1999.

Bronson, F.H., and Matherne, C.M. Exposure to anabolic-androgenic steroids shortens life span of male mice. *Medicine and Science in Sports and Exercise* 29(5): 615-619, 1997.

Brower, K.J. Withdrawal from anabolic steroids. Current *Therapy in Endocrinology and Metabolism* 6: 338-343, 1997.

Elliot, D., and Goldberg, L. Intervention and prevention of steroid use in adolescents. *The American Journal of Sports Medicine* 24(6): S46-S47, 1996.

Goldberg, L., et al. Anabolic steroid education and adolescents: Do scare tactics work? *Pediatrics* 87(3): 283-286, 1991.

Goldberg, L., et al. Effects of a multidimensional anabolic steroid prevention intervention: The Adolescents Training and Learning to Avoid Steroids (ATLAS) Program. *Journal of the American Medical Association* 276(19): 1555-1562, 1996.

Goldberg, L., et al. The ATLAS program: Preventing drug use and promoting health behaviors. *Archives of Pediatrics and Adolescent Medicine* 154: 332-338, 2000.

Gruber, A.J., and Pope, H.G., Jr. Compulsive weight lifting and anabolic drug abuse among women rape victims. *Comprehensive Psychiatry* 40(4): 273-277, 1999.

Gruber, A.J., and Pope, H.G., Jr. Psychiatric and medical effects of anabolic-androgenic steroid use in women. *Psychotherapy and Psychosomatics* 69: 19-26, 2000.

Hoberman, J.M., and Yesalis, C.E. The history of synthetic testosterone. *Scientific American* 272(2): 76-81, 1995.

Leder, B.Z., et al. Oral androstenedione administration and serum testosterone concentrations in young men. *Journal of the American Medical Association* 283(6): 779-782, 2000.

The Medical Letter on Drugs and Therapeutics. Creatine and androstenedione-two "dietary supplements." 40(1039): 105-106, 1998.

Middleman, A.B, et al. High-risk behaviors among high school students in Massachusetts who use anabolic steroids. *Pediatrics* 96(2): 268-272, 1995.

Pope, H.G., Jr., Kouri, E.M., and Hudson, M.D. Effects of supraphysiologic doses of testosterone on mood and aggression in normal men. *Archives of General Psychiatry* 57(2): 133-140, 2000.

Porcerelli, J.H., and Sandler, B.A. Anabolic-androgenic steroid abuse and psychopathology. *Psychiatric Clinics of North America* 21(4): 829-833, 1998.

Porcerelli, J.H., and Sandler, B.A. Narcissism and empathy in steroid users. *American Journal of Psychiatry* 152(11): 1672-1674, 1995.

Rich, J.D., Dickinson, B.P., Flanigan, T.P., and Valone, S.E. Abscess related to anabolic-androgenic steroid injection. *Medicine and Science in Sports and Exercise* 31(2): 207-209, 1999.

Su, T.-P., et al. Neuropsychiatric effects of anabolic steroids in male normal volunteers. *Journal of the American Medical Association* 269(21): 2760-2764, 1993.

Sullivan, M.L., Martinez, C.M., Gennis, P., and Gallagher, E.J. The cardiac toxicity of anabolic steroids. *Progress in Cardiovascular Diseases* 41(1): 1-15, 1998.

Yesalis, C.E. *Anabolic Steroids in Sports and Exercise, 2nd edition.* Champaign, IL: Human Kinetics. In press.

Yesalis, C.E. Androstenedione. *Sport Dietary Supplements Update, 2000,* E-SportMed.com.

Yesalis, C.E. Trends in anabolic-androgenic steroid use among adolescents. *Archives of Pediatrics and Adolescent Medicine* 151: 1197-1206, 1997.

Yesalis, C.E., Kennedy, N.J., Kopstein, A.N., and Bahrke, M.S. Anabolic-androgenic steroid use in the United States. *Journal of the American Medical Association* 270(10): 1217-1221, 1993.

Zorpette, G. Andro angst. *Scientific American* 279(6): 22-26, 1998.

Additional Information

National Institute on Drug Abuse (NIDA)
6001 Executive Boulevard, Room 5213
Bethesda, MD 20892-9561
Tel: 301-443-1124
Infofax: 888-644-6432
TTY: 888-889-6432
Website: www.drugabuse.gov
Website: www.steroidabuse.org

National Clearinghouse for Alcohol and Drug Information (NCADI)
11426-28 Rockville Pike, Suite 200
Rockville, MD 20852
Toll-Free: 800-729-6686
Website: www.health.org

Part Six

Preventing Common Sports Injuries

Chapter 45

Safety Gear Reduces Injuries

What do kissing, playing baseball and field hockey without a mouth guard, and chugging soda from a glass bottle have in common? They can all leave you with a chipped front tooth or, worse, no front tooth at all.

Drinking soda through a mouth guard can be rough going, and a face guard makes it next to impossible to enjoy kisses from the one you love. But it simply makes good sense to shield your face and head with protective gear when you play contact sports and sports where balls, bats, pucks, and other *missiles* fly in your face.

"Sports and recreational injuries are easily prevented," says Ruth Nowjack-Raymer, coauthor of a recent report on the use of protective head gear—mouth guards and helmets—in organized sports.[1] The strongest proof of this, she says, comes from the example of football. In the 1950s, a faculty member in the dental school at Ohio State University wrote a series of articles about mouth guards and their cushioning effects. Not only could a mouth guard protect the teeth and

This chapter includes "Sports Injuries: In Your Face," by Ruth Levy Guyer, Ph.D., *Research in the News*, National Institutes of Health; "Recommended Sports Eye Protectors," reprinted with permission from PREVENT BLIND-NESS AMERICA. Copyright 2000; "Tips for Buying Sports Eye Protectors," reprinted with permission from PREVENT BLINDNESS AMERICA. Copyright 2000; "Preventing Bicycle-Related Head Injuries," National Center for Injury Prevention and Control (NCIPC), 2000; and "National Campaign: Safety Equipment," © National Youth Sports Safety Foundation; this material is reprinted with permission of the National Youth Sports Safety Foundation, One Beacon Street, Suite 3333, Boston, Massachusetts 02108.

jaw but the custom-made style molded by dentists could even prevent a concussion, a form of brain injury. In the early 1960s, before rules and regulations governed the use of football gear, 50% of all injuries to high school football players involved their faces and heads. Then, guidelines were established for shielding those parts of the body, and football players suited up with helmets and mouth guards. Today, only 1.4% of all football injuries involve the head and face.

It is strange that the example set by football players has not been adopted by athletes who participate in other potentially dangerous sports. Fans and athletes alike readily accept and even admire the *armored* appearance of football players. Football players are, in fact, among the most popular athletes in high schools and colleges in the United States: the annual homecoming dance is always associated with a fall football game, the school's band and cheerleaders perform more often at football games than at other sporting events, and graduates typically return to their schools to see football games. There is no stigma attached to helmets, mouth guards, and padding in this sport.

But, for some reason, there is great resistance among athletes in other sports to wearing protective gear. Nine million students in the United States play baseball and softball (three million play football). But it is rare to see baseball and softball players sporting protective headgear in the field and not even all at-bat players wear helmets. Nowjack-Raymer found that only 35% of kids wear helmets most or all of the time when they play baseball and softball and only 7% wear mouth guards. In Little League ball games, 86% of injuries involve athletes in the field, and most of the injuries affect heads and faces.[2]

As students get older, says Nowjack-Raymer, they are more likely to wear protective gear. This may, in part, reflect their growing understanding of the physical risks they face. It may also have something to do with who sponsors and pays for a sport. Organized sports programs for little children are often run by community centers, parents chip in money to support them, and the organization is relatively low key. As kids grow, she says, more of the programs are coordinated by schools and governed by rules and regulations.

The survey documented some disturbing gender differences. "Girls are injured in sports too," notes Nowjack-Raymer, "and the injuries can be expensive and painful and cause problems that last a lifetime." But girls and women are much less likely to wear protective gear than are boys and men. Is this because they rarely see famous women athletes wearing mouth guards and helmets?

Nowjack-Raymer points to an example in her own family. Her sister, she says, is still dealing with problems that started years ago when she fractured her front teeth during a field hockey game. Field hockey, she notes, is a sport in which the disparity in safety practices between female and male athletes is striking. Male field hockey players at all levels wear headgear. Female hockey players typically do not, and whether they should is the subject of a raging debate. One group has been lobbying strongly for equal protection for female athletes. Another group is strongly opposed, arguing that, if girls and women wear protective gear, the nature and culture of the game will change toward more aggressive, violent play.

The data that Nowjack-Raymer analyzed were collected in a national health survey that was conducted in 1991. Nearly 10,000 parents and guardians of children in the 7 to 17 year old age range answered questions about the use of head gear and mouth guards in a number of organized sports. Nowjack-Raymer and her colleagues—epidemiologists, social scientists, health educators, behavioral scientists, and others—are now beginning to look at the research that has already been done to address the problems that exist and define what research should be conducted next. They are trying to determine what coalitions of students, parents, coaches, trainers, organizations, and others could actually establish educational programs and binding rules that will support the use of protective gear. They are assessing what approaches work best to get student athletes to protect themselves. They are considering looking at the design of protective gear—is it comfortable, well made, effective?—and what makes a product acceptable.

In the United States, says Nowjack-Raymer, the strategies that have proved most effective are those based on establishment of and compliance with regulations, and often these have been instituted at local levels. This country has no overarching authority that makes rules, as is true in other countries. In Australia, for example, public health agencies provide information about injuries and also develop rules and guidelines for enhancing the safety of sports.

Will headgear ever become stylish? It hasn't yet, notes Nowjack-Raymer, but it has come a long way. "When a new sport comes along," she says, "it is important to think about what gear really makes sense." For example, in-line skating is a newer sport in which both beginners and more experienced skaters routinely wear lots of protective gear. Why this has occurred is unclear; perhaps it stems from good training from the beginning, the ready availability of colorful gear, a general acceptance of protective equipment, or some combination of these.

Accidents happen not only during official games but also during informal play, so, warns Nowjack-Raymer, it is important for athletes to wear their gear even when they are just practicing at home. Over 14 million children and teens in the United States participate in at least one organized sport, and injuries are on the rise. Teeth are knocked out in basketball games by the elbows of other players; eye injuries are common for badminton and squash players not wearing protective goggles;[3] 144,000 children in the United States suffer annually from head injuries in bicycle accidents, and 85% of these injuries would not have occurred had the child worn a helmet.[4] Getting athletes to readily don their helmets and mouth guards may involve major changes in the cultures of some sports.

And yet, some cultures have really valued helmets and other protective gear, which have been around as long as people have participated in sports and engaged in battles. Some 5000 years ago, a prince of Ur named Meskalamdug apparently valued his gold and silver helmet so fully that he was buried in it. He also was buried with his bodyguards, all of whom were wearing helmets of copper.[5]

References

1. *Public Health Reports* 1996, 111:82-86.

2. *Pediatrics*, 1996, 98(3):445-448. J. R.

3. *Coll Surg*, Edinb, 1993 38(3):127-133.

4. *Public Health Reports* 1995, 110(3):251-259.

5. Aust. N.Z. *J. Surg.* 1996, 66:314-324.

Tips for Buying Sports Eye Protectors from Prevent Blindness America

Prevent Blindness America recommends that athletes wear sports eye guards when participating in sports. Prescription glasses, sunglasses, and even occupational safety glasses *do not* provide adequate protection. Sports eye guards come in a variety of shapes and sizes. Eye guards designed for use in racquet sports are now commonly used for basketball and soccer and in combination with helmets in football, hockey, and baseball. The eye guards you choose should fit securely and comfortably and allow the use of a helmet if necessary. Expect to spend between $20 and $40 for a pair of regular eye guards and $60 or more for eye guards with prescription lenses. The following guidelines can help you find a pair of eye guards right for you:

- If you wear prescription glasses, ask your eye doctor to fit you for prescription eye guards. If you're a monocular athlete (a person with only one eye that sees well), ask your eye doctor what sports you can safely participate in. *Monocular athletes should always wear sports eye guards.*

- Buy eye guards at sports specialty stores or optical stores. At the sports store, ask for a sales representative who's familiar with eye protectors to help you.

Table 45.1. Recommended Sports Eye Protectors. (Source: Prevent Blindness America)

Sport	Type of Eye Protection	Eye Injuries Prevented
Baseball	• Face guard (attached to helmet) made of poly-carbonate material • Sports eye guards	• Scratches on the cornea • Inflamed iris • Blood spilling into the eye's anterior chamber • Traumatic cataract • Swollen retina
Basketball	• Sports eye guards	• Fracture of the eye socket • Scratches on the cornea • Inflamed iris • Blood spilling into the eye's anterior chamber • Swollen retina
Soccer	• Sports eye guards	• Inflamed iris • Blood spilling into the eye's anterior chamber • Swollen retina
Football	• Polycarbonate shield attached to a face guard • Sports eye guards	• Scratches on the cornea • Inflamed iris • Blood spilling into the eye's anterior chamber • Swollen retina
Hockey	• Wire or polycarbonate mask • Sports eye guards	• Scratches on the cornea • Inflamed iris • Blood spilling into the eye's anterior chamber • Swollen retina

- Don't buy sports eye guards without lenses. Only "lensed" protectors are recommended for sports use. Make sure the lenses either stay in place or pop outward in the event of an accident. Lenses that pop in against your eyes can be very dangerous.

- Fogging of the lenses can be a problem when you're active. Some eye guards are available with anti-fog coating. Others have side vents for additional ventilation. Try on different types to determine which is most comfortable for you.

- Check the packaging to see if the eye protector you select has been tested for sports use. Also check to see that the eye protector is made of polycarbonate material. Polycarbonate eye guards are the most impact resistant.

- Sports eye guards should be padded or cushioned along the brow and bridge of the nose. Padding will prevent the eye guards from cutting your skin.

- Try on the eye protector to determine if it's the right size. Adjust the strap and make sure it's not too tight or too loose. If you purchased your eye guards at an optical store, an optical representative can help you adjust the eye protector for a comfortable fit. Until you get used to wearing a pair of eye guards, it may feel strange, but bear with it! It's a lot more comfortable than an eye injury.

Preventing Bicycle-Related Head Injuries

How Large a Problem Are Bicycle-Related Head Injuries in the United States?

- In 1997, 813 bicyclists were killed in crashes with motor vehicles, an increase of 7% over the previous year.[1] Of these, 31% were riders younger than 16 years old and 97% were not wearing helmets.[2]

- In 1997, an estimated 567,000 Americans sustained a bicycle-related injury that required emergency department care. Approximately two-thirds of these cyclists were children or adolescents.[3]

- An estimated 140,000 children are treated each year in emergency departments for head injuries sustained while bicycling.[4]

- In 1991, societal costs associated with bicycle-related head injury or death were estimated to exceed $3 billion.[5]

What Can Be Done?

- Riders should wear bicycle helmets every time they ride.

- In the event of a crash, wearing a bicycle helmet reduces the risk of serious head injury by as much as 85% and the risk for brain injury by as much as 88%.[6] Helmets have also been shown to reduce the risk of injury to the upper and mid-face by 65%.[7] In fact, if each rider wore a helmet, an estimated 500 bicycle-related fatalities and 151,000 nonfatal head injuries would be prevented each year—that's one death per day and one injury every four minutes.[8]

- Unfortunately, estimates on helmet usage suggest that only 25% of children ages 5-14 years wear a helmet when riding.[9] The percentage is close to zero when looking at teen riders. Children and adolescents' most common complaints are that helmets are not fashionable, or cool, their friends don't wear them, and/or they are uncomfortable (usually too hot). Riders also convey that they do not think about the importance of bike helmets, nor about the need to protect themselves from injury, particularly if they are not riding in traffic.

- Accordingly, the national health goal for 2010 is for 50% of teenage bicyclists in 9th-12th grade to wear helmets.[10]

What Strategies Are Available to Get Bicyclists to Wear Helmets?

- The primary strategies to increase bike helmet use include education, legislation, and helmet-distribution programs. Educational programs have been conducted in different communities and schools around the nation, with generally positive results. The most successful programs are multifaceted and often multisite campaigns that combine education with helmet giveaways or discount programs and state or local legislation requiring helmet use.

- Some evidence suggests that legislative efforts are more cost-effective than school- or community-based programs.[11]

What Is CDC Doing to Increase National Helmet Use?

- CDC developed and disseminated injury control recommendations on bicycle helmets.[12]

- CDC provides grant funding to state health departments to implement and evaluate programs that promote helmet use.

- CDC gives funds to selected injury control centers to promote helmet use. CDC funds research to improve helmet design.

- CDC collaborates with a host of other federal agencies and nonprofit organizations to promote helmet use and bicycle safety. For more information about this collaborative effort, visit the National Bicycle Safety Network website: www.cdc.gov/ncipc/bike.

How Many States Have Bicycle Helmet Laws?

- By early 1999, 15 states and more than 65 local governments had enacted some form of bicycle helmet legislation. Most of these laws pertain to children and adolescents.[13]

What Standards Exist to Ensure That Helmets Are Truly Protective?

- The U.S. Consumer Product Safety Commission issued a new safety standard for bike helmets in 1999. The new standard ensures that bike helmets will adequately protect the head and that chin straps will be strong enough to prevent the helmet from coming off in a crash, collision, or fall. In addition, helmets intended for children up to age five must cover a larger surface of the head than before. All bike helmets made or imported into the United States must meet the CPSC standard.[14]

How Can You Help Prevent Injuries While Bicycling?

- Wear a bicycle helmet every time you ride. A bicycle helmet is a necessity, not an accessory.

- Wear your bicycle helmet correctly. A bicycle helmet should fit comfortably and snugly, but not too tightly. It should sit on top of your head in a level position, and it should not rock forward and back or from side to side. Always keep the helmet straps buckled.

- Only buy a bicycle helmet if it meets or exceeds the safety standards developed by the U.S. Consumer Product Safety Commission.

- Learn the rules of the road and obey all traffic laws. Ride with the traffic, on the right side of the road. Use appropriate hand signals. Respect traffic signals, which are meant for riders as well as drivers. Stop at all intersections, not just those intersections with pedestrian markings. Stop and look both ways before entering a street.

- Children should not ride in the street until they are 10 years old, demonstrate good riding skills, and are able to observe the basic rules of the road. And, of course, children should always wear helmets when they ride.

References

1. *NHTSA Traffic Safety Facts, 1997: Bicyclists.* Washington, D.C.: National Highway Traffic Safety Administration

2. Insurance Institute for Highway Safety (IIHS). *1997 Fatality Facts: Bicycles.* Arlington (VA): IIHS, 1997.

3. U.S. Consumer Product Safety Commission. National Electronic Injury Surveillance System (NEISS). Washington, DC: Consumer Product Safety Commission; 1997.

4. Sosin DM, Sacks JJ, Webb KW. Pediatric head injuries and deaths from bicycling in the United States. *Pediatrics* 1996;98(5):868-70.

5. U.S. Consumer Products Safety Commission (CPSC). Bicycle-related head injury or death. Washington (DC): CPSC, 1994.

6. Thompson RS, Rivara FP, Thompson DC. A case-control study of the effectiveness of bicycle safety helmets. *N Engl J Med.* 1989; 320:1361-7.

7. Thompson DC, Nunn ME, Thompson RS, Rivara FP. Effectiveness of bicycle safety helmets in preventing serious facial injury. *JAMA* 1996; 276:1974-1975.

8. Sacks JJ, Holmgreen P, Smith S, Sosin D. Bicycle-associated head injuries and deaths in the United States from 1984-1988. *JAMA* 1991;266:3016-8.

9. Sacks JJ, Kresnow M, Houston B, Russell J. Bicycle helmet use among American children, 1994. *Injury Prevention* 1996;2:258-62.

10. Public Health Service (PHS). Healthy People 2010 Objectives: Draft for Public Comment. Washington (DC): US Department of Health and Human Services, PHS; 1999.

11. Hatziandreu EJ, Sacks JJ, Brown R, Taylor WR, Rosenberg ML, Graham JD. The cost effectiveness of three programs to increase use of bicycle helmets among children. *Public Health Reports* 1995 May-Jun;110(3):251-9.

12. CDC. Injury Control Recommendations: Bicycle Helmets. *MMWR* 44(RR-1)1995.

13. Bicycle Helmet Safety Institute (BHSI). *Mandatory helmet laws: summary*. Arlington (VA): BHSI, 1997.

14. Federal Register. U.S. Consumer Product Safety Commission. Safety standard for bicycle helmets; Final rule. FR Doc. 98-4214, February 13, 1998.

Safety Equipment for Sports

Protective safety equipment has been developed and recommended for many different sports. The purpose of the equipment is to help prevent and reduce the severity of injuries. The use of safety equipment is usually recommended as a result of research by health professionals that identified a high risk of injury in a particular sport or recreational activity. The use of safety equipment may be advocated by the government, national medical organizations, public health professionals, safety groups, national governing bodies of sports, or sports associations to prevent many different types of injuries, especially catastrophic injuries.

A national health objective in Healthy People 2000 regarding safety equipment states: "Extend requirements of the use of effective head, face, eye, and mouth protection to all organizations, agencies, and institutions sponsoring sporting and recreation events that pose risk of injury."

Standards for Safety Equipment

The following national organizations have developed standards for safety equipment:

American Society For Testing & Materials (ASTM)
P.O. Box C700
100 Barr Harbor Drive
West Conshohocken, PA 19428-2959
Tel: 610-832-9585
Fax: 610-832-9555
Website: www.astm.org
E-mail: service@astm.org

National Operating Committee on Standards for Athletic Equipment (NOCSAE)
P.O. Box 12290
Overland, KS 66282-2290
Tel: 913-888-1340
Fax: 913-888-1065
Website: www.nocsae.org
E-mail: mpo@op.wsabe.com

Snell Memorial Foundation (SNELL)
3628 Madison Avenue
Suite 11
North Highlands, CA 95660
Toll-Free: 888-SNELL99
Tel: 916-331-5073
Fax: 916-331-0359
Website: www.smf.org
E-mail: info@smf.org

American National Standards Institute (ANSI)
25 West 43rd Street, Fourth Floor
New York, NY 10036
Tel: 212-642-4900
Fax: 212-398-0023
Website: www.ansi.org
E-mail: info@ansi.org

Equipment Certifications

Protective Eyewear

Protective eyewear standards currently exist for racket sports, women's lacrosse, paintball, and youth baseball. They have been developed through voluntary consensus by subcommittees of the American Society for Testing and Materials (ASTM) which include concerned manufacturers, consumers, experts, and other interested parties. The following organization has been created to assist consumers, sports organizations, eye care professionals, manufacturers, and sports officials. The PECC seal on protective eyewear will assure that it protects adequately and has been tested and certified.

Protective Eyewear Certification Council (PECC)

c/o Paul F. Vinger, MD
297 Heath's Bridge Road
Concord, MA 01742
Website: www.protecteyes.org
E-mail: eyesafety@dtl-inc.com

Hockey Equipment

Hockey Equipment Certification Council (HECC)

3 Baker Hill Road
Great Neck, NY 11023
Tel.: 516-482-5374
Fax: 516-482-1231
Website: www.hecc-hockey.net/home.html
E-mail: CJAbraham1@aol.com

Helmets

Helmets have been proven effective in either preventing brain injury or reducing the severity of brain and head injuries. Helmets do not protect the neck.

Sport specific helmets have been designed to address different risk factors peculiar to each sport. Variables include different biomechanical forces on the skull and various possible impact sites. Forces differ because of distances to the ground associated with falls, playing surfaces, playing equipment, and speed of movement intrinsic to the sport.

Helmets have been either mandated or recommended for the following sports and recreational activities:

- auto and motor sports
- equestrian sports
- rollerblading
- snowmobiling
- football
- rugby
- women's softball
- bicycling
- skateboarding
- wrestling
- boxing
- lacrosse

- baseball
- hockey
- skiing

Standards for helmets have been developed by the American Society for Testing & Materials, National Operating Committee on Standards for Athletic Equipment, Snell Memorial Foundation, and the American National Standards Institute.

Mouth Guards

Mouth protectors help prevent injury to the mouth, teeth, lips, cheeks, and tongue. They also cushion blows that might cause concussions or jaw fractures. Even though a mouth protector is worn, it is still possible for a tooth to be knocked out; however, the wearing of a protector will reduce tooth injuries to a minimum. It is recommended that mouth guards be worn by all athletes during practice and competition of contact and collision sports.

The American Dental Association recommends mouth guards for the following sports:

- acrobatics
- football
- martial arts
- skiing
- volleyball
- basketball
- gymnastics
- racquetball

- skydiving
- water polo
- boxing
- handball
- rugby
- soccer
- weight lifting
- discus throwing

- ice hockey
- shot putting
- squash wrestling
- field hockey
- lacrosse
- skate boarding
- surfing

American Dental Association (ADA)

211 E. Chicago Avenue
Chicago, IL 60611
Tel: 312-440-2500
Fax: 312-440-2800
Website: www.ada.org

The American Society for Testing & Materials has developed standards for the care and use of mouth guards.

Face Protection

The American Society for Testing and Materials has developed standards for face protection for baseball and ice hockey.

Youth Baseball

In June, 1996, the United States Consumer Product Safety Commission (CPSC) issued findings of their research on baseball protective equipment.

The CPSC announced that safety equipment for baseball could significantly reduce the amount and severity of 58,000 (or almost 36 percent of) baseball-related injuries to children each year. Conclusions from the CPSC Study:

- Baseball protective equipment currently on the market may prevent, reduce, or lessen the severity of more than 58,000 injuries or almost 36 percent an estimated 162,100 hospital emergency-room-treated, baseball-related injuries occurring to children each year.

- Softer-than-standard balls may prevent, reduce, or lessen the severity of the 47,900 ball impact injuries to the head and neck.

- Batting helmets with face guards may prevent, reduce, or lessen the severity of about 3,900 facial injuries occurring to batters in organized play.

- Safety release bases that leave no holes in the ground or parts of the base sticking up from the ground when the base is released may prevent, reduce, or lessen the severity of the 6,600 base-contact sliding injuries occurring in organized play.

Additional Information

National Center for Injury Prevention and Control
Mailstop K63
4770 Buford Highway NE
Atlanta, GA 30341-3724
Tel: 770-488-4652
Fax: 770-488-1317
E-mail: OHCINFO@cdc.gov

National Youth Sports Safety Foundation
One Beacon Street
Suite 3333
Boston, MA 02108
Tel: 617-277-1771
Fax: 617-722-9999

Website: www.nyssf.org
E-mail: NYSSF@aol.com

U.S. Consumer Product Safety Commission
4330 East-West Highway
Bethesda, MD 20814-4408
Toll-Free: 800-638-2772
Tel: 301-504-0990
Fax: 301-504-0124 and 301-504-0025
Website: www.cpsc.gov
E-mail: info@cpsc.gov

Chapter 46

An Informed Parent Is the Best Protection against Kids' Sports Injuries

The participation of children in organized athletic activities raises many concerns in parents' mind:

- At what age is my child ready to participate in organized athletics?
- What is the risk of significant injury?
- What sports carry the highest likelihood of injury?
- Are there specific injuries related to specific sports?

The American Orthopaedic Society for Sports Medicine (AOSSM) has prepared this information to help provide parents with some answers.

Should My Child Participate in Organized Athletics?

Yes! Participating in sports is a fundamental part of our way of life. When kept in the proper perspective, athletic activities can become an important part of a healthy growth and development pattern. A child's participation in sports should be regarded as an extension of school time, playtime, or family time—coaches or parents should never view it as an end unto itself. Participating in sports is a very healthy way, both physically and socially, for a child to channel youthful energy in a positive manner.

"Youth in Sports," revised 2001 © The American Orthopaedic Society for Sports Medicine, reprinted with permission; and "Children and Adolescents Sports Safety," © SafeUSA™.

When Is a Child Mature Enough to Begin Participating in Organized Sports?

Understanding a child's social development is the first step in answering this question. Children under age six cannot compete in an adult sense. They live in a play world of their own where even play with other children is often incidental.

These youngsters have minimal ability to appreciate achievement in a sporting sense and are difficult, if not impossible, to organize. The adult measurements of competition are lost on pre-schoolers. Sports activities for children in this group are best promoted as playground opportunities.

Between ages six and ten, children come to appreciate interaction with their peer groups but, psychologically, still do not compete in the adult sense. Play and fun are the primary goals for these youngsters, with structure, organization, and scoring, at most of secondary importance. Children in this age group generally have very short attention spans and generally cannot perform in the adult-imposed structure of most sports activities. They are ready for group interaction but not for many restrictive rules or structure.

Between age ten and the onset of puberty, a youth develops increasing awareness of the goals, structure, and discipline required for team sports. The prime motivation of children this age is still joining in and having fun with their teammates. However, they will accept increasing amounts of structure and are becoming more goal oriented.

During and after puberty the aspiring athlete develops an increasing sophisticated perspective of the structure and organization of team sports, the post-pubescent athlete is ready to develop sports-related discipline.

When Is a Child Physically Capable of Participating in Organized Sports?

In terms of physical capabilities of the young athlete, participating in sports depends upon both chronological age and physiological maturation.

The positive effect of sports activity or training on the body is measurably less in the pre-pubescent (before puberty) athlete than in the post–pubescent (after puberty) athlete. The benefits of conditioning to the cardiopulmonary system (heart and lungs) are scientifically measurable in the younger athlete, but are of a much lower magnitude than in the older child. Training with weights also can have a positive effect in the pre-pubescent athlete, but it cannot result in the dramatic increase in muscle mass or strength that is seen in the post-pubescent athlete.

One of the major factors responsible for this lack of response to weight training is that the pre-pubescent child has not undergone the hormonal changes, which physiologically permit the muscle-bulking phenomenon to occur.

It should be noted that no matter what the form of specific training or sport activity, stretching and flexibility drills should be included in any pre-participation or warm-up program, even in the very young.

Is There Anything to Be Gained from Sports Activity and Training at an Early Age?

Given the fact that children have certain physiological and psychological limitations is there any reason for them to participate in sport before puberty? Once again, the answer is yes!

Youngsters involved in such activities develop motor skills, proper training habits, and a work ethic, which can carry over to life in general. They will also benefit from proper training with weights, cardiovascular conditioning, and from the non-parental discipline. Involved parents, coaches, and administrators should encourage such activities, while refraining from imposing adult performance standards.

How Should Organized Youth Sports Programs Be Structured?

The phenomenon of puberty is a troublesome period in any youngsters' life and athletic participation during this time may actually compound nature's built-in problems. A major reason is that most youth sports programs group participants according to chronological age.

Anatomic age (stage of body development), emotional age (maturity), and social age do not always coincide with calendar (chronological) age. An ideal system would be to group athletes by more than one standard. For example, arrange them not only by chronological age and weight, but also by emotional and physiological maturity.

The post-pubescent athlete can be thought of in near-adult terms. This athlete will practice with competitive goals in mind and can physically benefit from strength and endurance training. A youth in this age group should also participate in an aggressive stretching and flexibility program, which is sport specific.

However, the best system is only as good as the coach or parent who understands the psychosocial and physical maturity factors involved—and who will foster athletic participation at a level appropriate for each individual child.

What Type of Sports Should a Youngster Participate In?

The young athlete should participate in a variety of sports activities. Psychologically, the sports goal for a child under ten, and perhaps even the older pre-pubescent should be fun. Physically, the young athlete should be encouraged to acquire basic individual skills. There is no overriding reason to recommend participation in non-contact sports over contact sports.

Sports participation by these younger athletes should be an opportunity to develop motor skills and to have fun. These limited goals will give the child a healthy mental attitude as well as a healthy body, both of which will benefit him or her throughout life.

Above all, a pre-pubescent child-athlete must not become the focus of the personal athletic dreams of wishes of a parent or coach. While parental and coaching guidance is of immense value, the young athlete should not be pressured to swim or play football, for example, when another sport better fits his or her emotional and/or physical make-up. The post-pubescent athlete will usually select athletic endeavors based on a personal skill or through associations with a particular role model or peer group.

What Is the Risk of Injury in Youth Sports?

The question is not whether injuries accompany youth sports, but whether there is undue risk. Many studies have documented a very low incidence of injury in the total spectrum of youth sporting endeavors. Interestingly, the occurrence of injury in the pre-pubescent athlete has been documented as being much lower than in the post-pubescent athlete, and lower in the post-pubescent than the young adult.

This is probably due to the fact that the younger athlete has a lower ratio of kinetic energy to body mass—the more immature the physical body, the lower the speed and power.

Since the magnitude of injury is almost always directly related to energy expended in a traumatic event, the younger athlete is less likely to get injured then his older counterpart. The athletic injuries, which do occur, are usually minor contusions and sprains. Fractures, dislocations, and major ligament injuries can happen, but are more common in older age groups.

Parents have expressed concern about the potential for injuries to the growth areas of developing bones and muscle in the pre-pubescent athlete. This concern has proven to be more perceived than real, as several scientific studies have failed to document a significant increase in physeal injuries (damage to the growth areas of bones) in young athletes. Only in extreme cases, such as young gymnasts in intense training for long periods of time, are at some risk to growth plate injuries.

An argument against organized youth sporting activities, which is based on the potential for injury, is not realistic. Although documentation is not available, it is probable that injuries resulting from participation in organized sports are fewer than those suffered on the playgrounds, or by falling off bicycles or skateboards.

Young people have definite physical and emotional energies. It is probably less hazardous to release these energies in directed endeavors than through alternative means. Any traditional organized sport is certainly safer than riding a motorcycle, for instance.

Are There Specific Injuries Associated with Specific Sports?

While each of the individual and team sports has a family of injuries most common to it, listing of individual sports and injuries will be ignored here in favor of a generalized discussion based on contact versus non-contact sports.

The most notable examples of contact sports practiced in the United States are football, ice hockey, wrestling, and basketball. In each of these sports the athlete's body is used to physically control the opponent and, thus, to influence the play of the game. Using the body in this manner creates the opportunity for injury.

Fortunately, the majority of injuries in these contact sports are bruises and scrapes. The more significant injuries such as fractures, dislocations, or major ligament damage occur in the post-pubescent athlete. Parents should be responsive to complaints of pain and discomfort from athletes in all age groups and be aware that any athlete who is not playing up to skill level may be suffering from a significant injury.

In non-contact sports, major fractures, dislocations, or ligamentous injuries are usually associated with accidental rather than intended collisions. Minor sprains, muscle pulls, blisters, and overuse syndromes are commonly seen injuries in non-contact sports.

The overuse syndrome is usually related to sports requiring repetitive, high-stress motion such as tennis, swimming, track, golf, and baseball. Injury occurs as a result of constant repetition of a particular movement. Stress fractures, shin splints, and tendonitis are examples of overuse injuries.

The treatment in each case is early recognition of the problem, followed by abstinence from competition and at least a decrease or change in training until the affected area is totally symptom free. Training intensity and duration can then increase again. Return to the previous level of training should be gradual and well planned. If the symptoms of overuse persist beyond a few days of rest or it they recur, a physician should evaluate the athlete.

Are Youth Athletics Worthwhile?

Yes! While very few athletes participate on organized teams beyond high school, and even fewer beyond college, sports activity creates a physical fitness discipline and a positive learning experience which carries through to an active, healthy adult life.

Participation carries a risk of injury but, once again, the question is not whether the risk is present but whether the risk is undue. A question of similar importance is how best to direct the naturally occurring physical energies of youth.

The American Orthopaedic Society for Sports Medicine is convinced that appropriate sports and physical training are safe and healthy applications of these energies. Physical fitness is advisable throughout an entire lifetime and is achievable only through physical activity. The discipline, motivation, and training required to remain fit should begin as a youngster.

Sports Injury Prevention for Children and Adolescents

Each year, more than 775,000 children under age 15 are treated in hospital emergency rooms for sports injuries. In fact, sports injuries are the number one reason for emergency department visits among children. Many of these injuries can be prevented if parents get involved and make sure their children wear protective gear, follow the rules of play, and are physically and emotionally prepared to play the sport.

Tips for Preventing Sports Injuries

To help your child avoid sports injuries, follow these safety tips from the American Academy of Pediatrics, the American Academy of Orthopaedic Surgeons, the National SAFE KIDS Campaign, and other sports and health organizations.

- Before your child starts a training program or enters a competition, take him or her to the doctor for a physical exam. The doctor can help assess any special injury risks your child may have.

- Make sure your child wears all the required safety gear every time he or she plays and practices. Know how the sports equipment should fit your child and how to use it. If you're not sure, ask the coach or a sporting goods expert for help. Set a good example–if you play a sport, wear your safety gear, too.

- Insist that your child warm-up and stretch before playing, paying special attention to the muscles that will get the most use during play (for example, a pitcher should focus on warming-up the shoulder and arm).

- Teach your child not to play through pain. If your child gets injured, see your doctor. Follow all the doctor's orders for recovery, and get the doctor's approval before your child returns to play.

- Make sure first aid is available at all games and practices.

- Talk to and watch your child's coach. Coaches should enforce all the rules of the game, encourage safe play, and understand the special injury risks that young players face.

- If you're not sure if it's safe for your child to perform a certain technique or move (such as heading a soccer ball or diving off the highest platform), ask your pediatrician and the coach about it.

- Above all, keep sports fun. Putting too much focus on winning can make your child push too hard and risk injury.

How Do You Know if Your Child Is Ready to Play a Sport?

The American Academy of Pediatrics recommends that you wait until your child is six years old to play team sports. Most children younger than that don't understand the concept of team play. With older children, you should decide if it's okay for them to play based on their physical and emotional development and their eagerness to

485

play. Your child's doctor can help you make this decision. Remember, pushing children to play a sport before they're ready, or when they don't want to, can increase their risk of getting hurt.

Who Is Affected?

Close to 6 million high school students play team sports, and another 20 million children take part in recreational or competitive sports out of school. Sports activities help children and adolescents stay fit, learn about teamwork, and develop self-confidence. But playing a sport also brings the risk of injury. Each year, over 775,000 children under age 15 are treated in hospital emergency departments for sports-related injuries. About 80 percent of these injuries are from playing football, basketball, baseball, or soccer.

Most sports-related injuries in children—about two-thirds of them—are sprains (involving ligaments, which connect one bone to another) and strains (involving muscles). Only 5 percent of sports injuries involve broken bones. The majority of injuries are mild, but they can cause great inconveniences for both children and their parents during the healing process. And if not allowed to heal properly, a minor injury can become a more serious one that interferes with proper growth and causes lifelong problems.

References

American Academy of Ophthalmology. *Eye safety for children.* EyeNET web site. Available at (www.aao.org). Accessed July 7, 1999.

American Academy of Pediatrics. Fitness, activity, and sports participation in the preschool child. *Pediatrics* 1992;90(6):1002-1004.

American Academy of Pediatrics. *Sports and your child.* Available at www.aap.org/family/sports.htm. Accessed July 13, 1999.

American Academy of Pediatrics. *Sports Medicine: Health care for young athletes.* Elk Grove Village, IL: The Academy, 1991: 161-163.

Brain Injury Association. *Sports and concussion safety.* Available at www.biausa.org/Prevfacts.htm.

FIMS/WHO Ad Hoc Committee on Sports and Children. Sports and children: Consensus statement on "organized sports for children." *Sidelines* 1998;8(1):1-2, 4. (Sidelines is a publication of the National Youth Sports Safety Foundation.)

National Federation of State High School Associations. *The case for high school activities*. Available at www.nfhs.org. Accessed August 2, 1999.

National SAFE KIDS Campaign. *Sports and recreational activity injury*, December 1998. Available at www.safekids.org. Accessed July 30, 1999.

U.S. Consumer Product Safety Commission. Reducing youth baseball injuries with protective equipment. *Consumer Product Safety Review* 1996;1(1):1-4.

Zetaruk M, Mitchell W. Gymnastics injuries. *Sidelines* 1998;7(2):1-2.

Additional Information

American Academy of Ophthalmology
P.O. Box 7424
San Francisco, CA 94120
Tel: 415-561-8500
Fax: 415-561-8533
Website: www.aao.org
E-mail: customer_service@aao.org

American Academy of Orthopaedic Surgeons (AAOS)
6300 North River Road
Rosemont, IL 60018-4262
Toll-Free: 800-346-AAOS
Tel: 847-823-7186
Fax: 847-823-8125
AAOS Fax-on-Demand: 800-999-2939
Website: www.aaos.org
E-mail: custserv@aaos.org

American Academy of Pediatrics (AAP)
141 Northwest Point Boulevard
Elk Grove Village, IL 60007-1098
Tel: 847-434-4000
Fax: 847-434-8000
Website: www.aap.org
E-mail: kidsdocs@aap.org

Brain Injury Association
105 North Alfred St.
Alexandria, VA 22314
Toll-Free: 800-444-6443

Brain Injury Association (continued)
Tel: 703-236- 6000
Fax: 703-236-6001
Website: www.biausa.org
E-mail: familyhelpline@biausa.org

National Athletic Trainers Association
2952 Stemmons Freeway
Dallas, TX 75247-6916
Toll-Free: 800-879-6282
Tel: 214-637-6282
Fax: 214-637-2206
Website: www.nata.org
E-mail: natanews@nata.org

National Federation of State High School Associations (NFHS)
P.O. Box 690
Indianapolis, IN 46206
Tel: 317-972-6900
Fax: 317-822-5700
Website: www.nfhs.org

National SAFE KIDS Campaign
1301 Pennsylvania Ave NW, Suite 1000
Washington, DC 20004
Tel: 202-662-0600
Fax: 202-393-2072
Website: www.safekids.org
E-mail: info@safekids.org

National Youth Sports Safety Foundation
One Beacon Street, Suite 3333
Boston, MA 02108
Tel: 617-277-1171
Fax: 617-722-9999
Website: www.nyssf.org
E-mail: nyssf@aol.com

Chapter 47

Preventing Head Injuries in the "Extreme" World of Sports

Head Injuries in the "Extreme" World of Sports

A common thread that runs through all of the extreme sports is the risk of head injury. For sports physical therapists helping out at events of both conventional and extreme nature; it is a necessity to understand the recognition and treatment of these injuries. There are a number of classifications and severity grading schemes in the literature. I would refer the reader to the excellent summary article presented in the SPTS Newsletter published in the fall, 1998. This article reviews several classifications and the evaluation techniques used to identify and classify a concussion as well as an intracranial hemorrhage. This chapter will expand on this knowledge and discuss return to play considerations for the extreme athlete.

The basic recommendations regarding return to sports for the extreme athlete are the same as the conventional athlete. It is necessary to first classify the head injury and extent of severity in order to recommend treatment and return to play advice. In addition to these basic recommendations, there are a few other considerations when dealing with an athlete who may be participating in such activities as skateboarding, in-line skating, snowboarding in a halfpipe or extreme skiing. First, to what extent is the activity the individual is participating in a contact sport? Many of the extreme sports may not

"Head Injuries in the 'Extreme' World of Sports," Sports Physical Therapy Section of APTA, © 1999 American Physical Therapy Association (APTA), reprinted with permission.

be in contact with other individuals but likely will result in contact with the ground or playing surface such as a vertical ramp or wall. This contact occurs at extremely high speeds and with little if any protective equipment in place. The efficiency and skill of falling of the participant is something to consider. An individual who has been observed to fall incorrectly and thus precariously may be well served with the recommendation to give it a day despite having had only a minor concussion secondary to the likelihood of another such fall and increased risk of second-impact syndrome.

Another consideration is the potential risk to other participants. In many of the extreme sports such as skateboarding and snowboarding in a halfpipe, the competition as well as the recreational practice is completed in a confined area with the several participants doing their thing such as flipping and twisting in close proximity of each other. A head-injured participant who may be slowed or displaying questionable judgement may disrupt the normal flow of activity in this confined area; thus wreaking havoc on the whole scene. This disorder could potentially cause a series of crashes and ultimately injury to other participants. An astute sports physical therapist advising in such a situation may want to consider conservative management and recommend to the participant not to return to the activity if such conditions prevail. Ultimately, such advice will benefit not only the injured participant but also safeguard the other participants at the venue.

Helmet Use

The next consideration has already been alluded to, but I would like to expand on the idea. This item is the lack of protective equipment specifically headgear that is employed by extreme athletes. With the exception of mountain biking and motorcross, few of the extreme sports regularly utilize any sort of helmets. I was recently at the premier of a movie; "The Realm" produced and filmed by a local company, Teton Gravity Research. The film features many extreme feats of skiing and snowboarding around the mountains of the world. The participants literally outrun avalanches, jump off cliffs, and ski the "unski-able." Less than 2% of the featured participants wear a helmet. This illustrates the point that return to a head injured participant with even a mild level of severity may not be advised without the further recommendation to use protective head gear.

The final consideration that is the ability of the sports physical therapist to arrange adequate follow-up. In many cases, the participants at the local Skateboard Park are not going to be supervised by credible and responsible adults in case of a second impact or deterioration of the initial injury and symptoms. Therefore, recommendations regarding return to the activity in such an environment should be conservative in nature at the very least.

Much advice given to the local extreme crowd is not given in a direct fashion following a specific injury, but rather as general instruction in a preventive nature. Much of this instruction is in the form of local newspaper releases and articles to encourage the use of protective equipment and recommendations to seek medical care if an initial head injury is suspected. The opportunity to use expertise as a sports physical therapist may not present itself in a normal fashion, so some thought must be given to these considerations with the extreme athlete as well as some creative means of spreading the word to encourage safe and injury-free participation in and return to extreme sports.

Chapter 48

Running: Preventing Overuse Injuries

What Causes an Overuse Injury in a Runner?

Overuse injury in a runner most often occurs because of a training error (running too far, too fast, too soon). With every mile that is run, the feet must absorb 110 tons of energy. Therefore, it is not surprising that up to 70% of runners develop an injury every year.

How Can Overuse Injury Be Prevented?

You can decrease your risk of injury by following these recommendations:

- Do not increase running mileage by more than 10% per week.

- Do not run more than 45 miles per week. There is very little evidence that running more than 45 miles per week improves your performance, but there is a great deal of evidence that running more than 45 miles per week increases your risk for an overuse injury.

- Do not run on slanted or uneven surfaces. The best running surface is soft, flat terrain.

- Do not run through pain. Pain is a sign that should not be ignored, since it indicates that something is wrong.

- If you do have pain when you run, place ice on the area and rest for 2 or 3 days. If the pain continues for 1 week, see your doctor.

- Follow hard training or running days with easy days.

- Change your running shoes every 500 miles. After this distance shoes lose their ability to absorb the shock of running.

What about Orthotics to Reduce the Chance of Injury?

Orthotics are inserts that are placed in shoes to correct bad alignment between the foot and the lower leg. You will probably need orthotics if you have a problem called pronation, which means that the inside of the foot turns in. If you have bad alignment but no pain with running and you do not suffer from repeated injuries, you probably do not need orthotics. Many world class athletes with bad alignment do not wear orthotics. However, your doctor may suggest orthotics if you have bad alignment and become injured and do not get better with other measures, such as rest, ice, application, and cross-training.

What Exercises Help Prevent or Treat Injuries?

Before and after a run, perform specific stretching exercises. These exercises may also be part of your recovery from an injury. With each exercise, hold the stretch for at least 15 seconds, and do not bounce. Stretch until you feel tension but not pain.

If you do develop an injury, your doctor may suggest particular strengthening exercises. Every day you should do 3 sets of each exercise, with 10 repetitions in each set. For the exercises that involve straight-leg raises, you will want to add ankle weights as the exercises become easier for you to do. These exercises may also be done as part of your overall exercise program.

Stretching Exercises

Hamstring stretch. Sit with your injured leg straight and your other leg bent toward the straight leg. With your back straight and your head up, slowly lean forward at your waist. You should feel the stretch along the underside of your thigh. Hold the stretch for 10 to 15 seconds. Repeat the stretch 6 to 8 times. This stretching exercise may be helpful for patellofemoral syndrome, patellar tendinitis, and hamstring strain.

Iliotibial band stretch. Sit with your injured leg bent and crossed over your straightened opposite leg. Twist at your waist away from your injured leg, and slowly pull your injured leg across your chest. You should feel the stretch along the side of your hip. Hold the stretch for 10 to 15 seconds. Repeat the stretch 6 to 8 times. This stretching exercise may be helpful for iliotibial band syndrome and adductor strain.

Groin stretch. Sit with the soles of your feet together, your back straight, your head up, and your elbows on the inside of your knees. Then slowly push down on the inside of your knees with your elbows. You should feel the stretch along the inside of your thighs. Hold the stretch for 10 to 15 seconds. Repeat the stretch 6 to 8 times. This stretching exercise may be helpful for adductor strain.

Quadriceps stretch. Stand straight with your injured leg bent toward your back. Grasp the foot of your injured leg with your hand and slowly pull your heel to your buttocks. You should feel the stretch in the front of your thigh. Hold the stretch for 10 to 15 seconds. Repeat the stretch 6 to 8 times. This stretching exercise may be helpful for patellofemoral syndrome, iliotibial band syndrome, and patellar tendinitis.

Calf stretch. Stand with your hands against a wall and your injured leg behind your other leg. With your injured leg straight, your heel flat on the floor and your foot pointed straight ahead, lean slowly forward, bending the other leg. You should feel the stretch in the middle of your calf. Hold the stretch for 10 to 15 seconds. Repeat the stretch 6 to 8 times. This stretching exercise may be helpful for Achilles tendinitis, plantar fasciitis, and calcaneal apophysitis.

Plantar fascia stretch. Stand straight with your hands against a wall and your injured leg slightly behind your other leg. Keeping your heels flat on the floor, slowly bend both knees. You should feel the stretch in the lower part of your leg. Hold the stretch for 10 to 15 seconds. Repeat the stretch 6 to 8 times. This stretching exercise may be helpful for plantar fasciitis, Achilles tendinitis, and calcaneal apophysitis.

Strengthening Exercises

Straight-leg raise. Lie down on your back with your upper body supported on your elbows. Tighten the top of the thigh muscle of your injured leg. Raise your leg on a count of 4, hold for a 2 count and then lower the leg on a 4 count. Relax your thigh muscles. Then tighten the thigh and repeat. Do 3 sets of 10 repetitions each day. Once your leg gains strength, do the exercise with weights on your ankle. This strengthening exercise may be particularly helpful for patellofemoral syndrome or patellar tendinitis.

Straight-leg raise. Lie on your unaffected side, tighten the thigh muscle of your injured leg and then slowly raise the leg off the floor. Hold the leg up for a 2 count, and lower it on a 4 count. Relax your muscles. Then tighten the thigh and repeat. Do three sets of 10 repetitions each day. Once your leg gains strength, do the exercise with weights on your ankle. This strengthening exercise may be helpful for iliotibial band syndrome.

Straight-leg raise. Lie on your affected side with the unaffected leg crossed over the knee of your injured leg. Tighten your thigh muscles and raise the injured leg about 6 to 8 inches off the floor. Hold for 2 seconds, and then slowly lower your leg. Relax the muscles. Then tighten the thigh and repeat. Do 3 sets of 10 repetitions each day. Once your leg gains strength, do the exercise with weights on your ankle. This strengthening exercise may be helpful for adductor strain.

Standing wall slide. Stand with your back against the wall and your feet 6 to 8 inches away from the wall. Slowly lower your back and hips about one-third of the way down the wall. Hold the position for about 10 seconds or until you feel that the tops of your thigh muscles are becoming tired. Straighten up and repeat. Perform 10 repetitions each day. This strengthening exercise may be helpful for patellofemoral syndrome or patellar tendinitis.

Straight-leg raise. Lie on your stomach. Tighten your thigh muscles and slowly raise your injured leg off the floor on a 4 count. Hold the leg up for a 2 count, and then lower the leg on a 4 count. Relax your thigh muscles. Tighten the thigh and repeat. Do 3 sets of 10 repetitions each day. Once your leg gains strength, do the exercise with weights on your ankle. This strengthening exercise may be helpful for hamstring strain.

Lateral step-ups. Stand with your injured leg on a stair or platform that is 4 to 6 inches high. Slowly lower the other leg, striking the heel on the floor. Straighten the knee of the injured leg, allowing the foot of the other leg to raise off the floor. Repeat. Do 3 sets of 10 repetitions each day. This strengthening exercise may be helpful for patellofemoral syndrome and patellar tendinitis.

Chapter 49

Sports and Your Feet

Aerobics and Your Feet

What Is Aerobic Dancing?

From humble beginnings in the late 1960s, aerobic dance has become a major symbol of the fitness craze that exploded into American culture in the 1980s. It's still one of the most popular ways to get fit and stay fit around the world. More than 24 million people participate in aerobics. Once confined primarily to young women, aerobic dance has blossomed into a sport for both sexes and all age groups to have fun while losing weight and keeping in shape.

A typical hour aerobics program begins with 5-10 minutes of warm-ups and stretching, peaks with 20-30 minutes of target heart range dance, can include 20 minutes of a muscle stretching floor program known as body sculpting, and ends with 5-10 minutes of cool-down and more stretching. Programs typically run three to four times a week. The benefits of aerobics include increased cardiopulmonary efficiency, strengthened heart and lungs, improved circulation, lowered cholesterol levels, and stress and anxiety reduction.

It is a strenuous form of exercise, and thorough preparation, wise choice of routines, proper equipment, and consideration of floor surfaces are essential to avoid injury. It's a good idea to see a doctor of podiatric medicine specializing in sports medicine before beginning

"Aerobics & Your Feet," and "Winter Sports & Your Feet," both © American Podiatric Medical Association, reprinted with permission.

497

an aerobics regimen. The podiatrist will perform a biomechanical or gait analysis to assess your risk of injury.

Don't Forget the Feet

Because aerobic dancing involves quick lateral movements, jumping, and leaping for extended periods of time, proper care of the foot plays a crucial part in keeping the entire body fit to endure the pain that precedes the gain of a more fit physique and efficient heart and respiratory system. If your feet suffer from excess pronation or supination (your ankles tend to turn inward or outward too much), it's especially important to see a podiatric physician, who may recommend controlling the sometimes harmful motions with an orthotic shoe insert.

Proper shoes are crucial to successful, injury-free aerobics. Shoes should provide sufficient cushioning and shock absorption to compensate for pressure on the foot many times greater than found in walking. They must also have good medial-lateral stability. Impact forces from aerobics can reach up to six times the force of gravity, which is transmitted to each of the 26 bones in the foot. Because of the many side-to-side motions, shoes need an arch design that will compensate for these forces, and sufficiently thick upper leather or strap support to provide forefoot stability and prevent slippage of the foot and lateral shoe "breakup." Make sure shoes have a toe box that is high enough to prevent irritation of toes and nails.

According to the American Aerobics Association International (AAAI), the old sneakers in your closet are probably not proper shoes for aerobics. Major shoe companies today have designed special shoes for aerobics, which provide the necessary arch and side support; they also have soles that allow for the twisting and turning of an aerobics regimen.

Running shoes, perhaps the most popular athletic shoes, lack the necessary lateral stability and lift the heel too high to be considered proper for aerobics. They also often have an acute outside flare that may put the athlete at greater risk of injury in sports, like aerobics, that require side-by-side motion. Running shoes are not recommended by podiatric physicians for aerobics.

Once you've found the proper shoes, tie them securely, but not too tight, in the toe box to allow toes to spread, and tightly around the arch. Double-tie the laces to prevent accidental slippage in mid-routine. Purchase shoes in the afternoon, when the feet swell slightly. Wear the same socks (podiatrists recommend athletic socks made of an acrylic blend) that you will wear in training.

Prevention of Injuries

In a physically challenging sport such as aerobics, injuries are common, and often involve the foot, ankle, and lower leg. (Other susceptible parts of the body are the knee and back.) Physicians say most injuries from aerobics result from improper shoes, surfaces, or routines, and overuse of muscles through too vigorous a regimen.

New, properly tied, well-fitted aerobic-specific shoes will address the first problem, and common sense will help the with the others. The key to injury prevention is proper conditioning, which will provide muscles the flexibility and strength needed to avoid injury.

If you are attending an aerobics class, make sure it is led by a certified instructor. Hardwood floors, especially with padded mats, are the best surfaces possible. If you can, start with a multi-impact class, where you can start at a low-impact level and work your way up as your conditioning improves.

If your routine is at home with a video, be very careful. Read the label to determine whether the video is produced by certified aerobics instructors and whether you can handle the degree of impact. While it's safe to do low-to-moderate impact aerobics on the living room carpet, that's not a proper surface for high-impact routines. In addition, make sure the video includes a proper warm-up period. Make sure there are no rapid, violent movements. Do not bounce, use ballistic stretching, or stretches known as the Yoga plow or hurdler's stretch. Knees should always be loose during warm-up. A static stretch held for 10 seconds can help avoid over-stretching injury.

As you work out, monitor your heart rate to stay near the target heart range (start with 220, subtract your age, then multiply by 0.8 to find target heart range). You should be within five of the target range. Monitor pulse at peak and after final cool-off and compare. The difference is known as your cardiac reserve.

Drink lots of water to avoid dehydration during workouts; it can cause nausea, dizziness, muscle fatigue, and cramping.

Don't underestimate the importance of the cool-off period. It burns off lactic acid (which makes muscles feel tired) and adrenalin, while keeping blood from pooling in the extremities.

While fitness professionals exercise vigorously six times a week, it's best to start slower. Although it varies by the individual, it's safe to start exercising twice a week for several weeks, then gradually increase to a maximum of five times a week. Remember to pace yourself, and listen to your body. If you feel pain, stop. Don't attempt to exercise through pain, or you may aggravate an acute injury into a chronic or even permanent one. If you continue to be bothered by pain more than 24 hours after exercising, see a physician.

Common Aerobics Injuries

Plantar fasciitis (arch pain)—Arch pain is often caused by frequent stress on the plantar aspect, or bottom of the foot, in an aerobics routine. When the plantar fascia, a supportive, fibrous band of tissue running from the heel to the ball of the foot, becomes inflamed, pain on the bottom of the foot results. Forefoot and rear foot instability, with excessive pronation, may result in plantar fasciitis. Shoes with proper support in the arch often prevent plantar fasciitis; if not, see your podiatrist for a custom orthotic device or a recommendation for another shoe.

Heel spurs—Heel spur syndrome, related to plantar fasciitis, occurs after calcium deposits build up on the underside of the heel bone. Heel spurs form gradually over many months. Both plantar fasciitis and heel spurs can be avoided by a proper warm-up that includes stretching the band of tissue on the bottom of the foot.

Sesamoiditis—Sometimes referred to as the ball bearings of the foot, the sesamoids are a set of accessory bones found beneath the large first metatarsal bone. Incredible forces are exerted on the sesamoid bones during aerobics, and inflammation and fractures can occur. Proper shoe selection and custom orthotic devices can help avoid sesamoiditis.

Shin splints—Aside from ankle sprains, shin splints are perhaps the most common injury to the lower body, as the muscles attached to the shin bone bring the foot up and down. The pain is usually an inflammation of the shin muscle and tendon due to stress factors. Treat shin pain with cold compresses immediately after the workout to reduce inflammation. Proper stretching before the workout should prevent the onset of shin splints. Strengthening of muscles also helps reduce shin splints.

Achilles tendon and calf pain—The frequent rising on the toes of an aerobics routine often creates pain and tightness in the large muscles in the back of the legs, which can create pain and tightness in the calf and inflammation of the Achilles tendon. Again, stretching the calf muscles gently and gradually before and after the workout will ordinarily help alleviate the pain and stiffness.

Stress fractures—Probably the most common injuries to aerobics instructors, stress fractures are caused by poor shoe selection, hard surfaces, and overuse. Women are more likely to develop stress fractures, usually in the lesser metatarsal bones, than men. When swelling and pain surface, see a podiatrist. X-ray evaluation and early treatment can prevent a disabling injury.

If you experience any of these injuries, see a physician (a podiatrist can treat most of them), who will prescribe treatments to alleviate the pain, and make recommendations to prevent recurrence of any discomfort. As foot specialists trained in all aspects of foot care, podiatrists are also qualified to perform foot surgery if the condition requires it.

The Bottom Line

The bottom line when undertaking an aerobic dance program is to be careful and responsible. Aerobics may even provide a more vigorous workout than jogging, and injuries will inevitably occur if you don't listen to your body and exercise your common sense as well as your muscles.

Remember there are good aerobics programs and bad ones. Use discretion in choosing both a class to attend or home video to purchase that is right for you. Always pace yourself, and stop if you feel pain. Remember, foot pain is not normal, so don't ignore it. Chances are, a successful aerobics regimen will bring out the body you've always dreamed of, and a better feeling about yourself both physically and mentally.

Winter Sports and Your Feet

Winter's Own Sports

Under the pastoral beauty of a blanket of fresh-fallen snow, the outdoors beckons. For a while, winter doesn't feel quite so cold, and people of all ages feel a sense of youthful excitement about bundling up and getting outside. From the downhill rush of snow skiing or sledding, to rough-and-tumble ice hockey or placid casual skating, winter provides a fast track for fun and cardiovascular health.

In the absence of long, sunny days, winter sports provide the exercise active Americans otherwise couldn't get without being cooped up in a gym. High speeds attained on skis and skates make for exhilarating sports, but expose the body to injuries. Healthy feet and ankles, which act together as accelerators, steering, brakes, and shock absorbers in winter sports, are not only crucial to success in competition, but also help keep the body upright and out of the emergency room. Any problems with the foot or ankle could have serious repercussions for winter sports participants.

Preventing Cold Feet

Without warm, dry clothes, any wintertime outdoor activity is a potential health risk. Proper footwear—insulated, waterproof boots or shoes—is as important as coats, hats, or gloves in the outdoors during the winter. Socks are also important. Podiatric physicians recommend a single pair of thick socks made of acrylic fibers, or a blend including them, that wick away moisture caused by perspiration in the boot.

Feet soaked in snow should get back indoors quickly. In sub-freezing temperatures, soaked feet are in immediate danger of frostbite, a serious, painful condition that can result in loss of toes or fingers.

Impact Trauma

In skiing, particularly at an intermediate or advanced level, high speeds and force of gravity place tremendous levels of impact trauma on the lower extremity, especially on steep and bumpy runs. Skating also puts tremendous stress on the ankle. Hockey players change direction at speeds near 30 miles per hour, and even casual figure skating requires quick turns and stops negotiated by the lower extremity.

If any preexisting foot conditions, such as corns, calluses, bunions, or hammertoes are present, see a podiatric physician, a specialist of the foot and ankle, for evaluation before buckling or lacing up. A medical examination is also important if you have any preexisting circulatory problems, such as Raynaud's Disease or diabetes.

Before taking to the ice or slopes in cold weather, it's important to loosen up the muscles by stretching. Stretching helps to prevent muscle pulls and tears, and prepares the muscles for the flexing required by the constant forward lean stress of skiing and skating.

Ski Boots and Skates: A Perfect Fit, Please

Podiatric physicians specializing in sports medicine say properly fitted ski boots and skates are the single most important factor in safe and successful skiing and skating. Without a snug (but not too tight) and accurate fit, the pressure exerted by the constant forward motion and lateral movement of skiing and quick turns of skating will surely result in discomfort or injury. If boots and skates are too loose, toes quickly get irritated in the toe box. If they are too tight, pressure leads to blisters and abrasions that result in a host of painful problems and keep you indoors or, worse, compromise control and lead to an accident. Tight footwear also may inhibit circulation of the blood vessels of the lower extremity and cause cold feet, which both compromises performance and presents danger in the cold.

Ski boots are available in a forward-entry variety, a rear-entry style for easier entry and more comfort, or hybrids which incorporate both designs. Modern systems of cables and buckles make it possible to alter the boots to a near-perfect fit.

With ice skates, proper fit is equally important. Do not put children in hand-me-downs; skates that are too large or too small will cause blisters, inflammation of the foot, or nail irritation. The lack of proper ankle support in a too-large skate will leave the ankle susceptible to sprains, strains, or fractures. Whatever the style, skates should be laced snugly, using all the eyelets.

If you are not sure your ski boots or skates fit properly, or if an apparently proper-fitting pair still hurts, take them to a podiatric physician, who can evaluate the fit and make recommendations to improve both comfort and performance on the ice or slopes.

Cross-Country Skiing and Winter Running

Cross-country skiing is quite distinct from downhill skiing. An excellent way to maintain cardiovascular fitness in the winter, cross-country involves the entire body and requires different equipment. Cross-country footwear is more like a bicycle shoe than a downhill boot. Bound to the ski only at the ball of the foot, cross-country boots should not irritate the balls of the feet.

As with running in winter, proper stretching is vital before cross-country skiing. In cross-country, the heel goes up and down constantly. Without proper loosening up first, the motion can result in painful Achilles tendinitis and plantar fasciitis, among other problems. A podiatric physician can recommend proper stretching exercises.

Dedicated runners hate to give up their passion during the winter months. Remember, however, that muscles take longer to warm up in the cold, and the body is much more susceptible to muscle pulls and tear injuries. Again, proper stretching is essential. Whether consciously or unconsciously, runners may change their foot-strike pattern to protect themselves, which can lead to muscle strain or other overuse injuries. To increase traction, runners may land on slippery surfaces with the whole foot instead of the natural rolling action of the heel-to-toe strike. Lateral slippage could result in a painful groin pull.

It's best to avoid running on icy areas, but if that's impossible, podiatric physicians give a qualified endorsement to use of spikes slipped over running shoes. Spikes, however, have their own problems, so don't use them in winter if you're not familiar with their use on a running track.

Even though your feet are in motion while running, they're still susceptible to frostbite in thin nylon running shoes. Feet will sweat while running, and cold will permeate the thin material, inviting the condition. If shoes are too tight, there is an even greater chance of frostbite.

Biomechanics of Winter Sports

Keeping the ankle perpendicular to the ground and straight up and down while skiing brings out the best performance. Users of custom orthoses (shoe inserts) should transfer them to skis and skates to help maintain the best possible position. Skiers with minor biomechanical imbalances may encounter a frustrating phenomenon known as edging, in which the ski rolls to the inside or outside edge, inhibiting control going down the slopes.

Ski boots and skates can be canted internally to adjust the relationship between the boot and leg. For cases of rolling-in of the foot, or pronation, or rolling-out (supination), caused by flat feet or high arches, cants may be applied directly to the skis or within the boot. This improves edging and enhances performance and control, making the sport safer and more enjoyable. Ski shop technicians can work in conjunction with podiatric physicians on specific biomechanical adjustments to improve performance and safety.

Ice skates do not come in as many shapes and sizes as ski boots. Common side-to-side wobbling in the heel area can be remedied with shims, or pads, in the heel. Shims can also be added to the counter area, or middle of the skate, for a more snug fit.

Snowboarding

In recent years, skiers have shared the slopes with more snowboards—wide single skis that zigzag down the slopes. The feet are loosely bound perpendicular to the board. No special footwear is required for snowboarding, but podiatric physicians say large, sturdy, insulated boots flexible enough to accommodate the twisting of the lower body are best to safely control the board. Most popular with young people, snowboarding has become a bona fide alpine sport, and more snowboarders will share the slopes with skiers in the future.

Potential Foot Problems in Winter Sports

Frostbite. It's impossible to overstate the importance of understanding symptoms of frostbite. Skin-color changes, from blue to whitish, can't be seen under a boot, but if toes are extremely cold for a prolonged period, feel burning or numb, there is a danger of frostbite. People with a history of frostbite often get it again in the same place. New battery-powered heated ski boots are effective in preventing its occurrence. New exothermic packs are also effective in keeping the extremities warm and preventing frostbite.

Blisters. Friction in winter sports footwear often causes blisters. Do not pop a small blister, but if it breaks on its own, apply an antiseptic and cover with a sterile bandage.

Neuromas. Enlarged benign growths of nerves between the toes, called neuromas, are caused by friction in tight footwear and can result in pain, burning, tingling, or numbness. Neuromas require professional treatment, including an evaluation of skates and boots.

Sprains and strains. The stress of skiing and skating can result in sprains and strains of the foot and ankle. They can be treated with rest, ice, compression, and elevation (RICE). If pain persists, seek medical attention.

Subungual Hematoma. Pressure in the toe box of a ski or skate can cause bleeding under the toenail known as a subungual hematoma. Such a condition should be treated by a podiatric physician to prevent the loss of a toenail.

Bone Problems. Bunions and tailor's bunions, bony prominences at the joints on the inside or outside of the foot, often become irritated in ski boots or skates. Pain at these joints may indicate a need for a wider or better-fitting boot. Other preexisting conditions, such as hammertoes, and Haglund's Deformity (a bump on the back of the heel) can be irritated by an active winter sports regimen. If pain persists, consult a podiatric physician. Fractures caused by trauma require immediate medical attention.

Additional Information

The American Podiatric Medical Association
9312 Old Georgetown Road
Bethesda, MD 20814
Toll-Free: 800-366-8227
Tel: 301-571-9200
Fax: 301-530-2752
Website: www.apma.org
E-mail: askapma@apma.org

The American Academy of Podiatric Sports Medicine
4414 Ives Street
Rockville, MD 20853
Toll-Free: 800-438-3355
Tel: 301-962-1540
Website: wwwaapsm.org
E-mail: info@aapsm.org

Chapter 50

Prevent Baseball/Softball Injuries

Each year, more than 125,000 baseball and softball players under age 15 are injured badly enough to seek treatment in hospital emergency departments. Hundreds of thousands of adults receive minor injuries in these sports. Many of the injuries can be prevented if players wear safety gear and if additional safety measures are added to the game.

Tips for Preventing Baseball and Softball Injuries

To help your child avoid injuries while playing baseball or softball, follow these safety tips from the American Academy of Pediatrics, the Centers for Disease Control and Prevention (CDC), the Consumer Product Safety Commission, and other sports and health organizations. (Note: These tips apply to adult ball players, too.)

- Before your child starts a training program or plays competitive baseball or softball, take him or her to the doctor for a physical exam. The doctor can help assess any special injury risks your child may have.

- **Make sure your child wears all the required safety gear every time he or she plays and practices.** Insist that your child wear a helmet when batting, waiting to bat, or running the bases. Helmets should have eye protectors, either safety

"Baseball and Softball Safety," SafeUSA™, Centers for Disease Control and Prevention, updated February 2001.

goggles or face guards. Shoes with molded cleats are recommended (most youth leagues prohibit the use of steel spikes).

- If your child is a catcher, he or she will need additional safety gear: catcher's mitt, face mask, throat guard, long-model chest protector, and shin guards. If your child is a pitcher, make sure pitching time is limited. Little League mandates time limits and requires rest periods for young pitchers.

- Insist that your child warm-up and stretch before playing.

- Teach your child not to play through pain. If your child gets injured, see your doctor. Follow all the doctor's orders for recovery, and get the doctor's approval before your child returns to play.

- Make sure first aid is available at all games and practices.

- Talk to and watch your child's coach. Coaches should enforce all the rules of the game, encourage safe play, and understand the special injury risks that young players face. Make sure your child's coach teaches players how to avoid injury when sliding (prohibits headfirst sliding in young players), pitching, or dodging a ball pitched directly at them.

- Above all, keep baseball and softball fun. Putting too much focus on winning can make your child push too hard and risk injury.

Encourage your league to use breakaway bases. These bases, which detach when someone slides into them, can prevent many ankle and knee injuries in both children and adults. Leagues with players 10 years old and under should alter the rules of the game to include the use of adult pitchers or batting tees. Remember, you don't have to be on a baseball diamond to get hurt. Make sure your child wears safety gear and follows safety rules during informal baseball and softball games, too.

Who Is Affected?

In the United States, more than 33 million people participate in organized baseball and softball leagues. Nearly 6 million of these players are 5 to 14 years old. Even though these sports are not considered contact sports, they are associated with a large number of injuries. Hospital emergency departments treat more than 95,000 baseball-related injuries and 30,000 softball-related injuries among players under age 15 each year. The number of injuries among adults is also high, with as many as 8 percent of players sustaining injuries each year.

The majority of injuries in baseball and softball are minor, consisting mostly of abrasions (scrapes), sprains, strains, and fractures. Many of these injuries are to the ankle and knee. Eye injuries are also common in baseball. In fact, baseball is the leading cause of sports-related eye injuries in children. Catastrophic injuries in baseball and softball are rare. They occur most often when players are struck in the head or chest with a ball or a bat. On average, 3 children under age 15 die each year from baseball-related injuries.

Baseball can lead to injuries caused by overusing a certain body part. Pitchers commonly suffer overuse injuries in their elbows or shoulders. As many as 45 percent of pitchers under age 12 have chronic elbow pain, and among high school pitchers, the percentage rises to 58 percent. To prevent these injuries, Little League Baseball, Inc., has set a limit of six innings of pitching per week and requires pitchers to rest between appearances. Teaching proper pitching mechanics can also prevent serious overuse injuries.

Helmets and safety equipment for catchers have brought about reductions in injuries. Little League Rule 1.7 says *a catcher's helmet must meet NOCSAE specifications and standards.* Other safety gear has been added more recently, including eye protectors and face masks on helmets. Chest protectors and softer balls are also being studied for their protective effect.

Making changes to the playing field and the rules of the game can also prevent injuries. Sliding into the base causes more than 70 percent of recreational softball injuries and nearly one-third of baseball injuries. Using bases that break away upon impact can prevent 1.7 million injuries per year. Adding screens or fencing to the dugout and eliminating the on-deck circle protects players from wild pitches, foul balls, and flying bats.

Additional Information

American Academy of Orthopaedic Surgeons (AAOS)
6300 North River Road
Rosemont, IL 60018-4262
Toll-Free: 800-346-2267
Tel: 847-823-7186
Fax: 847-823-8125
AAOS Fax-on-Demand: 800-999-2939
Website: www.aaos.org
E-mail: custserv@aaos.org

American Academy of Pediatrics (AAP)
141 Northwest Point Boulevard
Elk Grove Village, IL 60007-1098
Tel: 847-434-4000
Fax: 847-434-8000
Website: www.aap.org/default/htm
E-mail: kidsdocs@aap.org

American Red Cross
P.O. Box 37243
Washington, DC 20013
Toll-Free: 800-435-7669
Website: www.redcross.org

Brain Injury Association
105 North Alfred Street
Alexandria, VA 22314
Toll-Free: 800-444-6443
Tel: 703-236-6000
Fax: 703-236-6001
Website: www.biausa.org
E-mail: familyhelpline@biausa.org

· BIA's fact sheet about sports and concussion safety provides data on brain injuries for several sports, including baseball.

U.S. Consumer Product Safety Commission
4330 East-West Highway
Bethesda, MD 20814-4408
Toll-Free: 800-638-2772
Tel: 301-504-0990
Fax: 301-504-0124 and 301-504-0025
Website: www.cpsc.gov
E-mail: info@cpsc.gov

Little League Baseball, Inc.
P.O. Box 3485
Williamsport, PA 17701
Tel: 570-326-1921
Website: www.littleleague.org

National SAFE KIDS Campaign
1301 Pennsylvania Ave. NW, Suite 1000
Washington, DC 20004

Tel: 202-662-0600
Fax: 202-393-2072
Website: www.safekids.org
E-mail: info@safekids.org

Fact sheets on sports and recreation injuries.

References

American Academy of Orthopaedic Surgeons. Baseball. Available at http://www.aaos.org/wordhtml/pat_educ/baseball.htm. Accessed July 8, 1999.

American Academy of Orthopaedic Surgeons Seminar (Sullivan J, Grana W, editors). The Pediatric Athlete. Park Ridge, IL: *The Academy*, 1990:141,149-151,259.

American Academy of Pediatrics. Risk of injury from baseball and softball in children 5 to 14 years of age. *Pediatrics* 1994;93(4):690-692.

American Academy of Pediatrics. Sports Medicine: Health care for young athletes. Elk Grove Village, IL: *The Academy*, 1991:148-150.

American Red Cross. *Red Cross gears up to help prevent sports injuries this spring: coaches advised on proper conditioning of young athletes.* News release, May 7, 1998.

Caine D, Caine C, Lindner K, editors. *Epidemiology of Sports Injuries.* Champaign, IL: Human Kinetics, 1996:63-85.

CDC. Sliding-associated injuries in college and professional baseball - 1990-1991. *Morbidity and Mortality Weekly Report* 1993;42(12):223,229-230.

Institute for Preventative Sports Medicine. *Softball injuries: Phase I of a study on the costs, causes and prevention of recreational softball injuries.* Available at http://users.aol.com/wwwipsm/pubs/softball_I.html. Accessed July 7, 1999.

U.S. Consumer Product Safety Commission. *Baseball safety.* CPSC publication #329. Washington, DC: The Commission.

U.S. Consumer Product Safety Commission. Reducing youth baseball injuries with protective equipment. *Consumer Product Safety Review* 1996;1(1):1-4.

Chapter 51

Heading Off Soccer Injuries

Soccer Safety

More than 200,000 youths under age 15 are treated each year in hospital emergency departments, doctors' offices, clinics, and outpatient centers for injuries related to soccer. Many injuries can be prevented if players wear proper safety gear and follow the rules of the game. Increasing the safety of the goal posts can also reduce the number of injuries.

Tips for Preventing Soccer Injuries

To help your child avoid injury while playing soccer, follow these safety tips from the American Academy of Pediatrics, the American Academy of Orthopaedic Surgeons, the U.S. Consumer Product Safety Commission, and other sports health organizations. (Note: Adults should heed this safety guidance, too.)

- Before your child starts a training program or enters a competition, take him or her to the doctor for a physical exam. The doctor can help assess any special injury risks your child may have.

- Make sure your child wears all the required safety gear every time he or she plays and practices. Your child should wear shin

"Soccer Safety," SafeUSA™, Centers for Disease Control and Prevention, updated July 2001.

guards during every game and every practice. Shoes with molded cleats or ribbed soles are recommended.

- Insist that your child warm up and stretch before playing. Don't allow your child to shoot goals before warming up.

- Teach your child not to play through pain. If your child gets injured, see your doctor. Follow all the doctor's orders for recovery, and get the doctor's approval before your child returns to play.

- Make sure first aid is available at all games and practices.

- Insist that your child follow and that coaches and referees enforce all the rules of the game. For example, most leagues prohibit sliding tackles from behind, which can result in serious injury to players.

- Talk to and watch your child's coach. Coaches should enforce all the rules of the game, encourage safe play, and understand the special injury risks that young players face.

- Ask your child's doctor and coach whether it's safe for your child to head the ball and, if so, make sure your child knows how to head the ball correctly to avoid head and neck injury.

- Don't let your child climb on the goal posts or hang or swing from the crossbar.

- Above all, keep soccer fun. Putting too much focus on winning can make your child push too hard and risk injury.

Make sure the field and equipment are safe. Work with coaches, city officials, and other parents to improve safety.

- Encourage your child's league to use waterproof, synthetic balls instead of leather ones. Leather balls can become waterlogged and very heavy, making them dangerous for play.

- Make sure movable soccer goals are anchored to the ground at all times, not just during play. Goals have been known to tip over in strong winds or when climbed on, causing severe injuries.

If the goal posts on your field(s) don't have padding, talk to school or park authorities about adding pads. Studies have shown that padding on goal posts greatly reduces the risk of serious injury caused by a player's head hitting the post.

Who Is Affected?

With about 40 million amateur players, soccer is the most popular sport worldwide. It is also a sport associated with a fairly high rate of injury. In the U.S., more than 200,000 young people each year are injured badly enough to seek medical treatment.

For players under 12 years old, the injury rate in soccer is very low—less than 1 percent—but the injury rate rises with age. Nearly 8 percent of high school soccer players are injured in a season, and among community leagues, nearly 9 percent of players 19 years old and younger sustain injuries. Older participants sustain more frequent and severe injuries than young players, and girls are injured more often than boys. Most injuries are caused by illegal plays, poor field conditions, or heading the ball incorrectly.

Injuries in soccer are usually mild—sprains, strains, and contusions (bruises)—and mostly affect the lower extremities. The most common site of injury is the ankle, followed closely by the knee. Acute head injuries are rare, accounting for about 5 percent of injuries. Many of the most severe injuries are related to soccer goal posts. Goal posts have been responsible for at least 22 deaths in the last 20 years, and hospital emergency departments treat about 90 goal-related injuries each year. Most of these deaths and injuries have been caused by hitting one's head on the goal post or being hit or crushed by a falling goal post.

Injuries can be prevented if players wear shin guards, warm up before play, and follow the rules of the game. Changes in equipment can also greatly enhance injury prevention efforts. Most notably, the addition of padding to goal posts can reduce the number and severity of head injuries. Laboratory testing has shown that padding reduces the force of hitting the post by 31 to 63 percent. Anchoring movable goal posts to the ground at all times, even when not in use, can also greatly reduce some of the most serious injuries. The National Federation of State High School Associations' Soccer Rules Committee now requires that soccer goals be anchored. The international soccer association (FIFA) is also considering making this change to its rules.

Additional Information

American Academy of Orthopaedic Surgeons
6300 North River Road
Rosemont, IL 60018-4262
Toll-Free: 800-346-AAOS (2267)
Tel: 847-823-7186

American Academy of Orthopaedic Surgeons (continued)
Fax: 847-823-8125
AAOS Fax-on Demand: 800-999-2939
Website: www.aaos.org
E-mail: custserv@aaos.org

Brain Injury Association
105 North Alfred Street
Alexandria, VA 22314
Toll-Free: 800-444-6443
Tel: 703-236-6001
Website: www.biausa.org
E-mail: familyhelpline@biausa.org

National Athletic Trainers Association
2952 Stemmons Freeway
Dallas, TX 75247-6916
Toll-Free: 800-879-6282
Tel: 214-637-6282
Fax: 214-637-2206
Website: www.nata.org
E-mail: natanews@nata.org

National Youth Sports Safety Foundation
One Beacon Street, Suite 3333
Boston, MA 02108
Tel: 617-277-1771
Fax: 617-722-9999
Website: www.nyssf.org
E-mail: NYSSF@aol.com

U.S. Consumer Product Safety Commission
4330 East-West Highway
Bethesda, MD 20814-4408
Toll-Free: 800-638-2772
Fax: 301-504-0124 and 301-504-0025
Website: www.cpsc.gov
E-mail: info@cpsc.gov

References

American Academy of Orthopaedic Surgeons. *Public information on soccer.* Available at www.aaos.org/wordhtml/pat_educ/soccer.htm. Accessed July 1999.

American Academy of Orthopaedic Surgeons Seminar (Sullivan J, Grana W, editors). *The Pediatric Athlete.* Park Ridge, IL: The Academy, 1990:141.

American Academy of Pediatrics. *Sports Medicine: Health care for young athletes.* Elk Grove Village, IL: The Academy, 1991:154-155.

Bir C, Cassatta S, Janda D. *An analysis and comparison of soccer shin guards (abstract).* The Institute for Preventative Sports Medicine web site. Available at www.ipsm.org. Accessed July 1999.

Caine D, Caine C, Lindner K, editors. Epidemiology of Sports Injuries. Champaign, IL: *Human Kinetics,* 1996:387-398.

CDC. Injuries associated with soccer goalposts–United States, 1979-1993. *Morbidity and Mortality Weekly Report* 1994;43(9):153-155.

Janda D, Bir C, Wild B, Olson S, Hensinger R. *A laboratory and field testing analysis of a preventive intervention (abstract).* The Institute for Preventative Sports Medicine web site. Available at www.ipsm.org.

U.S. Consumer Product Safety Commission. *New standard for soccer goals helps prevent tip-over deaths linked to unanchored goals.* News release, May 4, 1999.

U.S. Consumer Product Safety Commission. *CPSC warns consumers: anchor soccer goals to prevent tip-over.* News release, March 29, 1996.

Chapter 52

Winter Sports Injury Prevention

For many children, winter is not the end of outdoor fun. From sledding to skiing, snowmobiling to ice skating, children find lots to do when the snow starts to fall. Unfortunately, the cold season can also lead to tragedy.

For 10-year-old Joshua of Minnesota, it was a deadly snowmobile incident. Five-year-old Jonathan from Massachusetts nearly drowned. Frostbite affected 3-year-old Nicole of Colorado. Winter does not need to be a tragic time for children. When properly prepared, they can enjoy a safe and fun-filled winter wonderland.

"The inviting snow draws children to ice-covered lakes and ski slopes each winter, regardless of the frigid temperatures and the risks," says Heather Paul, Ph.D., executive director of the National SAFE KIDS Campaign. "Parents should watch their children closely, limit their outdoor playtime, and make sure that they are dressed appropriately for the weather." The National SAFE KIDS Campaign recommends the following tips to help keep your children safe.

Winter Drowning

Most parents associate drowning with summer months, but the increased use of hot tubs and whirlpools as well as the danger of hidden bodies of water or weak ice make winter drowning a risk as well. To minimize drowning dangers, parents and caregivers should:

"Stay Safe in Your Winter Wonderland," National SAFE KIDS Campaign, 2000; and "Winter Sports Injury Prevention," SafeUSA, 2000.

- Supervise children in or near a pool, hot tub, or any open body of water.

- Make sure pools and spas are secure. If you have a pool or spa, install four-sided isolation fencing that is at least 5 feet high. The fence should have a self-closing and self-latching gate. Do not use the exterior of the house as one side of the fence.

- Allow children to skate only on ponds or lakes that have been approved for skating.

Frostbite

Exposure to cold without adequate protection can result in frostbite. Parents can protect their children by following these precautions:

- Dress children warmly. Several thin layers will help keep children dry as well as warm. Clothing should consist of thermal long johns, turtlenecks, one or two shirts, pants, sweater, coat, warm socks, boots, gloves or mittens, and a hat.

- Set reasonable time limits on outdoor play. Call children in periodically to warm up with drinks such as hot chocolate.

- When possible, avoid taking infants outdoors when it is colder than 40 degrees Fahrenheit. Infants lose body heat quickly.

If a child complains of numbness or pain in the fingers, toes, nose, cheeks, or ears while playing in the snow, or if his skin is blistered, hard to the touch or glossy, be alerted to the possibility of frostbite and take the following steps:

- Take the child indoors.

- Call a doctor.

- Tell the child to wiggle the affected body part(s) to increase blood supply to that area.

- Warm the frozen part(s) against the body. Hold fingers to the chest, for example.

- Immerse frozen part(s) in warm, not hot, water. Frozen tissue is fragile and can be damaged easily. Avoid warming with high heat from radiators, fireplaces, or stoves, and avoid rubbing or breaking blisters.

Pedestrian Safety

Slippery driveways and sidewalks can be particularly hazardous in the winter. Keep them well shoveled, and apply materials such as rock salt or sand to improve traction.

- Make sure that children under age 10 do not cross streets alone, and make sure children wear appropriate shoes and brightly colored (not white) clothing while walking in snowy conditions.

- Use retro-reflective clothing or stickers for maximum protection, especially at dawn and dusk.

Winter Sports and Activities

Parents and caregivers should inspect equipment and the environment for possible hazards before children engage in winter activities such as sledding, ice skating, and skiing. Remind children not to push, shove, or roughhouse while engaging in sports, and tell them always to wait their turn.

Ice Skating

In 1999, more than 16,000 children ages 5 to 14 were treated in emergency rooms for injuries related to ice skating. But with extra care, even children as young as age 4, as long as they are steady walkers, can enjoy the sport. Allow children to skate only on approved surfaces. Check for signs posted by local police or recreation departments, or call your local police department to find out which areas have been approved. Children should be taught to:

- Skate in the same direction as the crowd.

- Avoid darting across the ice.

- Never skate alone.

- Never go out on ice that an adult has not approved.

- Throw away chewing gum or candy before skating onto the ice.

- If a child falls through the ice, he should stretch his arms over the ice and kick as if swimming, in an attempt to crawl back onto the solid ice.

Sledding

More than 14,000 children ages 5 to 14 were treated in emergency rooms in 1999 for injuries related to sledding. Parents and caregivers should remember the following tips:

- Make sure terrain is free of obstacles and far from traffic. Children should sled on packed snow (not ice) that is free of debris. Check carefully for snow-covered hazards such as rocks, tree limbs, and stumps that could endanger sledders or skiers.

- Use equipment that is sturdy and safely constructed. Avoid equipment with sharp and jagged edges.

- Look for energy absorbing pads on sled seats.

- Examine handholds on sleds to be sure they are secure.

- Ensure sleds and toboggans have easy steering, non-jamming devices.

Parents should remind children to:

- Sled only on terrain that is free of obstacles.

- Make sure the bottom of the slope is far from streets and traffic.

- Always use a sled with a steering mechanism. Avoid makeshift sleds.

- Avoid lying flat on the sled while riding down hill. Always sit up with feet forward—lying flat increases the chance of head and abdominal injuries.

- Never ride in a sled that is being pulled by a motorized vehicle.

- Make sure the number of children riding on the sled does not exceed the manufacturer's recommendations.

Snow Skiing and Snowboarding

According to the National Sporting Goods Association, nearly 10 million persons participate in alpine skiing more than once a year and up to 2.5 million snowboard each year. Skiing, snowboarding, and sledding can be great fun and are terrific ways to exercise. But they can also be risky. The U.S. Consumer Product Safety Commission (CPSC) estimates that 84,200 skiing injuries and 37,600 snowboarding injuries were treated in hospital emergency rooms in the United States in 1997, including approximately 17,500 head injuries. However, the most common skiing-related injuries are knee and ankle sprains and fractures. While most skiing and snowboarding injuries occur among adults, the majority of sledding-related injuries are among children 5-14 years old. More than 14,500 children in this age group were treated for sledding-related injuries in the United States in 1997.

The estimated number of skiing-related injuries declined by more than 25 percent from 1993 to 1997, partly because of improvements in ski equipment, such as redesigned bindings. However, during that same period, snowboarding injuries nearly tripled and the number of head injuries from snowboarding increased five-fold.

A CPSC study found there were 17,500 head injuries associated with skiing and snowboarding in 1997. This study estimated that 7,700 head injuries, including 2,600 head injuries to children, could be prevented or reduced in severity each year by using skiing or snowboarding helmets. The study also showed that helmet use could prevent about 11 skiing- and snowboarding-related deaths annually. As a result of these findings, CPSC recommends skiers and snowboarders wear helmets specifically designed for these activities to prevent head injuries from falls and collisions.

Preparation

- Before you get out on the slopes, be sure you're in shape. You'll enjoy the sports more and have lower risk of injury if you're physically fit.

- Take a lesson (or several) from a qualified instructor. Like anything, you'll improve the most when you receive expert guidance. And be sure to learn how to fall correctly and safely to reduce the risk of injury.

- Don't start jumping maneuvers until you've had proper instruction on how to jump and have some experience. Jumps are the most common cause of spinal injuries among snowboarders.

- Obtain proper equipment. Be sure that your equipment is in good condition and have your ski or snowboard bindings adjusted correctly at a local ski shop. (Extra tip for snowboarders: wrist guards and knee pads can help protect you when you fall.)

- Wear a helmet to prevent head injuries from falls or collisions. (One study showed that helmet use by skiers and snowboarders could prevent or reduce the severity of nearly half of head injuries to adults and more than half of head injuries to children less than 15 years old.) Skiers and snowboarders should wear helmets specifically designed for these sports.

- When buying ski wear, look for fabric that is water and wind-resistant. Look for wind flaps to shield zippers, snug cuffs at wrists and ankles, collars that can be snuggled up to the chin, and drawstrings that can be adjusted for comfort and to keep the wind out.

- Dress in layers. Layering allows you to accommodate your body's constantly changing temperature. For example, dress in polypropylene underwear (top and bottoms), which feels good next to the skin, dries quickly, absorbs sweat, and keeps you warm. Wear a turtleneck, sweater, and jacket.

- Be prepared for changes in the weather. Bring a headband or hat with you to the slopes (60 percent of heat loss is through the head) and wear gloves or mittens.

- Protect your skin from the sun and wind by using a sun screen or sun block. The sun reflects off the snow and is stronger than you think, even on cloudy days!

- Always use appropriate eye protection. Sunglasses or goggles will help protect your vision from glare, help you to see the terrain better, and help shield your eyes from flying debris.

When You're on the Slopes

- The key to successful skiing and snowboarding is control. To have it, you must be aware of your technique and level of ability, the terrain, and the skiers and snowboarders around you.

- Take a couple of slow ski or snowboard runs to warm up at the start of each day.

- Ski or snowboard with partners and stay within sight of each other, if possible. If one partner loses the other, stop, and wait.

- Stay on marked trails and avoid potential avalanche areas such as steep hillsides with little vegetation. Begin a run slowly. Watch out for rocks and patches of ice on the trails.

- Be aware of the weather and snow conditions and how they can change. Make adjustments for icy conditions, deep snow powder, wet snow, and adverse weather conditions.

- If you find yourself on a slope that exceeds your ability level, always leave your skis or snowboard on and sidestep down the slope.

- If you find yourself skiing or snowboarding out of control, fall down on your rear end or on your side, the softest parts of your body.

- Drink plenty of water to avoid becoming dehydrated.

- Avoid alcohol consumption. Skiing and snowboarding do not mix well with alcohol or drugs. Beware of medicines or drugs that impair the senses or make you drowsy.

- If you're tired, stop, and rest. Fatigue is a risk factor for injuries.

The National Ski Areas Association endorses a responsibility code for skiers. This code can be applied to snowboarders also. The following are the code's seven safety rules of the slopes:

1. Always stay in control and be able to stop or avoid other people or objects.

2. People ahead of you have the right of way. It is your responsibility to avoid them.

3. You must not stop where you obstruct a trail or are not visible from above.

4. Whenever starting downhill or merging into a trail, look uphill, and yield to others.

5. Always use devices to help prevent runaway equipment.

6. Observe all posted signs and warnings.

7. Keep off closed trails and out of closed areas. Prior to using any lift, you must have the knowledge and ability to load, ride, and unload safely.

Snowmobiling

Snowmobiles can weigh up to 600 pounds and travel at speeds in excess of 90 mph. Head injuries are the leading cause of snowmobile-related deaths. In 1999, nearly 1,500 children ages 14 and under were treated in emergency rooms for snowmobile-related injuries. The American Academy of Pediatrics has stated that operating snowmobiles is inappropriate for children under age 16. If a child is riding as a passenger on a snowmobile, be sure he is wearing an approved helmet. Children ages 5 and under should never ride on snowmobiles.

References

American Academy of Orthopaedic Surgeons. *Skiing*. Available at www. aaos.org/wordhtml/pat_educ/skiing.htm. Accessed December 10, 1999.

American Academy of Orthopaedic Surgeons. *Sledding Safety*. Available at www.aaos.org/wordhtml/papers/position/sledding.htm. Accessed December 10, 1999.

Caine D, Caine C, Lindner K, editors. Epidemiology of Sports Injuries. Champaign, IL: *Human Kinetics*, 1996:29-40.

National Ski Areas Association. *Ski and Snowboarding Tips*. Available at www.nsaa.org/MemberUpdate/skitips.htm. Accessed December 13, 1999.

National Ski Areas Association. *Your Responsibility Code*. Available at www.nsaa.org/MemberUpdate/thecode.htm. Accessed December 13, 1999.

SAFE KIDS. *Sports and Recreational Activity Injury*. Available at www.safekids.org/fact99/sports99.html. Accessed December 10, 1999.

U.S. Consumer Product Safety Commission. *CPSC Staff Recommends Use of Helmets for Skiers, Snowboarders to Prevent Head Injuries*. Available at www.cpsc.gov/cpscpub/prerel/prhtm199/99046.html. Accessed December 10, 1999.

Safety Resources

American Academy of Orthopaedic Surgeons
6300 North River Road
Rosemont, IL 60018-4262
Toll-Free: 800-346-AAOS (2267)
Tel: 847-823-7186
Fax: 847-823-8125
Fax on Demand: 800-999-2939
Website: www.aaos.org
E-mail: custserv@aaos.org

Through the public information link to patient education on the AAOS home page www.aaos.org, you can access fact sheets on injury prevention for many sports, including skiing and sledding.

American Academy of Pediatrics

141 Northwest Point Boulevard
Elk Grove Village, IL 60007-1098
Tel: 847-434-4000
Fax: 847-434-8000
Website: www.aap.org
E-mail: kidsdocs@aap.org

AAP has safety tips for the winter holidays (including tips on outdoor sports).

National Safety Council

1121 Spring Lake Drive
Itasca, IL 60143-3201
Tel: 630-285-1121
Fax: 630-285-1315
Website: www.nsc.org
E-mail: customerservice@nsc.org

National Ski Areas Association

133 S. Van Gordon Street
Suite 300
Lakewood, CO 80228
Tel: 303-987-1111
Fax: 303-986-2345
Website: www.nsaa.org
E-mail: nsaa@nsaa.org

NSAA is the trade association for ski area owners and operators. Suggestions for safe skiing and snowboarding can be found on their website at www.nsaa.org/MemberUpdate/skitips.htm.

National Ski Patrol

133 S. Van Gordon Street
Suite 100
Lakewood, CO 80228
Tel: 303-987-1111
Fax: 303-988-3005
Website: www.nsp.org
E-mail: nsp@nsp.org

NSP is a nonprofit membership association providing education services about emergency care and safety to the public and mountain recreation industry.

National SAFE KIDS Campaign
1301 Pennsylvania Ave., N.W.
Suite 1000
Washington, DC 20004
Tel: 202-662-0600
Fax: 202-393-2072
Website: www.safekids.org
E-mail: info@safekids.org

U.S. Consumer Product Safety Commission
4330 East-West Highway
Washington, DC 20207-0001
Toll-Free: 800-638-2772
Tel: 301-504-0990
Fax: 301-504-0124 and 301-504-0025
Website: www.cpsc.gov
E-mail: info@cpsc.gov

Chapter 53

Rules for Water Safety

In 1996, nearly 1,000 children younger than 15 years of age drowned in the United States. It is surprising to many parents that young children tend not to splash or make noise when they get into trouble in the water and thus usually drown silently. An adult should always be watching young children playing, swimming, or bathing in water.

Tips for General Water Safety

You can greatly reduce the chances of you and your children becoming a drowning victim or being injured if you follow a few simple safety tips:

1. Make sure an adult is constantly watching young children swimming, playing, or bathing in water. Do not read, play cards, talk on the phone, mow the lawn, or do any other distracting activity while supervising children around water.

2. Never swim alone or in unsupervised places. Teach your children to always swim with a buddy.

3. Keep small children away from buckets containing liquid: 5-gallon industrial containers are a particular danger. Be sure

---

"Water Safety," SafeUSA™; and "Executive Summary Boating Statistics–2000," U.S. Coast Guard, Commandant Publication P16754.14, 2001.

to empty buckets of all liquid when household chores are done. An infant or toddler can drown in as little as one inch of water.

4. Never drink alcohol before or during swimming, boating, or water skiing. Never drink alcohol while supervising children around water. Teach teenagers about the danger of drinking alcohol and swimming, boating, or water skiing.

5. To prevent choking, never chew gum or eat while swimming, diving, or playing in water.

6. Learn to swim. Enroll yourself and your children aged 4 and older in swimming classes. Swimming classes are not recommended for children under age 4.

7. Learn CPR (cardio-pulmonary resuscitation). This applies particularly to pool owners and water sports enthusiasts.

8. Do *not* use air-filled swimming aids (such as water wings) in place of life jackets or life preservers with children. Using air-filled swimming aids can give parents and children a false sense of security, which may increase the risk of drowning. These air-filled aids are toys and are not designed to be personal flotation devices (life jackets). Air-filled plastic tubes can deflate because they become punctured or unplugged.

9. Check the water depth before entering. The American Red Cross recommends nine feet as a minimum depth for diving or jumping.

If You Have a Swimming Pool at Your Home

1. Install a four-sided, isolation pool-fence with self-closing and self-latching gates around the pool. Such a fence should be at least four feet tall and completely separate the pool from the house and play area of the yard.

2. Prevent children from having direct access to the swimming pool.

3. Install a telephone near the pool. Know how to contact local emergency medical services. Post the emergency number, 911, in an easy-to-see place.

4. Remove toys from pool immediately after use. Floats, balls, and other toys may tempt children to lean into pool, and they may fall in.

5. Remember always to closely supervise children using the pool and insist that others do too.

Tips for Open Water

1. Know the local weather conditions and forecast before swimming or boating. Thunderstorms and strong winds are dangerous to swimmers and boaters.

2. Restrict activities to designated swimming areas, usually marked by buoys.

3. Use U.S. Coast Guard-approved personal flotation devices (life jackets) when boating, regardless of distance to be traveled, size of boat, or swimming ability of boaters.

4. Remember that open water usually has limited visibility, and conditions can sometimes change from hour to hour. Currents are often unpredictable, moving rapidly and quickly changing direction. A strong water current can carry even expert swimmers far from shore.

5. Watch for dangerous waves and signs of rip currents—water that is discolored, unusually choppy, foamy, or filled with debris.

6. If you are caught in a rip current, swim parallel to the shore. Once you are out of the current, swim toward the shore.

Boating Statistics–2000 from the United States Coast Guard

Life jackets could have saved the lives of approximately 445 boaters who drowned of the 519 drowned in 2000. In 2000, approximately eight out of every 10 victims in fatal boating accidents were not wearing life jackets. Boaters continue to be at greater risk of dying when involved in an accident during the fall and winter months than in the summer. Besides the colder weather and water, there are fewer boaters and patrol officers in the area to rescue boaters in distress. When waters are below 60 degrees Fahrenheit, hypothermia can set in quickly. Those who hunt and fish from boats, especially in colder weather, need to dress for possible immersion and wear their life jackets. Boaters in larger bodies of water should also take advantage of using available distress alerting and position indicating technologies to improve their chances of survival if a mishap occurs.

Fatalities by known boat length include 83% of fatalities which occurred on boats less than 26 feet in length. Seventy-five percent of those victims drowned. Specifically, 337 fatalities occurred on boats less than 16 feet in length and 245 occurred on boats 16 to less than 26 feet in length.

Alcohol involvement in reported boating accidents accounted for 31 percent of all boating fatalities—up five percent from 1999. A Coast Guard study estimates that boat operators with a blood alcohol concentration above .10 percent are estimated to be more than 10 times as likely to be killed in a boating accident than boat operators with zero blood alcohol concentration.

Fatalities by known boat operator education showed that 84% of all boating fatalities occurred on boats where the operator had not completed a boating safety education course.

The primary causes of accidents are operator inattention, careless/ reckless operation, operator inexperience, operating at an unsafe speed, and no proper lookout. Nearly 70 percent of all reported accidents involve operator controllable factors.

Types of boating accidents. Capsizing and falls overboard accounted for 418 fatalities, almost two-thirds of all reported boating fatalities. Nearly nine out of every 10 of those victims drowned. Collision with another vessel was the most reported type of accident. These accidents resulted in 1,413 injuries and accounted for 8.7 million dollars in property damage.

Age of boating fatality victims. Twenty-eight children age 12 and under lost their lives while boating in 2000. One hundred and thirty-four boaters died in the 30-39 age group category—the highest number reported for any age group.

Types of boating injuries. Approximately eighty percent of all reported injuries were associated with the use of open motorboats (45%) and personal watercraft (36%). Lacerations were the most reported type of injury for open motorboats. For personal watercraft, broken bones accounted for the highest number of injuries.

Who Is Affected?

Water sports—like swimming, wading, boating, and water skiing—are fun and exciting. But they can also be dangerous for people of all ages. In 1996, nearly 4,000 people drowned in the United States, including almost 1,000 children younger than 15 years of age. Among children aged 1-9, drowning is the second leading cause of death from injuries. Near-drowning can result in brain damage.

Childhood drowning and near-drowning often occur when a child is left alone, even for a few seconds. It is surprising to many parents that young children tend not to splash or make noise when they get into trouble in the water and thus usually drown silently. Most children who drown in pools were last seen inside the home, had been out of sight less than five minutes, and were in the care of one or both parents at the time.

How young children drown tends to vary by age. For example:

- Children under age one most often drown in bathtubs, buckets, and toilets.

- Children aged 1-4 most often drown in swimming pools, hot tubs, and spas.

- Children aged 5-14 most often drown in swimming pools and open water, such as lakes and rivers.

Many people don't realize that alcohol use is involved in many drownings: 25-50% of adolescent and adult drowning involves alcohol use. In 40-50% of drownings among adolescent boys, alcohol is a major contributing factor.

Chapter 54

Gymnastics Injury Prevention

Gymnastics Safety

Hospital emergency departments treat more than 25,000 injured gymnasts under age 15 each year. Many of these injuries can be prevented if athletes and trainers know about the special injury risks associated with the sport and if safety measures and equipment are put into place.

Tips for Preventing Gymnastics Injuries

To help your child avoid gymnastics injuries, follow these safety tips from the American Academy of Pediatrics, the American Academy of Orthopaedic Surgeons, the National SAFE KIDS Campaign, and other sports and health organizations.

- Before your child starts a gymnastics training program, take him or her to the doctor for a physical exam. The doctor can help assess any special injury risks your child may have.

- *Make sure your child wears all the required safety gear every time he or she competes or practices.* Gymnasts may need wrist guards and hand grips; special footwear and pads may also be required.

"Gymnastics Safety," SafeUSA™, Centers for Disease Control and Prevention, updated February 2001.

- Teach your child not to play through pain. If your child gets injured, see your doctor. Follow all the doctor's orders for recovery, and get the doctor's approval before your child returns to the sport.

- Make sure first aid is available at all competitions and practices.

- Talk to and watch your child's coach. Coaches should emphasize safety and understand the special injury risks that young gymnasts face.

- Inspect the facilities where your child trains and competes. Equipment should be in good condition and spaced far enough apart to avoid collisions. Floors should be padded, and mats should be secured under every apparatus. Safety harnesses should be used when your child does new or difficult moves.

- Insist that your child have spotters when learning new skills or doing difficult moves. Spotters should be present during practice and competition—they can help catch your child if he or she falls.

- Encourage your child to express concern about doing difficult moves. Don't let the coach push your child to do things he or she is not ready for.

- Above all, keep gymnastics fun. Putting too much focus on winning can make your child push too hard and risk injury.

Who Is Affected?

In the U.S., more than 600,000 children take part in school-sponsored and club-level gymnastics competitions. Some gymnasts start training at an early age (as young as 4 or 5 years old) and practice for several hours each day. With the high physical demands of gymnastics—and the increasing levels of difficulty—comes a high risk of injury. In a study of high school athletes, gymnastics was the fourth leading cause of injury, with an injury rate of 56 percent. Club gymnastics programs had a rate of injury as high as 22 percent.

The majority of gymnastics-related injuries are mild to moderate, with sprains, strains, and stress fractures being most common. Ankles and knees are the most frequent sites of injury, typically resulting from landings and dismounts. Injuries to the lower back are also common. Although acute injuries are rarely severe, as many as half of all injuries lead to chronic pain, and bone fractures in young athletes can cause long-term physical problems.

Floor exercises are the most common cause of injury, due to the large number of bends, twists, and landings required in those routines. Other factors that increase the risk of injury are trying moves that are too complicated for one's skill level, not using safety harnesses or spotters, getting over-tired, and spending long hours practicing.

Of special concern among female gymnasts is improper diet and eating disorders, such as anorexia nervosa and bulimia. The emphasis on a slender physique can lead some female gymnasts to lower their food intake so much that they deprive their bodies of essential nutrients. Studies have found that these athletes have lower bone density and a greater incidence of stress fractures.

Additional Information

American Academy of Pediatrics
141 Northwest Point Boulevard
Elk Grove Village, IL 60007-1098
Tel: 847-434-4000
Fax: 847-434-8000
Website: www.aap.org
E-mail: kidsdoc@asp.org

American Academy of Orthopaedic Surgeons
6300 North River Road
Rosemont, IL 60018-4262
Toll-Free: 800-346-AAOS (2267)
Tel: 847-823-7186
Fax: 847-823-8125
AAOS Fax-on Demand: 800-999-2939
Website: www.aaos.org
E-mail: custserv@aaos.org

National Athletic Trainers Association
2952 Stemmons Freeway
Dallas, TX 75247-6916
Toll-Free: 800-879-6282
Tel: 214-637-6282
Fax: 214-637-2206
Website: www.nata.org
E-mail: natanews@nata.org

National SAFE KIDS Campaign
1301 Pennsylvania Ave., N.W., Suite 1000
Washington, DC 20004
Tel: 202-662-0600
Fax: 202-393-2072
Website: www.safekids.org
E-mail: info@safekids.org

National Youth Sports Safety Foundation
One Beacon Street, Suite 3333
Boston, MA 02108
Tel: 617-277-1771
Fax: 617-722-9999
Website: www.nyssf.org
E-mail: NYSSF@aol.com

References

American Academy of Orthopaedic Surgeons Seminar (Sullivan J, Grana W, editors). *The Pediatric Athlete*. Park Ridge, IL: The Academy, 1990:138.

American Academy of Pediatrics. *Sports Medicine: Health care for young athletes*. Elk Grove Village, IL: The Academy, 1991:158-159.

Caine D, Caine C, Lindner K, editors. Epidemiology of Sports Injuries. Champaign, IL: *Human Kinetics*, 1996:213-246.

Raney E. *Child and adolescent gymnastics: How to avoid injury*. Hughston Health Alert. Available at http://www.hughston.com/hha/a.gym.htm. Accessed July 9, 1999.

Zetaruk M, Mitchell W. Gymnastics injuries. *Sidelines* 1998;7(2):1-2. (Sidelines is a publication of the National Youth Sports Safety Foundation.)

Chapter 55

Baby Boomer Sports Injury Prevention Tips

While there may be no single fountain of youth, you can slow down the process by staying physically active. Regular exercise enhances muscle and joint function, keeps bones strong, and decreases your risk of heart attack or stroke. The following tips have been developed by the American Orthopaedic Society for Sports Medicine and the American Academy of Orthopaedic Surgeons.

- **Always take time to warm-up and stretch before physical activity.** Research studies have shown that cold muscles are more prone to injury. Warm-up with jumping jacks, stationary cycling, or by running or walking in place for three to five minutes. Then slowly and gently stretch, holding each stretch for 30 seconds.

- **Don't succumb to the *weekend warrior* syndrome.** Compressing your physical activity into two days sets you up for trouble and does not increase your fitness level. Try to get at least 30 minutes of moderate physical activity every day. If you're truly pressed for time, you can break it up into ten-minute chunks. Remember that moderate physical activity includes things like walking the dog, working in the garden, playing with the kids, and taking the stairs instead of the elevator.

- **Take lessons and invest in good equipment.** Whether you're a beginner or have been playing a sport for a long time, lessons are a worthwhile investment. Proper form and instruction reduce the chance of developing an overuse injury like tendinitis or stress fractures. Lessons at varying levels of play for many sports are offered by local park districts and athletic clubs. Select the proper shoes for your sport and use them only for that sport. When the treads start to look worn the shoes are no longer as supportive as they were, it's time to replace them.

- **Listen to your body.** As you age, you may find that you are not as flexible as you were, or that you cannot tolerate the same types of activities that you did years ago. While no one is happy about getting older, you will be able to prevent injury by modifying your activity to accommodate your body's needs.

- **Use the 10% rule.** When changing your activity level, increase it in increments of no more than ten percent per week. If you normally do two miles a day and want to increase your fitness level, don't try to suddenly walk four miles. Slowly build up to more miles each week until you reach you higher goal. Use the ten percent rule as your guide as well for strength training and increase your weights gradually.

- **Develop a balanced fitness program that incorporates cardiovascular exercise, strength training, and flexibility**. In addition to providing a total body workout, a balanced program will keep you from getting bored and lessen your chance of injury.

- **Add activity and new exercises cautiously.** No matter if you've been sedentary or are very fit, don't try to take on too many activities at a time. It's best to add no more than one or two new activities per workout.

If you have, or have had sports or orthopaedic injuries or problems such as tendinitis, arthritis, stress fractures, or low back pain, in the past, consult an orthopaedic surgeon who can help you design a fitness routine to promote wellness and minimize the chance of injury.

Chapter 56

Fitness Facts for Older Americans

During the lifetime of older Americans there have been revolutionary changes in how we live and work and what we eat. Even more importantly, there has been a revolution in what we know about living long and living well. Today, our scientific knowledge regarding exercise, nutrition, and other areas of health is being added to and revised so rapidly that unless you have the latest facts, you can easily be following outmoded recommendations.

Boning Up on the Latest Facts about Musculoskeletal and Cardiovascular Systems

"Take it easy you're not as young as you used to be" is not so sage advice. Yet, the majority of middle-aged and older Americans seem to adhere to this outmoded dictate. Surveys show that only 30 percent of Americans aged 45 to 64 exercise regularly, while 32 percent of adults 65 and older follow a regular plan of exercise.

We now know that the human body repairs itself and performs more efficiently with proper conditioning that is achieved through a program of regular exercise and good nutrition. This is particularly true for the musculoskeletal system and the cardiovascular-pulmonary system, which is made up of our lungs, heart, and the miles of veins, arteries, and capillaries that traverse our bodies.

"Fitness Facts for Older Americans," *Elder Action: Action Ideas for Older Persons and Their Families*, Administration on Aging; available online at http://www.aoa.dhhs.gov/aoa/eldractn/; modified July 2000.

With exercise, our bones, particularly our joint bones and the bones of the spinal column, rebuild and repair themselves as they should. Without exercise, they tend to become thin and porous—a condition known as osteoporosis.

When we do not exercise, fat displaces muscle, muscles become smaller and weaker—a process known as atrophy, and we gain weight more easily because even at rest muscles burn more calories than does fat. Added weight puts added stress on our heart and lungs, and on the weight bearing joints of the knees, hips, ankles, and feet. It becomes more difficult to climb stairs, get out of a chair, and even to walk and to maintain our balance. Weak muscles cannot protect our joints or help to provide needed strength and balance so that we are more prone to falls. Frail bones and weak muscles limit our ability to care for ourselves and our homes, and to enjoy the later years-years that can and should be a time of productivity and enjoyment.

When you exercise, however, you help to reduce fat tissue, while building muscle and bone. Muscle is heavier than fat but takes up half the space, so you can actually reduce your body measurements without losing weight. Strong muscles help to protect your joints and spinal column, improve your posture and balance, increase your mobility, reduce the likelihood of falls and other accidents, and give you a younger body image.

An Ounce of Prevention Is Worth a Pound of Cure

When it comes to our health and fitness this is sage advice indeed. But being out of shape does not mean that you cannot get in shape and this is true not only for people in their 40s, 50s, and 60s, but also people in their 90s.

Recent research has found that when it comes to exercise you need a combination of three types—weight training for strength; aerobic exercise for strength and endurance; and calisthenics (stretching, bending, and twisting exercises) for flexibility. Studies have found that violent physical exertion is no more useful to gaining and maintaining fitness than is moderate exercise. Also, violent physical exertion can result in an increased risk of injury or heart attacks for those who are not in prime physical condition. So start off slow and go slow with your new exercise program.

Walking and other aerobic exercises done at a pace which makes you breathe a little harder and work up a mild sweat for a half-hour to one hour three days a week will keep your heart, lungs, and vascular system in good working order and strengthen your bones and muscles. Exercise intensity for aerobic conditioning is measured by heart rate. A good activity level is 70 percent of your maximum heart rate, which is determined by subtracting your age from 220. Thus the recommended exercise heart rate for a 60-year-old person is 112 beats per minute. People who have not been exercising should begin using 60 percent of their maximum heartbeat as the target heart rate and can ultimately move up to 80 percent when they have reached their maximum fitness level.

Do not attempt a strenuous workout during hot, humid weather and wait until at least two hours after eating before engaging in moderate to heavy exercise. Warning signs of overexertion include an inability to talk, dizziness or disorientation, nausea, or pains in your chest, upper back, left shoulder, or arm. If you have any of these symptoms check with your physician as soon as possible.

To avoid excess strain on the heart, and injury to your muscles, warm up for about five minutes before working out, and cool down after exercises. Never abruptly stop exercising, since the sudden stop in motion can cause lightheadedness or muscle cramping.

Walking is a good exercise because it can be done at a pace that you can easily set for yourself, it takes no equipment other than a pair of good walking shoes, and it can be done at virtually any time, and on your own. Walking strengthens muscles in the lower body, helps to build new joint bone and tissue, and helps to ward off or slow osteoporosis. Since walking only works the lower half of the body, other aerobic exercises as well as exercises that increase flexibility should be included in your routine. Other good aerobic exercises for weight bearing joints include dancing, tennis, racquetball, basketball, and biking.

Before beginning an exercise program, check with your personal physician and start off slow to avoid overexertion and accidents—and stick with it. Varying the type of physical activity you engage in will help to use all the major muscle groups in your body, and avoid overuse of any one major muscle group. It will also prevent boredom.

Aerobic exercise not only strengthens your bones and muscles and helps to prevent osteoporosis, it also strengthens your heart and helps to maintain your lung capacity. Aerobic exercise slows or prevents the buildup of cholesterol plaque in the veins and arteries (atherosclerosis) and helps to ward off arteriosclerosis or hardening of the arteries by keeping them flexible, thus reducing high blood pressure which plays a major role in heart disease and strokes. Exercise also improves the functioning of the liver, pancreas, and other vital organs.

Sustained aerobic exercise can help to control Late Onset, or Type II, diabetes mellitus since it aids in the metabolism of sucrose. Also, exercise helps to spur the production of human growth hormone which otherwise ceases to be produced after about age fifty. Human growth hormone helps to maintain the size and strength of muscles which diminish as we age.

If you have arthritis and other joint or motion impeding conditions, swimming is an excellent aerobic exercise. It offers many of the benefits of other aerobic exercises without putting undue stress on joints which because of arthritis or injury, are unable to repair and rebuild themselves in the normal manner. Swimming, however, unlike weight bearing aerobic exercises, does not aid in the rebuilding of bone and therefore is not helpful in preventing or slowing osteoporosis, nor does it appear to be helpful in reducing weight.

Physical exercise not only increases the metabolic rate so that more calories are burned during the activity, but benefits continue for several hours after you have stopped. What is more, as you improve your muscle tone and enlarge your muscles, they will burn more calories even when you are engaged in sedentary activities.

If You Do Not Use It, You Will Lose It

Not long ago, it was accepted knowledge that older people could not increase their muscle strength nor their muscle mass. Now, happily, this myth has been dispelled. In 1989, researchers from Tufts and Harvard Universities undertook a study of older people in their late 80s and 90s. The researchers worked with a group of frail elderly residents at Boston's Hebrew Rehabilitation Center for the Aged. These residents had multiple functional problems, chronic conditions, and were very sedentary.

At the beginning of the project, the project participants, whose average age was 90, were tested to determine the heaviest weights that they could lift with their legs. Following this initial test, they began a program of weight training. They did three sets composed of eight weight lifting repetitions each for three days a week. They worked out with weights that were 80 percent of the maximum weight that they could lift.

After two weeks, they were re-tested and the weights were increased. At the end of six weeks, these frail older people had increased their muscle strength on average by 180 percent. None of the participants had reached a plateau. As a result of their increased muscle strength, their average walking speed increased 48 percent, two participants no longer needed their canes, and one participant was able to rise from a chair without using the chair arms.

All of the participants resumed their sedentary lifestyles at the end of the program. The researchers then re-tested them, and found a 32 percent loss in maximum strength after only 4 weeks of detraining. The moral of this story is, "if you don't use it, you'll lose it," but the happy ending is that you can regain your fitness and strength at almost any age which will help you to retain or regain your independence, freedom, and add to your good looks.

Weight training is as essential to good physical health in your later years as aerobic exercise is. It strengthens your muscles and bones, and there are indications that it is helpful in lowering cholesterol levels. Weight training also increases the strength of ligaments and tendons so that less stress is placed on your joints. In the past, people with high blood pressure, heart diseases, and conditions such as arthritis were warned to avoid using weights. But researchers in the Tufts and Harvard study found that weight training had no adverse effect on blood pressure or heart function and advise that strengthening your muscles, tendons, and ligaments actually helps to ease pressure on the joints.

Weight training can either be with free weights such as barbells and dumbbells, or with specially designed equipment which works various parts of the body. Weight training can be used to increase your muscle strength or your muscle endurance.

If you have not worked with weights before be sure to have a qualified person instruct you in their use and have them set up a program of exercises which includes the specified number of repetitions to be done in each set as you progress toward your goal. Muscle strengthening exercises should be done for at least 20 minutes three times a week.

A program of calisthenics, isometric, and stretching exercises combined with dance will enable you to develop muscle strength and endurance as well as flexibility and cardio-pulmonary fitness. Joining a class or renting or buying videos made by qualified instructors (not just movie stars) is a good way to get in shape and avoid mishaps. Many dance classes especially those in ballet, modern, and aerobic dance include calisthenics, isometric, and stretching exercises as part of the routine.

Staying physically fit can give you a body that performs and looks like those of persons years younger than your chronological age. At the VA Medical Center in Salt Lake City Utah, physically fit men in their mid-fifties were compared to inactive men in their mid-20s. The results were astounding. Active older men had lower resting heart rates—64 beats per minute versus 85 beats per minute for the younger men, higher oxygen uptake during maximum exercise, and slower heart beats in the first minute after exercise than the men in their 20s who did not keep fit. The older men weighed an average of 166 pounds compared to 192 pounds for the younger sedentary men.

Get Moving

Before you begin an exercise program, be prudent and be prepared. Check with your physician and make sure that you begin your exercise program by the book or with a qualified instructor. In so doing you will gain the maximum benefit from the program and avoid strains, sprains, and other mishaps.

Even if you have been exercising on a regular basis, it does not hurt to take a refresher class every so often, since new exercises are added and older, less effective ones are dropped. Make sure that your instructor is licensed or certified to provide instruction. If no classes are available in your area and you want to start an exercise program on your own, obtain the latest publications and/or videos available. Some calisthenics and isometric exercises recommended a decade or two ago are no longer considered safe, so it is important to have current information.

Many agencies and organizations including the YMCA and YWCA, junior colleges and universities, senior and community centers, adult and continuing education, health clubs, and spas offer classes in sports, exercise, dance, and weight training that provide instruction that will enable you to gain the maximum result and avoid injuries and mishaps.

Get Moving and Discover a New, Revitalized You

If you are retired you now have the time it takes to get in shape. If you are not retired, make the time. Remember weight training should be done three times a week for a minimum of 20 minutes under a trained instructor, while bending and stretching exercises should be done every day for about 10 minutes and aerobic exercise for 30 to 60 minutes three times a week.

Part Seven

Additional Help and Information

Chapter 57

Glossary of Sports Injury Terms

A

Accident: An occurrence in a sequence of events that produces un-intended injury, death, or property damage. Accident refers to the event, not the result of the event (see unintentional injury).

Acute: An illness or injury that lasts for a short time and may be intense.

Addiction: A chronic, relapsing disease, characterized by compulsive drug-seeking and use.

Aerobics: Exercises that develop the strength and endurance of heart and lungs.

Amenorrhea: The absence of menstrual periods.

Anabolic effects: Drug-induced growth or thickening of the body's nonreproductive tract tissues—including skeletal muscle, bones, the larynx, and vocal cords—and a decrease in body fat.

Analgesics: A group of medications that reduce pain.

This chapter includes excerpts from "National Safety Council Statistics Glossary," © National Safety Council, July 25, 2000, reprinted with permission; and "Questions and Answers about Sprains and Strains," National Institute of Arthritis and Musculoskeletal and Skin Diseases (NIAMS), December 1999.

Androgenic effects: A drug's effects upon the growth of the male reproductive tract and the development of male secondary sexual characteristics.

Antidepressants: A group of drugs used in treating depressive disorders.

Arthroplasty: Shoulder joint replacement. In this operation, a surgeon replaces the shoulder joint with an artificial ball for the top of the humerus and a cap (glenoid) for the scapula.

Arthroscopy: The doctor manipulates a small, lighted optic tube (arthroscope) that has been inserted into the joint through a small incision typically in the knee or shoulder. Images of the inside of the joint are projected onto a television screen. While the arthroscope is inside the joint, removal of loose pieces of bone or cartilage or the repair of torn ligaments is possible.

B

Biopsy: The doctor removes a small amount of tissue to examine under a microscope.

Bone scan (radionuclide scanning): A very small amount of radioactive material is injected into the patient's bloodstream and detected by a scanner. This test detects blood flow to the bone and cell activity within the bone and can show abnormalities in these processes that may aid diagnosis.

Bruise: Bleeding under the skin.

C

Cardiovascular system: The heart and blood vessels.

Chronic: An illness or injury that lasts for a long time.

Computerized axial tomography (CAT) scan: X-rays lasting a fraction of a second are passed through the body at different angles, detected by a scanner, and analyzed by a computer. This produces a series of clear cross-sectional images (slices) of the tissues on a computer screen. CAT scan images show soft tissues such as ligaments or muscles more clearly than conventional x-rays. The computer can combine individual images to give a three-dimensional view.

D

Death from accident: A death that occurs within one year of an accident.

Dehydration: A deficit in body fluids caused by lack of drinking enough fluids It can occur quickly during exercise or hot weather.

Direct sport injury: Those injuries which resulted directly from participation in the skills of a specific sport.

Disabling injury: An injury causing death, permanent disability, or any degree of temporary total disability beyond the day of the injury.

E

Electrostimulation: Provides pain relief by preventing nerve cells from transmitting pain impulses to the brain and is used to make a muscle contract, which helps prevent muscle atrophy and maintain or increase muscle strength.

Exercise: A type of physical activity that is planned, repetitive, and designed to improve or maintain at least one of the health-related components of physical fitness.

F

Fatal accident: An accident that results in one or more deaths within one year.

Femur: The upper leg or thigh bone, which extends into the hip socket at its upper end and down to the knee at its lower end.

Fibula: The thin, outer bone of the leg that forms part of the ankle joint at its lower end.

G

Gait: Pattern of walking or running.

Growth plate: The growth plate, also known as the physis, is the area of developing tissue near the end of the long bones in children and adolescents.

H

Heat exhaustion: Heat-related illness with possible symptoms including nausea, dizziness, weakness, headache, pale and moist skin, heavy perspiration, normal or low body temperature, weak pulse, dilated pupils, disorientation, or fainting spells.

Heat stroke: Heat-related illness with symptoms that may include headache, dizziness, confusion, and hot dry skin, possibly leading to vascular collapse, coma, and death.

Hormone: A chemical substance formed in glands in the body and carried in the blood to organs and tissues where it influences function, structure, and behavior.

I

Incidence rate, as defined by OSHA: The number of occupational injuries and/or illnesses or lost workdays per 100 full-time employees.

Indirect sport injury: Those injuries which were caused by systemic failure as a result of exertion while participating in a sport activity or by a complication which was secondary to a non-fatal injury.

Inflammation: A characteristic reaction of tissues to disease or injury; it is marked by four signs: swelling, redness, heat, and pain.

Injury: A physical harm or damage to the body resulting from an exchange, usually acute, of mechanical, chemical, thermal, or other environmental energy that exceeds the body's tolerance.

J

Joint: A junction where two bones meet.

L

Ligament: A band of tough, fibrous tissue that connects two or more bones at a joint and prevents excessive movement of the joint.

Lost workdays: Those days on which, because of occupational injury or illness, the employee was away from work or limited to restricted work activity. The number of lost workdays (consecutive or not) does not include the day of injury or onset of illness or any days on which the employee would not have worked even though able to work.

M

Magnetic resonance imaging (MRI): Energy from a powerful magnet (rather than x-rays) stimulates tissue to produce signals that are detected by a scanner and analyzed by a computer. This creates a series of cross-sectional images of a specific part of the body. A MRI is particularly useful for detecting soft tissue damage or disease. Like a CAT scan, a computer is used to produce three-dimensional views during MRI.

Motor vehicle accident: An unstabilized situation that includes at least one harmful event (injury or property damage) involving a motor vehicle in transport (in motion, in readiness for motion, or on a roadway, but not parked in a designated parking area) that does not result from discharge of a firearm or explosive device and does not directly result from a cataclysm.

Motor vehicle nontraffic accident: Any motor vehicle accident that occurs entirely in any place other than a trafficway.

Motor vehicle traffic accident: A motor vehicle accident that occurs on a trafficway—a way or place, any part of which is open to the use of the public for the purposes of vehicular traffic.

Muscle: Tissue composed of bundles of specialized cells that contract and produce movement when stimulated by nerve impulses.

Musculoskeletal system: The body's muscles, bones, tendons, and ligaments.

N

Nonfatal injury accident: An accident in which at least one person is injured, and no injury results in death.

O

Occupational injury: Any such injury such as a cut, fracture, sprain, amputation, etc., which results from a work accident or from a single instantaneous exposure in the work environment.

Orthopaedic surgeons: Doctors who treat disorders of the bones, muscles, and related structures.

Orthotics: Inserts that are placed in shoes to correct bad alignment between the foot and the lower leg.

Osteoporosis: A disease in which bone density is decreased, leaving your bones vulnerable to fracture (breaking).

P

Pedalcycle: A vehicle propelled by human power and operated solely by pedals; excludes mopeds.

Pedestrian: Any person involved in a motor vehicle accident who is not in or upon a motor vehicle or nonmotor vehicle. Includes persons injured while using a coaster wagon, child's tricycle, roller skates, etc. Excludes persons boarding, alighting, jumping, or falling from a motor vehicle in transport who are considered occupants of the vehicle.

Permanent disability (or permanent impairment): Includes any degree of permanent nonfatal injury . It includes any injury that results in the loss, or complete loss of use, of any part of the body, or any permanent impairment of functions of the body or a part thereof.

Physical activity: Movement created by skeletal muscle contractions, resulting in energy expenditure.

Physical fitness: Can be categorized into five health-related components: a) cardiorespiratory endurance (aerobic fitness), b) muscle endurance, c) strength, d) flexibility, and e) body composition.

Physical therapy: Is used to increase the range of motion and strength after an injury. Physical therapy includes various exercise and physical fitness programs that can be customized to meet each patient's needs.

Physical training (as used in the military): An organized exercise intended to enhance fitness. The terms exercise and physical training are used interchangeably.

Placebo: An inactive substance, used in experiments to distinguish between actual drug effects and effects that are expected by the volunteers in the experiments.

Property damage accident: An accident that results in property damage, but in which no person is injured.

Public accident: Any accident other than motor vehicle that occurs in the public use of any premises. Includes deaths in recreation (swimming, hunting, etc.), transportation except motor vehicle, public buildings, etc., and from widespread natural disasters even though some may have happened on home premises. Excludes accidents to persons in the course of gainful employment.

R

Range-of-motion: The arc of movement of a joint from one extreme position to the other; range-of-motion exercises help increase or maintain flexibility and movement in muscles, tendons, ligaments, and joints.

Repetitive motion injuries: Painful injuries such as stress fractures (where the ligament pulls off small pieces of bone) and tendinitis (inflammation of a tendon) can occur from overuse of muscles and tendons.

RICE: Rest, Ice, Compression, and Elevation

- **Rest**—Reduce or stop using the injured area for 48 hours.
- **Ice**—Put an ice pack on the injured area for 20 minutes at a time, 4 to 8 times per day. Use a cold pack, ice bag, or a plastic bag filled with crushed ice that has been wrapped in a towel.
- **Compression**—Compression may help reduce the swelling. Compress the area with bandages, such as an elastic wrap, to help stabilize the shoulder.
- **Elevation**—Keep the injured area elevated above the level of the heart. Use a pillow to help elevate the injury.

S

Sex hormones: Hormones that are found in higher quantities in one sex than in the other. Male sex hormones are the androgens, which include testosterone; and the female sex hormones are the estrogens and progesterone.

Snowboarder's ankle: A fracture of the lateral process of the talus. The mechanism of injury is a forcing of the ankle into dorsiflexion and inversion, which may occur during a landing from an aerial maneuver or a jump, especially when the landing has been over-rotated.

Source of injury: The principal object such as tool, machine, or equipment involved in the accident and is usually the object inflicting injury or property damage. Also called agency or agent.

Sprain: An injury to a ligament—a stretching or a tearing. One or more ligaments can be injured during a sprain.

Strain: An injury to either a muscle or a tendon.

Sunburn: An injury to the skin.

T

Temporary total disability: An injury that does not result in death or permanent disability, but that renders the injured person unable to perform regular duties or activities on one or more full calendar days after the day of the injury.

Tendons: Tough, fibrous cords of tissue that connect muscle to bone.

Tibia: The thick, long bone of the lower leg (also called the shin) that forms part of the knee joint at its upper end and the ankle joint at its lower end.

U

Ultrasound rehabilitation: Uses the vibrations from sound waves to stimulate blood flow to soft tissue such as muscles and ligaments. Stimulation of blood flow helps reduce swelling and aids healing.

Unintentional injury: The preferred term for accidental injury in the public health community. It refers to the result of an accident.

W

Withdrawal: Symptoms that occur after chronic use of a drug is reduced or stopped.

X

X-ray (radiography): An x-ray beam is passed through the body to produce a two-dimensional picture of the bones.

Chapter 58

Directory of Sports Injury Resources

Organizations with Information about Sports-Related Injuries and Injury Prevention

Alzheimer's Disease Education & Referral Center (ADEAR)
P.O. Box 8250
Silver Spring, MD 20907-8250
Toll-Free: 800-438-4380
Website: www.alzheimers.org
E-mail: adear@alzheimers.org

American Academy of Allergy, Asthma and Immunology
611 E. Wells Street
Milwaukee, WI 53202-3889
Toll-Free Physician Referral and Information Line: 800-822-2762
Tel: 414-272-6071
Website: www.aaaai.org
E-mail: info@aaaai.org

American Academy of Ophthalmology
P.O. Box 7424
San Francisco, CA 94120
Tel: 415-561-8500
Fax: 415-561-8533
Website: www.aao.org
E-mail: customer_service@aao.org

American Academy of Orthopaedic Surgeons (AAOS)
6300 North River Road
Rosemont, IL 60018-4262
Toll-Free: 800-346-AAOS (2267)
Tel: 847-823-7186
Fax: 847-823-8125
Fax-on-Demand: 800-999-2939
Website: www.aaos.org
E-mail: custserv@aaos.org

Resources in this chapter were compiled from many sources including: "Librarian Picks: Traumatic Brain Injury," April 2001, and "Librarian Picks: Spinal Cord Injury," April 1999, from the National Rehabilitation Information Center. All information was verified to be correct as of June 2002.

557

American Academy of Otolaryngology-Head and Neck Surgery
One Prince St.
Alexandria, VA 22314-3357
Tel: 703-836-4444
Website: www.entnet.org

American Academy of Pediatrics (AAP)
141 Northwest Point Boulevard
Elk Grove Village, IL 60007-1098
Tel: 847-434-4000
Fax: 847-434-8000
Website: www.aap.org
E-mail: kidsdocs@aap.org

American Academy of Podiatric Sports Medicine
4414 Ives Street
Rockville, MD 20853
Toll-Free: 800-438-3355
Tel: 301-962-1540
Website: www.aapsm.org
E-mail: info@aapsm.org

American Chronic Pain Association (ACPA)
P.O. Box 850
Rocklin, CA 95677-0850
Tel: 916-632-0922
Fax: 916-632-3208
Website: www.theacpa.org
E-mail: ACPA@pacbell.net

American College of Rheumatology
1800 Century Place, Suite 250
Atlanta, GA 30345
Tel: 404-633-3777
Fax: 404-633-1870
Website: www.rheumatology.org
E-mail: acr@rheumatology.org

American Dental Association (ADA)
211 E Chicago Avenue
Chicago, IL 60611
Tel: 312-440-2500
Fax: 312-440-2800
Website: www.ada.org

American Medical Society for Sports Medicine
11639 Earnshaw
Overland Park, KS 66210
Tel: 913-327-1415
Fax: 913-327-1491
Website: www.amssm.org
E-mail: office@amssm.org

American National Standards Institute (ANSI)
Fourth Floor
25 West 43rd Street
New York, NY 10036
Tel: 212-642-4900
Fax: 212-398-0023
Website: www.ansi.org
E-mail: info@ansi.org

American Orthopaedic Society for Sports Medicine
6300 N. River Road, Suite 200
Rosemont, IL 60018
Tel: 847-292-4900
Fax: 847-292-4905
Website: www.sportsmed.org

American Physical Therapy Association (APTA)
1111 North Fairfax Street
Alexandria, VA 22314-1488
Toll-Free: 800-999-2782
Tel: 703-684-2782
TDD: 703-683-6748
Fax: 703-684-7343
Website: www.apta.org

American Podiatric Medical Association
9312 Old Georgetown Road
Bethesda, MD 20814
Toll-Free: 800-366-8227
Tel: 301-571-9200
Fax: 301-530-2752
Website: www.apma.org
E-mail: askapma@apma.org

American Red Cross
P.O. Box 37243
Washington, DC 20013
Toll-Free: 800-435-7669
Website: www.redcross.org

American Society for Testing & Materials (ASTM)
100 Barr Harbor Drive
West Conshocken, PA 19428
Tel: 610-832-9585
Fax: 610-832-9555
Website: www.astm.org
E-mail: service@astm.org

American Sport Education Program (ASEP)
Box 5076
Champaign, IL 61825-5076
Toll-free: 800-747-3698

Arizona Sports Summit Accord
Josephson Institute
4640 Admiralty Way, Suite 1001
Marina del Rey, CA 90292
Tel: 310-306-1868
Fax: 310-306-2140
Website: www.charactercounts.org/sports/accord.htm

Arthritis Foundation
1330 West Peachtree Street
Atlanta, GA 30309
Toll-Free: 800-283-7800
Tel: 404-872-7100 or call your local chapter (listed in the local telephone directory)
Website: www.arthritis.org

Brain Injury Association
105 North Alfred Street
Alexandria, VA 22314
Toll-Free: 800-444-6443
Tel: 703-236-6000
Fax: 703-236-6001
Website: www.biausa.org
E-mail: familyhelpline@biausa.org

Centers for Disease Control and Prevention (CDC)
Division of Data Services
National Center for Health Statistics
6525 Belcrest Road
Hyattsville, MD 20782-2003
Tel: 301-458-4636
Website: www.cdc.gov/nchs

559

Disabled Sports USA
451 Hungerford Dr., Suite 100
Rockville, MD 20850
Tel: 301-217-0960
Fax: 301-217-0968
Website: www.dsusa.org
E-mail: dsusa@dsusa.org

***Hockey Equipment
Certification Council***
3 Baker Hill Road
Great Neck, New York 11023
Tel: 516-482-5374
Fax: 516-482-1231
Website: www.hecc-hockey.org

Little League Baseball, Inc.
P.O. Box 3485
Williamsport, PA 17701
Tel: 570-326-1921
Website: www.littleleague.org

***Minnesota Amateur Sports
Commission***
1700 105th Ave. N.E.
Blaine, MN 55449
Tel: 763-785-5630
Fax: 763-785-5699
Website: www.masc.state.mn.us/
resources/index.html

***National Alliance for Youth
Sports***
2050 Vista Parkway
West Palm Beach, FL 33411
Toll-Free: 800-729-2057 or 800-
688-KIDS
Tel: 561-684-1141
Fax: 561-684-2546
Website: www.nays.org
E-mail: nays@nays.org

***National Athletic Trainers
Association (NATA)***
2952 Stemmons Freeway
Dallas, TX 75247-6916
Toll-Free: 800-879-6282
Tel: 214-637-6282
Fax: 214-637-2206
Website: www.nata.org
E-mail: natanews@nata.org

***National Center for Injury
Prevention and Control***
Mailstop K65
4770 Buford Highway N.E.
Atlanta, GA 30341-3724
Tel: 770-488-1506
Fax: 770-488-1667
Website: www.cdc.gov/ncipc
E-mail: OHCINFO@cdc.gov

***National Children's Center
for Rural and Agricultural
Health and Safety***
National Farm Medicine Center
1000 North Oak Avenue
Marshfield, WI 54449
Toll-Free: 888-924-SAFE (7233)
Fax: 715-389-4996
Website: http://research.marsh
fieldclinic.org/children/Resources/
Equestrian/FactSheet.htm
E-mail: nccrahs@mfldclin.edu

***National Chronic Pain
Outreach Association
(NCPOA)***
7979 Old Georgetown Road
Suite 100
Bethesda, MD 20814-2429
Tel: 301-652-4948
Fax: 301-907-0745
E-mail: ncpoa@cfw.com

National Clearinghouse for Alcohol and Drug Information (NCADI)
11426-28 Rockville Pike
Suite 200
Rockville, MD 20852
Toll-Free: 800-729-6686
Website: www.health.org

National Federation of State High School Associations
P.O. Box 690
Indianapolis, IN 46206
Tel: 317-972-6900
Fax: 317-822-5700
Website: www.nfhs.org

National Headache Foundation
Second Floor
428 W. St. James Pl.
Chicago IL 60614-2750
Toll-Free: 888-NHF-5552 (643-5552)
Tel: 773-388-6399
Fax: 773-525-7357
Website: www.headaches.org
E-mail: info@headaches.org

National Institute of Arthritis and Musculoskeletal and Skin Diseases
NIAMS/National Institutes of Health
1 AMS Circle
Bethesda, MD 20892-3675
Toll-Free: 877-22-NIAMS (64267)
Tel: 301-495-4484
TTY: 301-565-2966
Fax: 301-718-6366
Website: www.nih.gov/niams
E-mail: NIAMSinfo@mail.nih.gov

National Institute of Child Centered Coaching
3160 Pinebrook Road
Park City, UT 84060
Toll-Free: 801-649-5822

National Institute on Drug Abuse (NIDA)
6001 Executive Boulevard
Room 5213
Bethesda, MD 20892-9561
Tel: 301-443-1124
Infofax: 888-644-6432
TTY: 888-889-6432
Website: www.drugabuse.gov
Website: www.steroidabuse.org

National Operating Committee on Standards for Athletic Equipment (NOCSAE)
P.O. Box 12290
Overland, KS 66282
Tel: 913-888-1340
Fax: 913-888-1065
Website: www.nocsae.org

National Osteoporosis Foundation
1232 22nd Street, N.W.
Washington, D.C. 20037-1292
Tel: 202-223-2226
Website: www.nof.org
E-mail: patientinfo@nof.org

National Program for Playground Safety

School for Health, Physical Education and Leisure Services
WRC 205
University of Northern Iowa
Cedar Falls, IA 50614-0618
Toll-Free: 800-554-PLAY (7529)
Tel: 319-273-2416
Fax: 319-273-7308
Website: www.uni.edu/playground
E-mail: playground-safety@uni.edu

National Rehabilitation Information Center (NARIC)

4200 Forbes Boulevard, Suite 202
Lanham, MD 20706
Toll-Free: 800-346-2742
Tel: 301-459-5900
Website: www.naric.com
E-mail: naricinfo@heitechservices.com

National SAFE KIDS Campaign

1301 Pennsylvania Ave. N.W.
Suite 202
Washington, DC 20004
Tel: 202-662-0600
Fax: 202-393-2072
Website: www.safekids.org
E-mail: info@safekids.org

National Safety Council

1121 Spring Lake Drive
Itasca, IL 60143-3201
Tel: 630-285-1121
Fax: 630-285-1315
Website: www.nsc.org
E-mail: customerservice@nsc.org

National Ski Areas Association

133 S. Van Gordon Street
Suite 300
Lakewood, CO 80228
Tel: 303-987-1111
Fax: 303-986-2345
Website: www.nsaa.org
E-mail: nsaa@nsaa.org

National Ski Patrol

133 S. Van Gordon Street
Suite 100
Lakewood, CO 80228
Tel: 303-987-1111
Fax: 303-988-3005
Website: www.nsp.org
E-mail: nsp@nsp.org

National Youth Sports Safety Foundation

One Beacon Street, Suite 3333
Boston, MA 02108
Tel: 617-277-1771
Fax: 617-722-9999
Website: www.nyssf.org
E-mail: NYSSF@aol.com

Osteoporosis and Related Bone Diseases–National Resource Center

1232 22nd Street, N.W.
Washington, D.C. 20037-1292
Toll-Free: 800-624-BONE (2663)
Tel: 202-223-0344
TTY: 202-466-4315
Fax: 202-293-2356
Website: www.osteo.org
E-mail: orbdnrc@nof.org

Positive Coaching Alliance
c/o Stanford Athletic Department
Stanford, CA 94305
Tel: 650-725-0024
Fax: 650-725-7242
Website: www.positivecoach.org
E-mail: pca@positivecoach.org

Protective Eyewear
Certification Council (PECC)
c/o Paul F. Vinger, MD
297 Heath's Bridge Road
Concord, MA 01742
Website: www.protecteyes.org
E-mail: eyesafety@dtl-inc.com

SafeUSA™
P.O. Box 8189
Silver Springs, MD 20907-8189
Toll-Free: 888-252-7751
Website: www.cdc.gov/safeusa
E-mail: sainfo@cdc.gov

Snell Memorial Foundation
(SNELL)
3628 Madison Avenue, Suite 11
North Highlands, CA 95660
Toll-Free: 888-SNELL99
Tel: 916-331-5073
Fax: 916-331-0359
Website: www.smf.org
E-mail: info@smf.org

USA Hockey
Toll-Free: 800-667-0781
Website: www.usahockey.com
E-mail: comments@usahockey.org

U.S. Consumer Product
Safety Division
4330 East-West Highway
Bethesda, MD 20814-4408
Toll-Free: 800-638-2772
Tel: 301-504-0990
Fax: 301-504-0124 and 301-504-0025
Website: www.cpsc.gov/kids/skate.html
E-mail: info@cpsc.gov

Information Sources on Traumatic Brain Injury (TBI)

Brain Injury Association
105 North Alfred Street
Alexandria, VA 22314
Toll-Free: 800-444-6443
Tel: 703-236-6000
Fax: 703-236-6001
Website: www.biausa.org
E-mail: familyhelpline@biausa.org

Provides education and information on TBI, support groups, advocacy, and local resources. Website contains definitions to medical terminology, details of the rehabilitation process, and information on state affiliates.

Head Injury Hotline
212 Pioneer Building
Seattle, WA 98104
Tel: 206-621-8558
Website: www.headinjury.com
E-mail: brain@headinjury.com

Provides callers with information on living with brain injury, including consultations and referrals to health care, legal professionals, and support groups. Established by the Phoenix Project, a TBI information clearinghouse.

Family Caregiver Alliance
690 Market Street
Suite 600
San Francisco, CA 94104
Toll-Free: 800-245-6686 (California only)
Tel: 415-434-3388
Fax: 415-434-3508
Website: www.caregiver.org
E-mail: info@caregiver.org

Assists families of persons with chronic or progressive brain disorders. Distributes information on caregiving and care of people with cognitive impairments.

Coma Recovery Association
100 East Old Country Rd., Suite 9
Mineola, NY 11501
Tel: 516-746-7714
Fax: 516-997-1613
Website: www.comarecovery
E-mail: office@comarecovery.org

Provides information and referrals regarding treatment, rehabilitation, and support, to those affected by coma and head injury. Website includes reports and a listing of available materials.

A Chance to Grow
1800 Second Street, N.E.
Minneapolis, MN 55418
Tel: 612-789-1236
Fax: 612-706-5555
Website: www.actg.org
E-mail: actg@mail.actg.org

Provides neurophysiological rehabilitation services to the brain injured. Maintains a library on brain injury. Programs can be made available on an in-home basis.

The National Resource Center for Traumatic Brain Injury
P.O. Box 980542
Richmond, VA 23298-0542
Tel: 804-828-9055
Fax: 804-828-2378
Website: http://neuro.pmr.vcu.edu

Provides practical and relevant information, including videotapes. Develops educational materials including intervention and assessment tools. Website contains lists of materials available, a question and answer column, and relevant links.

National Easter Seal Society
230 West Monroe Street, Suite 1800
Chicago, IL 60606
Toll-Free: 800-221-6827
Tel: 312-726-6200
TTY: 312-726-4258
Fax: 312-726-1494
Website: www.easter-seals.org
E-mail: info@easter-seals.org

Provides multiple services including physical, occupational and speech therapy, adult day care, and vocational rehabilitation. Call for information on offices in your area. Website includes program information listed by city and state.

Additional Online Information about Traumatic Brain Injury

The Brain Information Page
Toll-Free: 800-992-9477
Tel: 920-361-9447
Website: www.tbilaw.com

Wide variety of information on TBI.

The Perspectives Network
P.O. Box 121012
W. Melbourne, FL 32912-1012
Website: www.tbi.org
E-mail: tpn@tbi.org

Information on peer communication networks.

Case Management Resource Guide
1500 Walnut Street, Suite 1000
Philadelphia, PA 19102
Toll-Free: 800-784-2332
Tel: 215-875-1212
Fax: 215-735-3966
Website: www.cmrg.com
E-mail: cmrg@cmrg.com

Search for rehab facilities and numerous other healthcare providers.

Institute on Community Integration
University of Minnesota
102 Pattee Hall
150 Pillsbury Drive, S.E.
Minneapolis, MN 55455
Tel: 612-624-6300
Fax: 612-624-9344
Website: http://ici/umn.edu/default.html
E-mail: info@icimail.education.umn.edu

Information on life after TBI.

Information Sources on Spinal Cord Injury (SCI)

Marketing Health Promotion, Wellness, and Risk Information to Spinal Cord Injury Survivors in the Community
Craig Hospital
3425 South Clarkson Street
Englewood, CO 80110
Tel: 303-789-8308
Fax: 303-789-8699
Website: www.craighospital.org
E-mail: admissions@craighospital.org

Project offers information to assist SCI survivors, caregivers, and researchers in the areas of health maintenance, lifestyle choices, and improving quality of life. Website features the Wellness and Risk Assessment Profile, which can be completed online.

Spinal Cord Injury Information Network
Department of Physical Medicine and Rehabilitation
University of Alabama/Birmingham
Spain Rehabilitation Center
619 19th Street, South
Birmingham, AL 35249-7300
Tel: 205-934-3283
TTY: 205-934-4642
Fax: 205-975-4691
Website: www.spinalcord.uab.edu
E-mail: rtc@uab.edu

Center disseminates information based on research activities surrounding the prevention and treatment of secondary complications of SCI. Topics include urology, respiratory health, and treatments for pain and depression. Website contains an extensive variety of reports and fact sheets.

ABLEDATA
8630 Fenton Street, Suite 930
Silver Spring, MD 20910
Toll-Free: 800-227-0216
TTY: 301-608-8912
Fax: 301-608-8958
Website: www.abledata.com
E-mail abledata@macroint.com

Provides computerized searches for assistive devices, products, and equipment. Searches include distributor information and product descriptions. Fact sheets and information on catalogs are also available. The database can be searched from the ABLEDATA website.

National Spinal Cord Injury Association
6701 Democracy Boulevard, Suite 300-9
Bethesda, MD 20817
Toll-Free: 800-962-9629
Tel: 301-588-6959
Fax: 301-588-9414
Website: www.spinalcord.org
E-mail: nscia2@aol.com

Serves as a comprehensive information source for anyone effected by spinal cord injury. Referrals and consultations are available through the national office or one of the many state chapters. Website includes fact sheets, rehabilitation centers by state, and state chapter information.

National Institute of Neurological Disorders and Stroke
National Institutes of Health
Bethesda, MD 20892
Toll-Free: 800-352-9424
Website: www.ninds.nih.gov

Provides scientific documents, research reports, and publications. Website includes up-to-date research findings, health information, and a publications guide.

National Center for Medical Rehabilitation Research (NCMRR)

Executive Building, Room 2A03
MSC 7510
6100 Executive Blvd.
Bethesda, MD 20892-7510
Tel: 301-402-2242
Website: www.nichd.nih.gov/about/ncmrr/ncmrr.htm

Funds and supports research projects and fosters the development of scientific knowledge needed to enhance the quality of life of persons with disabilities. Website includes mission statement and information on funding activities.

The Miami Project to Cure Paralysis University of Miami School of Medicine

P.O. Box 016960
Miami, FL 33101-6960
Toll-Free: 800-782-6387
Tel: 305-243-6001
Fax: 305-243-6017
Website: www.miamiproject.miami.edu

A science and clinical research effort dedicated to finding new treatments and ultimately, a cure for paralysis. Project offers research and rehabilitation information packets. Website includes project overview, newsletter, and latest research findings.

Paralyzed Veterans of America (PVA)

801 18th Street, N.W.
Washington, DC 2000-3517
Toll-Free: 800-424-8200
Website: www.pva.org
E-mail: info@pva.org

Advocacy and information association with brochures covering such topics as accessibility, legislation, assistive technology, and sports. Website includes SCI related news, research and treatment guides, chapter information, and Internet links.

Additional Online Information on Spinal Cord Injury

Case Management Resource Guide
1500 Walnut Street, Suite 1000
Philadelphia, PA 19102
Toll-Free: 800-784-2332
Tel: 215-875-1212
Fax: 215-735-3966
Website: www.cmrg.com
E-mail: cmrg@cmrg.com

Search for rehab facilities and numerous other healthcare providers.

New Mobility Magazine
Website: www.mobility.com

Latest SCI news, jobline, bookstore, chat rooms, other resources.

Spinal Cord Injury Update
Website: http://depts.washington.edu/rehab/sci/update.shtml

Info on medical care, rehabilitation, living with SCI.

Back and Neck Injury Links
http://backandneck.about.com/msubsci.htm

Resources and information

Index

Index

M

magnetic resonance imaging (MRI)
ankle injuries 288
brain injury 81
defined 553
described 380
growth plate injuries 161
knee problems 129
shoulder problems 148
sports injuries 374
stress fractures 113
Malone, T. 125n
Mangine, R. 125n
Marketing Health Promotion,
Wellness, and Risk Information to
Spinal Cord Injury Survivors in the
Community, contact information
567
Marshfield Clinic, horses and children
publication 315n
Massachusetts Governor's Committee
on Physical Fitness and Sports, contact information 446
Matava, Matthew 213n
McAdam, C. 351n
MCL *see* medial collateral ligament
mechanical knee problems, described
126
medial collateral ligament (MCL), described 128
medial tibial stress syndrome, running 217
meniscus
described 127
injuries 131–33
soccer injury 204
metaphysis, described 161
metatarsalgia, running 216
methandrostenolone 448
methylprednisolone 361
Metzl, Jordan D. 17n
The Miami Project to Cure
Paralysis University of Miami
School of Medicine, contact
information 569
micro-traumatic knee injury, described 140

Miller, D. 351n
Miller full-body splint, described
358–59
mineral supplements 432–34
Minnesota Amateur Sports Commission, contact information 173, 560
Monitoring the Future study, steroid
abuse 447, 449
motorized scooters 323–26
motor vehicle accidents, defined 553
motor vehicle nontraffic accidents,
defined 553
motor vehicle traffic accidents, defined 553
mountain biking injuries 221–30,
225, 226, 227, 228
"Mountain Biking Injuries: Fitting
Treatment to the Causes"
(Kronisch) 221n
mouth guards 464, 475
MRI *see* magnetic resonance imaging
Mueller, Frederick O. 31n, 181n, 181–
82, 193
muscle
defined 123, 553
exercise 431
protein intake 434
muscular strength evaluation 439–
40
musculoskeletal injuries
exercise 235
statistics 17–18
musculoskeletal system
defined 458, 553
older adults 541–42
steroid abuse 454

N

nandrolone decanoate 448
nandrolone phenpropionate 448
naproxen, shoulder problems 151
NARIC *see* National Rehabilitation
Information Center
NATA *see* National Athletic Trainers
Association
National Alliance for Youth Sports,
contact information 173, 560

O

withdrawal, defined 458, 556
wrestling, catastrophic injuries 37–
39, 42–43, 53
wrist guards
skating 76
snowboarding 289, 297, *298*
wrist injuries, snowboarding *286–87,*
288–89, *290,* 295–97

X

X-rays
defined 556
knee problem diagnosis 128
shoulder problem diagnosis 147
sports injuries 374
see also computerized axial tomography

Y

Young, Craig C. 283n
youth endurance, development guidelines 443–44
youth fitness, development guidelines
440–43
youth flexibility, development guidelines 444–45
"Youth in Sports" (AOSSM) 479n

Z

Zigman, Cary 343n
Zoltan, Donald 203n
zygapophyseal joints, described 362

Health Reference Series
COMPLETE CATALOG

Adolescent Health Sourcebook

Basic Consumer Health Information about Common Medical, Mental, and Emotional Concerns in Adolescents, Including Facts about Acne, Body Piercing, Mononucleosis, Nutrition, Eating Disorders, Stress, Depression, Behavior Problems, Peer Pressure, Violence, Gangs, Drug Use, Puberty, Sexuality, Pregnancy, Learning Disabilities, and More

Along with a Glossary of Terms and Other Resources for Further Help and Information

Edited by Chad T. Kimball. 658 pages. 2002. 0-7808-0248-9. $78.

■

AIDS Sourcebook, 1st Edition

Basic Information about AIDS and HIV Infection, Featuring Historical and Statistical Data, Current Research, Prevention, and Other Special Topics of Interest for Persons Living with AIDS

Along with Source Listings for Further Assistance

Edited by Karen Bellenir and Peter D. Dresser. 831 pages. 1995. 0-7808-0031-1. $78.

"One strength of this book is its practical emphasis. The intended audience is the lay reader . . . useful as an educational tool for health care providers who work with AIDS patients. Recommended for public libraries as well as hospital or academic libraries that collect consumer materials."
— *Bulletin of the Medical Library Association, Jan '96*

"This is the most comprehensive volume of its kind on an important medical topic. Highly recommended for all libraries."
— *Reference Book Review, '96*

"Very useful reference for all libraries."
— *Choice, Association of College and Research Libraries, Oct '95*

"There is a wealth of information here that can provide much educational assistance. It is a must book for all libraries and should be on the desk of each and every congressional leader. Highly recommended."
— *AIDS Book Review Journal, Aug '95*

"Recommended for most collections."
— *Library Journal, Jul '95*

■

AIDS Sourcebook, 2nd Edition

Basic Consumer Health Information about Acquired Immune Deficiency Syndrome (AIDS) and Human Immunodeficiency Virus (HIV) Infection, Featuring Updated Statistical Data, Reports on Recent Research and Prevention Initiatives, and Other Special Topics of Interest for Persons Living with AIDS, Including New Antiretroviral Treatment Options, Strategies for Combating Opportunistic Infections, Information about Clinical Trials, and More

Along with a Glossary of Important Terms and Resource Listings for Further Help and Information

Edited by Karen Bellenir. 751 pages. 1999. 0-7808-0225-X. $78.

"Highly recommended."
— *American Reference Books Annual, 2000*

"Excellent sourcebook. This continues to be a highly recommended book. There is no other book that provides as much information as this book provides."
— *AIDS Book Review Journal, Dec-Jan 2000*

"Recommended reference source."
— *Booklist, American Library Association, Dec '99*

"A solid text for college-level health libraries."
— *The Bookwatch, Aug '99*

Cited in *Reference Sources for Small and Medium-Sized Libraries, American Library Association, 1999*

■

Alcoholism Sourcebook

Basic Consumer Health Information about the Physical and Mental Consequences of Alcohol Abuse, Including Liver Disease, Pancreatitis, Wernicke-Korsakoff Syndrome (Alcoholic Dementia), Fetal Alcohol Syndrome, Heart Disease, Kidney Disorders, Gastrointestinal Problems, and Immune System Compromise and Featuring Facts about Addiction, Detoxification, Alcohol Withdrawal, Recovery, and the Maintenance of Sobriety

Along with a Glossary and Directories of Resources for Further Help and Information

Edited by Karen Bellenir. 613 pages. 2000. 0-7808-0325-6. $78.

"This title is one of the few reference works on alcoholism for general readers. For some readers this will be a welcome complement to the many self-help books on the market. Recommended for collections serving general readers and consumer health collections."
— *E-Streams, Mar '01*

"This book is an excellent choice for public and academic libraries."
— *American Reference Books Annual, 2001*

"Recommended reference source."
— *Booklist, American Library Association, Dec '00*

"Presents a wealth of information on alcohol use and abuse and its effects on the body and mind, treatment, and prevention." — *SciTech Book News, Dec '00*

"Important new health guide which packs in the latest consumer information about the problems of alcoholism." — *Reviewer's Bookwatch, Nov '00*

SEE ALSO Drug Abuse Sourcebook, Substance Abuse Sourcebook

Allergies Sourcebook, 1st Edition

Basic Information about Major Forms and Mechanisms of Common Allergic Reactions, Sensitivities, and Intolerances, Including Anaphylaxis, Asthma, Hives and Other Dermatologic Symptoms, Rhinitis, and Sinusitis

Along with Their Usual Triggers Like Animal Fur, Chemicals, Drugs, Dust, Foods, Insects, Latex, Pollen, and Poison Ivy, Oak, and Sumac; Plus Information on Prevention, Identification, and Treatment

Edited by Allan R. Cook. 611 pages. 1997. 0-7808-0036-2. $78.

■

Allergies Sourcebook, 2nd Edition

Basic Consumer Health Information about Allergic Disorders, Triggers, Reactions, and Related Symptoms, Including Anaphylaxis, Rhinitis, Sinusitis, Asthma, Dermatitis, Conjunctivitis, and Multiple Chemical Sensitivity

Along with Tips on Diagnosis, Prevention, and Treatment, Statistical Data, a Glossary, and a Directory of Sources for Further Help and Information

Edited by Annemarie S. Muth. 598 pages. 2002. 0-7808-0376-0. $78.

■

Alternative Medicine Sourcebook, First Edition

Basic Consumer Health Information about Alternatives to Conventional Medicine, Including Acupressure, Acupuncture, Aromatherapy, Ayurveda, Bioelectromagnetics, Environmental Medicine, Essence Therapy, Food and Nutrition Therapy, Herbal Therapy, Homeopathy, Imaging, Massage, Naturopathy, Reflexology, Relaxation and Meditation, Sound Therapy, Vitamin and Mineral Therapy, and Yoga, and More

Edited by Allan R. Cook. 737 pages. 1999. 0-7808-0200-4. $78.

"Recommended reference source."
—*Booklist, American Library Association, Feb '00*

"A great addition to the reference collection of every type of library." —*American Reference Books Annual, 2000*

■

Alternative Medicine Sourcebook, Second Edition

Basic Consumer Health Information about Alternative and Complementary Medical Practices, Including Acupuncture, Chiropractic, Herbal Medicine, Homeopathy, Naturopathic Medicine, Mind-Body Interventions, Ayurveda, and Other Non-Western Medical Traditions

Along with Facts about such Specific Therapies as Massage Therapy, Aromatherapy, Qigong, Hypnosis, Prayer, Dance, and Art Therapies, a Glossary, and Resources for Further Information

Edited by Dawn D. Matthews. 618 pages. 2002. 0-7808-0605-0. $78.

Alzheimer's, Stroke & 29 Other Neurological Disorders Sourcebook, 1st Edition

Basic Information for the Layperson on 31 Diseases or Disorders Affecting the Brain and Nervous System, First Describing the Illness, Then Listing Symptoms, Diagnostic Methods, and Treatment Options, and Including Statistics on Incidences and Causes

Edited by Frank E. Bair. 579 pages. 1993. 1-55888-748-2. $78.

"Nontechnical reference book that provides reader-friendly information."
—*Family Caregiver Alliance Update, Winter '96*

"Should be included in any library's patient education section." —*American Reference Books Annual, 1994*

"Written in an approachable and accessible style. Recommended for patient education and consumer health collections in health science center and public libraries." —*Academic Library Book Review, Dec '93*

"It is very handy to have information on more than thirty neurological disorders under one cover, and there is no recent source like it." —*Reference Quarterly, American Library Association, Fall '93*

SEE ALSO Brain Disorders Sourcebook

■

Alzheimer's Disease Sourcebook, 2nd Edition

Basic Consumer Health Information about Alzheimer's Disease, Related Disorders, and Other Dementias, Including Multi-Infarct Dementia, AIDS-Related Dementia, Alcoholic Dementia, Huntington's Disease, Delirium, and Confusional States

Along with Reports Detailing Current Research Efforts in Prevention and Treatment, Long-Term Care Issues, and Listings of Sources for Additional Help and Information

Edited by Karen Bellenir. 524 pages. 1999. 0-7808-0223-3. $78.

"Provides a wealth of useful information not otherwise available in one place. This resource is recommended for all types of libraries."
—*American Reference Books Annual, 2000*

"Recommended reference source."
—*Booklist, American Library Association, Oct '99*

■

Arthritis Sourcebook

Basic Consumer Health Information about Specific Forms of Arthritis and Related Disorders, Including Rheumatoid Arthritis, Osteoarthritis, Gout, Polymyalgia Rheumatica, Psoriatic Arthritis, Spondyloarthropathies, Juvenile Rheumatoid Arthritis, and Juvenile Ankylosing Spondylitis

Along with Information about Medical, Surgical, and Alternative Treatment Options, and Including Strategies for Coping with Pain, Fatigue, and Stress

Edited by Allan R. Cook. 550 pages. 1998. 0-7808-0201-2. $78.

". . . accessible to the layperson."
—Reference and Research Book News, Feb '99

Asthma Sourcebook

Basic Consumer Health Information about Asthma, Including Symptoms, Traditional and Nontraditional Remedies, Treatment Advances, Quality-of-Life Aids, Medical Research Updates, and the Role of Allergies, Exercise, Age, the Environment, and Genetics in the Development of Asthma

Along with Statistical Data, a Glossary, and Directories of Support Groups, and Other Resources for Further Information

Edited by Annemarie S. Muth. 628 pages. 2000. 0-7808-0381-7. $78.

"A worthwhile reference acquisition for public libraries and academic medical libraries whose readers desire a quick introduction to the wide range of asthma information." *— Choice, Association of College & Research Libraries, Jun '01*

"Recommended reference source."
— Booklist, American Library Association, Feb '01

"Highly recommended." *— The Bookwatch, Jan '01*

"There is much good information for patients and their families who deal with asthma daily."
— American Medical Writers Association Journal, Winter '01

"This informative text is recommended for consumer health collections in public, secondary school, and community college libraries and the libraries of universities with a large undergraduate population."
— American Reference Books Annual, 2001

Attention Deficit Disorder Sourcebook, First Edition

Basic Consumer Health Information about Attention Deficit/Hyperactivity Disorder in Children and Adults, Including Facts about Causes, Symptoms, Diagnostic Criteria, and Treatment Options Such as Medications, Behavior Therapy, Coaching, and Homeopathy

Along with Reports on Current Research Initiatives, Legal Issues, and Government Regulations, and Featuring a Glossary of Related Terms, Internet Resources, and a List of Additional Reading Material

Edited by Dawn D. Matthews. 470 pages. 2002. 0-7808-0624-7. $78.

Back & Neck Disorders Sourcebook

Basic Information about Disorders and Injuries of the Spinal Cord and Vertebrae, Including Facts on Chiropractic Treatment, Surgical Interventions, Paralysis, and Rehabilitation

Along with Advice for Preventing Back Trouble

Edited by Karen Bellenir. 548 pages. 1997. 0-7808-0202-0. $78.

"The strength of this work is its basic, easy-to-read format. Recommended."
— Reference and User Services Quarterly, American Library Association, Winter '97

Blood & Circulatory Disorders Sourcebook

Basic Information about Blood and Its Components, Anemias, Leukemias, Bleeding Disorders, and Circulatory Disorders, Including Aplastic Anemia, Thalassemia, Sickle-Cell Disease, Hemochromatosis, Hemophilia, Von Willebrand Disease, and Vascular Diseases

Along with a Special Section on Blood Transfusions and Blood Supply Safety, a Glossary, and Source Listings for Further Help and Information

Edited by Karen Bellenir and Linda M. Shin. 554 pages. 1998. 0-7808-0203-9. $78.

"Recommended reference source."
—Booklist, American Library Association, Feb '99

"An important reference sourcebook written in simple language for everyday, non-technical users. "
—Reviewer's Bookwatch, Jan '99

Brain Disorders Sourcebook

Basic Consumer Health Information about Strokes, Epilepsy, Amyotrophic Lateral Sclerosis (ALS/Lou Gehrig's Disease), Parkinson's Disease, Brain Tumors, Cerebral Palsy, Headache, Tourette Syndrome, and More

Along with Statistical Data, Treatment and Rehabilitation Options, Coping Strategies, Reports on Current Research Initiatives, a Glossary, and Resource Listings for Additional Help and Information

Edited by Karen Bellenir. 481 pages. 1999. 0-7808-0229-2. $78.

"Belongs on the shelves of any library with a consumer health collection." *— E-Streams, Mar '00*

"Recommended reference source."
— Booklist, American Library Association, Oct '99

SEE ALSO *Alzheimer's, Stroke & 29 Other Neurological Disorders Sourcebook, 1st Edition*

Breast Cancer Sourcebook

Basic Consumer Health Information about Breast Cancer, Including Diagnostic Methods, Treatment Options, Alternative Therapies, Self-Help Information, Related Health Concerns, Statistical and Demographic Data, and Facts for Men with Breast Cancer

Along with Reports on Current Research Initiatives, a Glossary of Related Medical Terms, and a Directory of Sources for Further Help and Information

Edited by Edward J. Prucha and Karen Bellenir. 580 pages. 2001. 0-7808-0244-6. $78.

"Recommended reference source."
— *Booklist, American Library Association, Jan '02*

"This reference source is highly recommended. It is quite informative, comprehensive and detailed in nature, and yet it offers practical advice in easy-to-read language. It could be thought of as the 'bible' of breast cancer for the consumer." — *E-Streams, Jan '02*

"The broad range of topics covered in lay language make the *Breast Cancer Sourcebook* an excellent addition to public and consumer health library collections." — *American Reference Books Annual 2002*

"From the pros and cons of different screening methods and results to treatment options, *Breast Cancer Sourcebook* provides the latest information on the subject." — *Library Bookwatch, Dec '01*

"This thoroughgoing, very readable reference covers all aspects of breast health and cancer. . . . Readers will find much to consider here. Recommended for all public and patient health collections." — *Library Journal, Sep '01*

SEE ALSO *Cancer Sourcebook for Women, 1st and 2nd Editions, Women's Health Concerns Sourcebook*

■

Breastfeeding Sourcebook

Basic Consumer Health Information about the Benefits of Breastmilk, Preparing to Breastfeed, Breastfeeding as a Baby Grows, Nutrition, and More, Including Information on Special Situations and Concerns Such as Mastitis, Illness, Medications, Allergies, Multiple Births, Prematurity, Special Needs, and Adoption

Along with a Glossary and Resources for Additional Help and Information

Edited by Jenni Lynn Colson. 388 pages. 2002. 0-7808-0332-9. $78.

SEE ALSO *Pregnancy & Birth Sourcebook*

■

Burns Sourcebook

Basic Consumer Health Information about Various Types of Burns and Scalds, Including Flame, Heat, Cold, Electrical, Chemical, and Sun Burns

Along with Information on Short-Term and Long-Term Treatments, Tissue Reconstruction, Plastic Surgery, Prevention Suggestions, and First Aid

Edited by Allan R. Cook. 604 pages. 1999. 0-7808-0204-7. $78.

"This is an exceptional addition to the series and is highly recommended for all consumer health collections, hospital libraries, and academic medical centers." — *E-Streams, Mar '00*

"This key reference guide is an invaluable addition to all health care and public libraries in confronting this ongoing health issue." — *American Reference Books Annual, 2000*

"Recommended reference source." — *Booklist, American Library Association, Dec '99*

SEE ALSO *Skin Disorders Sourcebook*

■

Cancer Sourcebook, 1st Edition

Basic Information on Cancer Types, Symptoms, Diagnostic Methods, and Treatments, Including Statistics on Cancer Occurrences Worldwide and the Risks Associated with Known Carcinogens and Activities

Edited by Frank E. Bair. 932 pages. 1990. 1-55888-888-8. $78.

Cited in *Reference Sources for Small and Medium-Sized Libraries, American Library Association, 1999*

"Written in nontechnical language. Useful for patients, their families, medical professionals, and librarians." — *Guide to Reference Books, 1996*

"Designed with the non-medical professional in mind. Libraries and medical facilities interested in patient education should certainly consider adding the *Cancer Sourcebook* to their holdings. This compact collection of reliable information . . . is an invaluable tool for helping patients and patients' families and friends to take the first steps in coping with the many difficulties of cancer." — *Medical Reference Services Quarterly, Winter '91*

"Specifically created for the nontechnical reader . . . an important resource for the general reader trying to understand the complexities of cancer." — *American Reference Books Annual, 1991*

"This publication's nontechnical nature and very comprehensive format make it useful for both the general public and undergraduate students." — *Choice, Association of College and Research Libraries, Oct '90*

■

New Cancer Sourcebook, 2nd Edition

Basic Information about Major Forms and Stages of Cancer, Featuring Facts about Primary and Secondary Tumors of the Respiratory, Nervous, Lymphatic, Circulatory, Skeletal, and Gastrointestinal Systems, and Specific Organs; Statistical and Demographic Data; Treatment Options; and Strategies for Coping

Edited by Allan R. Cook. 1,313 pages. 1996. 0-7808-0041-9. $78.

"An excellent resource for patients with newly diagnosed cancer and their families. The dialogue is simple, direct, and comprehensive. Highly recommended for patients and families to aid in their understanding of cancer and its treatment."

— *Booklist Health Sciences Supplement,*
American Library Association, Oct '97

"The amount of factual and useful information is extensive. The writing is very clear, geared to general readers. Recommended for all levels." — *Choice,*
Association of College & Research Libraries, Jan '97

Cancer Sourcebook, 3rd Edition

Basic Consumer Health Information about Major Forms and Stages of Cancer, Featuring Facts about Primary and Secondary Tumors of the Respiratory, Nervous, Lymphatic, Circulatory, Skeletal, and Gastrointestinal Systems, and Specific Organs

Along with Statistical and Demographic Data, Treatment Options, Strategies for Coping, a Glossary, and a Directory of Sources for Additional Help and Information

Edited by Edward J. Prucha. 1,069 pages. 2000. 0-7808-0227-6. $78.

"This title is recommended for health sciences and public libraries with consumer health collections."
— *E-Streams, Feb '01*

". . . can be effectively used by cancer patients and their families who are looking for answers in a language they can understand. Public and hospital libraries should have it on their shelves."
— *American Reference Books Annual, 2001*

"Recommended reference source."
—*Booklist, American Library Association, Dec '00*

Cancer Sourcebook for Women, 1st Edition

Basic Information about Specific Forms of Cancer That Affect Women, Featuring Facts about Breast Cancer, Cervical Cancer, Ovarian Cancer, Cancer of the Uterus and Uterine Sarcoma, Cancer of the Vagina, and Cancer of the Vulva; Statistical and Demographic Data; Treatments, Self-Help Management Suggestions, and Current Research Initiatives

Edited by Allan R. Cook and Peter D. Dresser. 524 pages. 1996. 0-7808-0076-1. $78.

". . . written in easily understandable, non-technical language. Recommended for public libraries or hospital and academic libraries that collect patient education or consumer health materials."
— *Medical Reference Services Quarterly, Spring '97*

"Would be of value in a consumer health library. . . . written with the health care consumer in mind. Medical jargon is at a minimum, and medical terms are explained in clear, understandable sentences."
— *Bulletin of the Medical Library Association, Oct '96*

"The availability under one cover of all these pertinent publications, grouped under cohesive headings, makes this certainly a most useful sourcebook." — *Choice,*
Association of College & Research Libraries, Jun '96

"Presents a comprehensive knowledge base for general readers. Men and women both benefit from the gold mine of information nestled between the two covers of this book. Recommended."
—*Academic Library Book Review, Summer '96*

"This timely book is highly recommended for consumer health and patient education collections in all libraries." — *Library Journal, Apr '96*

SEE ALSO *Breast Cancer Sourcebook, Women's Health Concerns Sourcebook*

Cancer Sourcebook for Women, 2nd Edition

Basic Consumer Health Information about Gynecologic Cancers and Related Concerns, Including Cervical Cancer, Endometrial Cancer, Gestational Trophoblastic Tumor, Ovarian Cancer, Uterine Cancer, Vaginal Cancer, Vulvar Cancer, Breast Cancer, and Common Non-Cancerous Uterine Conditions, with Facts about Cancer Risk Factors, Screening and Prevention, Treatment Options, and Reports on Current Research Initiatives

Along with a Glossary of Cancer Terms and a Directory of Resources for Additional Help and Information

Edited by Karen Bellenir. 604 pages. 2002. 0-7808-0226-8. $78.

SEE ALSO *Breast Cancer Sourcebook, Women's Health Concerns Sourcebook*

Cardiovascular Diseases & Disorders Sourcebook, 1st Edition

Basic Information about Cardiovascular Diseases and Disorders, Featuring Facts about the Cardiovascular System, Demographic and Statistical Data, Descriptions of Pharmacological and Surgical Interventions, Lifestyle Modifications, and a Special Section Focusing on Heart Disorders in Children

Edited by Karen Bellenir and Peter D. Dresser. 683 pages. 1995. 0-7808-0032-X. $78.

". . . comprehensive format provides an extensive overview on this subject." — *Choice,*
Association of College & Research Libraries, Jun '96

". . . an easily understood, complete, up-to-date resource. This well executed public health tool will make valuable information available to those that need it most, patients and their families. The typeface, sturdy non-reflective paper, and library binding add a feel of quality found wanting in other publications. Highly recommended for academic and general libraries. "
—*Academic Library Book Review, Summer '96*

SEE ALSO *Healthy Heart Sourcebook for Women, Heart Diseases & Disorders Sourcebook, 2nd Edition*

Caregiving Sourcebook

Basic Consumer Health Information for Caregivers, Including a Profile of Caregivers, Caregiving Responsibilities and Concerns, Tips for Specific Conditions, Care Environments, and the Effects of Caregiving

Along with Facts about Legal Issues, Financial Information, and Future Planning, a Glossary, and a Listing of Additional Resources

Edited by Joyce Brennfleck Shannon. 600 pages. 2001. 0-7808-0331-0. $78.

"Essential for most collections."
—Library Journal, Apr 1, 2002

"An ideal addition to the reference collection of any public library. Health sciences information professionals may also want to acquire the *Caregiving Sourcebook* for their hospital or academic library for use as a ready reference tool by health care workers interested in aging and caregiving."   *—E-Streams, Jan '02*

"Recommended reference source."
—Booklist, American Library Association, Oct '01

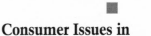

Colds, Flu & Other Common Ailments Sourcebook

Basic Consumer Health Information about Common Ailments and Injuries, Including Colds, Coughs, the Flu, Sinus Problems, Headaches, Fever, Nausea and Vomiting, Menstrual Cramps, Diarrhea, Constipation, Hemorrhoids, Back Pain, Dandruff, Dry and Itchy Skin, Cuts, Scrapes, Sprains, Bruises, and More

Along with Information about Prevention, Self-Care, Choosing a Doctor, Over-the-Counter Medications, Folk Remedies, and Alternative Therapies, and Including a Glossary of Important Terms and a Directory of Resources for Further Help and Information

Edited by Chad T. Kimball. 638 pages. 2001. 0-7808-0435-X. $78.

"A good starting point for research on common illnesses. It will be a useful addition to public and consumer health library collections."
—American Reference Books Annual 2002

"Will prove valuable to any library seeking to maintain a current, comprehensive reference collection of health resources. . . . Excellent reference."
—The Bookwatch, Aug '01

"Recommended reference source."
—Booklist, American Library Association, July '01

Communication Disorders Sourcebook

Basic Information about Deafness and Hearing Loss, Speech and Language Disorders, Voice Disorders, Balance and Vestibular Disorders, and Disorders of Smell, Taste, and Touch

Edited by Linda M. Ross. 533 pages. 1996. 0-7808-0077-X. $78.

"This is skillfully edited and is a welcome resource for the layperson. It should be found in every public and medical library."   *—Booklist Health Sciences Supplement, American Library Association, Oct '97*

Congenital Disorders Sourcebook

Basic Information about Disorders Acquired during Gestation, Including Spina Bifida, Hydrocephalus, Cerebral Palsy, Heart Defects, Craniofacial Abnormalities, Fetal Alcohol Syndrome, and More

Along with Current Treatment Options and Statistical Data

Edited by Karen Bellenir. 607 pages. 1997. 0-7808-0205-5. $78.

"Recommended reference source."
—Booklist, American Library Association, Oct '97

SEE ALSO Pregnancy & Birth Sourcebook

Consumer Issues in Health Care Sourcebook

Basic Information about Health Care Fundamentals and Related Consumer Issues, Including Exams and Screening Tests, Physician Specialties, Choosing a Doctor, Using Prescription and Over-the-Counter Medications Safely, Avoiding Health Scams, Managing Common Health Risks in the Home, Care Options for Chronically or Terminally Ill Patients, and a List of Resources for Obtaining Help and Further Information

Edited by Karen Bellenir. 618 pages. 1998. 0-7808-0221-7. $78.

"Both public and academic libraries will want to have a copy in their collection for readers who are interested in self-education on health issues."
—American Reference Books Annual, 2000

"The editor has researched the literature from government agencies and others, saving readers the time and effort of having to do the research themselves. Recommended for public libraries."
—Reference and User Services Quarterly, American Library Association, Spring '99

"Recommended reference source."
—Booklist, American Library Association, Dec '98

Contagious & Non-Contagious Infectious Diseases Sourcebook

Basic Information about Contagious Diseases like Measles, Polio, Hepatitis B, and Infectious Mononucleosis, and Non-Contagious Infectious Diseases like Tetanus and Toxic Shock Syndrome, and Diseases Occurring as Secondary Infections Such as Shingles and Reye Syndrome

Along with Vaccination, Prevention, and Treatment Information, and a Section Describing Emerging Infectious Disease Threats

Edited by Karen Bellenir and Peter D. Dresser. 566 pages. 1996. 0-7808-0075-3. $78.

Death & Dying Sourcebook

Basic Consumer Health Information for the Layperson about End-of-Life Care and Related Ethical and Legal Issues, Including Chief Causes of Death, Autopsies, Pain Management for the Terminally Ill, Life Support Systems, Insurance, Euthanasia, Assisted Suicide, Hospice Programs, Living Wills, Funeral Planning, Counseling, Mourning, Organ Donation, and Physician Training

Along with Statistical Data, a Glossary, and Listings of Sources for Further Help and Information

Edited by Annemarie S. Muth. 641 pages. 1999. 0-7808-0230-6. $78.

"Public libraries, medical libraries, and academic libraries will all find this sourcebook a useful addition to their collections."
— *American Reference Books Annual, 2001*

"An extremely useful resource for those concerned with death and dying in the United States."
— *Respiratory Care, Nov '00*

"Recommended reference source."
— *Booklist, American Library Association, Aug '00*

"This book is a definite must for all those involved in end-of-life care." — *Doody's Review Service, 2000*

■

Depression Sourcebook

Basic Consumer Health Information about Unipolar Depression, Bipolar Disorder, Postpartum Depression, Seasonal Affective Disorder, and Other Types of Depression in Children, Adolescents, Women, Men, the Elderly, and Other Selected Populations

Along with Facts about Causes, Risk Factors, Diagnostic Criteria, Treatment Options, Coping Strategies, Suicide Prevention, a Glossary, and a Directory of Sources for Additional Help and Information

Edited by Karen Belleni. 625 pages. 2002. 0-7808-0611-5. $78.

■

Diabetes Sourcebook, 1st Edition

Basic Information about Insulin-Dependent and Non-insulin-Dependent Diabetes Mellitus, Gestational Diabetes, and Diabetic Complications, Symptoms, Treatment, and Research Results, Including Statistics on Prevalence, Morbidity, and Mortality

Along with Source Listings for Further Help and Information

Edited by Karen Bellenir and Peter D. Dresser. 827 pages. 1994. 1-55888-751-2. $78.

". . . very informative and understandable for the layperson without being simplistic. It provides a comprehensive overview for laypersons who want a general understanding of the disease or who want to focus on various aspects of the disease."
— *Bulletin of the Medical Library Association, Jan '96*

Diabetes Sourcebook, 2nd Edition

Basic Consumer Health Information about Type 1 Diabetes (Insulin-Dependent or Juvenile-Onset Diabetes), Type 2 (Noninsulin-Dependent or Adult-Onset Diabetes), Gestational Diabetes, and Related Disorders, Including Diabetes Prevalence Data, Management Issues, the Role of Diet and Exercise in Controlling Diabetes, Insulin and Other Diabetes Medicines, and Complications of Diabetes Such as Eye Diseases, Periodontal Disease, Amputation, and End-Stage Renal Disease

Along with Reports on Current Research Initiatives, a Glossary, and Resource Listings for Further Help and Information

Edited by Karen Bellenir. 688 pages. 1998. 0-7808-0224-1. $78.

"An invaluable reference." — *Library Journal, May '00*

Selected as one of the 250 "Best Health Sciences Books of 1999." — *Doody's Rating Service, Mar-Apr 2000*

"This comprehensive book is an excellent addition for high school, academic, medical, and public libraries. This volume is highly recommended."
— *American Reference Books Annual, 2000*

"Provides useful information for the general public."
— *Healthlines, University of Michigan Health Management Research Center, Sep/Oct '99*

". . . provides reliable mainstream medical information . . . belongs on the shelves of any library with a consumer health collection." — *E-Streams, Sep '99*

"Recommended reference source."
— *Booklist, American Library Association, Feb '99*

■

Diet & Nutrition Sourcebook, 1st Edition

Basic Information about Nutrition, Including the Dietary Guidelines for Americans, the Food Guide Pyramid, and Their Applications in Daily Diet, Nutritional Advice for Specific Age Groups, Current Nutritional Issues and Controversies, the New Food Label and How to Use It to Promote Healthy Eating, and Recent Developments in Nutritional Research

Edited by Dan R. Harris. 662 pages. 1996. 0-7808-0084-2. $78.

"Useful reference as a food and nutrition sourcebook for the general consumer." — *Booklist Health Sciences Supplement, American Library Association, Oct '97*

"Recommended for public libraries and medical libraries that receive general information requests on nutrition. It is readable and will appeal to those interested in learning more about healthy dietary practices."
— *Medical Reference Services Quarterly, Fall '97*

"An abundance of medical and social statistics is translated into readable information geared toward the general reader." — *Bookwatch, Mar '97*

"With dozens of questionable diet books on the market, it is so refreshing to find a reliable and factual reference book. Recommended to aspiring professionals, librari-

ans, and others seeking and giving reliable dietary advice. An excellent compilation." —*Choice, Association of College and Research Libraries, Feb '97*

SEE ALSO *Digestive Diseases & Disorders Sourcebook, Gastrointestinal Diseases & Disorders Sourcebook*

∎

Diet & Nutrition Sourcebook, 2nd Edition

Basic Consumer Health Information about Dietary Guidelines, Recommended Daily Intake Values, Vitamins, Minerals, Fiber, Fat, Weight Control, Dietary Supplements, and Food Additives

Along with Special Sections on Nutrition Needs throughout Life and Nutrition for People with Such Specific Medical Concerns as Allergies, High Blood Cholesterol, Hypertension, Diabetes, Celiac Disease, Seizure Disorders, Phenylketonuria (PKU), Cancer, and Eating Disorders, and Including Reports on Current Nutrition Research and Source Listings for Additional Help and Information

Edited by Karen Bellenir. 650 pages. 1999. 0-7808-0228-4. $78.

"This book is an excellent source of basic diet and nutrition information." —*Booklist Health Sciences Supplement, American Library Association, Dec '00*

"This reference document should be in any public library, but it would be a very good guide for beginning students in the health sciences. If the other books in this publisher's series are as good as this, they should all be in the health sciences collections." —*American Reference Books Annual, 2000*

"This book is an excellent general nutrition reference for consumers who desire to take an active role in their health care for prevention. Consumers of all ages who select this book can feel confident they are receiving current and accurate information." —*Journal of Nutrition for the Elderly, Vol. 19, No. 4, '00*

"Recommended reference source." —*Booklist, American Library Association, Dec '99*

SEE ALSO *Digestive Diseases & Disorders Sourcebook, Gastrointestinal Diseases & Disorders Sourcebook*

∎

Digestive Diseases & Disorders Sourcebook

Basic Consumer Health Information about Diseases and Disorders that Impact the Upper and Lower Digestive System, Including Celiac Disease, Constipation, Crohn's Disease, Cyclic Vomiting Syndrome, Diarrhea, Diverticulosis and Diverticulitis, Gallstones, Heartburn, Hemorrhoids, Hernias, Indigestion (Dyspepsia), Irritable Bowel Syndrome, Lactose Intolerance, Ulcers, and More

Along with Information about Medications and Other Treatments, Tips for Maintaining a Healthy Digestive Tract, a Glossary, and Directory of Digestive Diseases Organizations

Edited by Karen Bellenir. 335 pages. 2000. 0-7808-0327-2. $78.

"This title would be an excellent addition to all public or patient-research libraries." —*American Reference Books Annual, 2001*

"This title is recommended for public, hospital, and health sciences libraries with consumer health collections." —*E-Streams, Jul-Aug '00*

"Recommended reference source." —*Booklist, American Library Association, May '00*

SEE ALSO *Diet & Nutrition Sourcebook, 1st and 2nd Editions, Gastrointestinal Diseases & Disorders Sourcebook*

∎

Disabilities Sourcebook

Basic Consumer Health Information about Physical and Psychiatric Disabilities, Including Descriptions of Major Causes of Disability, Assistive and Adaptive Aids, Workplace Issues, and Accessibility Concerns

Along with Information about the Americans with Disabilities Act, a Glossary, and Resources for Additional Help and Information

Edited by Dawn D. Matthews. 616 pages. 2000. 0-7808-0389-2. $78.

"It is a must for libraries with a consumer health section." —*American Reference Books Annual 2002*

"A much needed addition to the Omnigraphics *Health Reference Series*. A current reference work to provide people with disabilities, their families, caregivers or those who work with them, a broad range of information in one volume, has not been available until now.... It is recommended for all public and academic library reference collections." —*E-Streams, May '01*

"An excellent source book in easy-to-read format covering many current topics; highly recommended for all libraries." —*Choice, Association of College and Research Libraries, Jan '01*

"Recommended reference source." —*Booklist, American Library Association, Jul '00*

"An involving, invaluable handbook." —*The Bookwatch, May '00*

∎

Domestic Violence & Child Abuse Sourcebook

Basic Consumer Health Information about Spousal/ Partner, Child, Sibling, Parent, and Elder Abuse, Covering Physical, Emotional, and Sexual Abuse, Teen Dating Violence, and Stalking; Includes Information about Hotlines, Safe Houses, Safety Plans, and Other Resources for Support and Assistance, Community Initiatives, and Reports on Current Directions in Research and Treatment

Along with a Glossary, Sources for Further Reading, and Governmental and Non-Governmental Organizations Contact Information

Edited by Helene Henderson. 1,064 pages. 2001. 0-7808-0235-7. $78.

"This is important information. The Web has many resources but this sourcebook fills an important societal need. I am not aware of any other resources of this type." —*Doody's Review Service, Sep '01*

"Recommended for all libraries, scholars, and practitioners." —*Choice, Association of College & Research Libraries, Jul '01*

"Recommended reference source." —*Booklist, American Library Association, Apr '01*

"Important pick for college-level health reference libraries." —*The Bookwatch, Mar '01*

"Because this problem is so widespread and because this book includes a lot of issues within one volume, this work is recommended for all public libraries." —*American Reference Books Annual, 2001*

■

Drug Abuse Sourcebook

Basic Consumer Health Information about Illicit Substances of Abuse and the Diversion of Prescription Medications, Including Depressants, Hallucinogens, Inhalants, Marijuana, Narcotics, Stimulants, and Anabolic Steroids

Along with Facts about Related Health Risks, Treatment Issues, and Substance Abuse Prevention Programs, a Glossary of Terms, Statistical Data, and Directories of Hotline Services, Self-Help Groups, and Organizations Able to Provide Further Information

Edited by Karen Bellenir. 629 pages. 2000. 0-7808-0242-X. $78.

"Containing a wealth of information, this book will be useful to the college student just beginning to explore the topic of substance abuse. This resource belongs in libraries that serve a lower-division undergraduate or community college clientele as well as the general public." —*Choice, Association of College and Research Libraries, Jun '01*

"Recommended reference source." —*Booklist, American Library Association, Feb '01*

"Highly recommended." —*The Bookwatch, Jan '01*

"Even though there is a plethora of books on drug abuse, this volume is recommended for school, public, and college libraries." —*American Reference Books Annual, 2001*

SEE ALSO *Alcoholism Sourcebook, Substance Abuse Sourcebook*

■

Ear, Nose & Throat Disorders Sourcebook

Basic Information about Disorders of the Ears, Nose, Sinus Cavities, Pharynx, and Larynx, Including Ear Infections, Tinnitus, Vestibular Disorders, Allergic and Non-Allergic Rhinitis, Sore Throats, Tonsillitis, and Cancers That Affect the Ears, Nose, Sinuses, and Throat

Along with Reports on Current Research Initiatives, a Glossary of Related Medical Terms, and a Directory of Sources for Further Help and Information

Edited by Karen Bellenir and Linda M. Shin. 576 pages. 1998. 0-7808-0206-3. $78.

"Overall, this sourcebook is helpful for the consumer seeking information on ENT issues. It is recommended for public libraries." —*American Reference Books Annual, 1999*

"Recommended reference source." —*Booklist, American Library Association, Dec '98*

■

Eating Disorders Sourcebook

Basic Consumer Health Information about Eating Disorders, Including Information about Anorexia Nervosa, Bulimia Nervosa, Binge Eating, Body Dysmorphic Disorder, Pica, Laxative Abuse, and Night Eating Syndrome

Along with Information about Causes, Adverse Effects, and Treatment and Prevention Issues, and Featuring a Section on Concerns Specific to Children and Adolescents, a Glossary, and Resources for Further Help and Information

Edited by Dawn D. Matthews. 322 pages. 2001. 0-7808-0335-3. $78.

"Recommended for health science libraries that are open to the public, as well as hospital libraries. This book is a good resource for the consumer who is concerned about eating disorders." —*E-Streams, Mar '02*

"This volume is another convenient collection of excerpted articles. Recommended for school and public library patrons; lower-division undergraduates; and two-year technical program students." —*Choice, Association of College & Research Libraries, Jan '02*

"Recommended reference source." —*Booklist, American Library Association, Oct '01*

■

Emergency Medical Services Sourcebook

Basic Consumer Health Information about Preventing, Preparing for, and Managing Emergency Situations, When and Who to Call for Help, What to Expect in the Emergency Room, the Emergency Medical Team, Patient Issues, and Current Topics in Emergency Medicine

Along with Statistical Data, a Glossary, and Sources of Additional Help and Information

Edited by Jenni Lynn Colson. 494 pages. 2002. 0-7808-0420-1. $78.

Endocrine & Metabolic Disorders Sourcebook

Basic Information for the Layperson about Pancreatic and Insulin-Related Disorders Such as Pancreatitis, Diabetes, and Hypoglycemia; Adrenal Gland Disorders Such as Cushing's Syndrome, Addison's Disease, and Congenital Adrenal Hyperplasia; Pituitary Gland Disorders Such as Growth Hormone Deficiency, Acromegaly, and Pituitary Tumors; Thyroid Disorders Such as Hypothyroidism, Graves' Disease, Hashimoto's Disease, and Goiter; Hyperparathyroidism; and Other Diseases and Syndromes of Hormone Imbalance or Metabolic Dysfunction

Along with Reports on Current Research Initiatives

Edited by Linda M. Shin. 574 pages. 1998. 0-7808-0207-1. $78.

"Omnigraphics has produced another needed resource for health information consumers."
—American Reference Books Annual, 2000

"Recommended reference source."
—Booklist, American Library Association, Dec '98

■

Environmentally Induced Disorders Sourcebook

Basic Information about Diseases and Syndromes Linked to Exposure to Pollutants and Other Substances in Outdoor and Indoor Environments Such as Lead, Asbestos, Formaldehyde, Mercury, Emissions, Noise, and More

Edited by Allan R. Cook. 620 pages. 1997. 0-7808-0083-4. $78.

"Recommended reference source."
—Booklist, American Library Association, Sep '98

"This book will be a useful addition to anyone's library." *—Choice Health Sciences Supplement, Association of College and Research Libraries, May '98*

". . . a good survey of numerous environmentally induced physical disorders . . . a useful addition to anyone's library."
—Doody's Health Sciences Book Reviews, Jan '98

". . . provide[s] introductory information from the best authorities around. Since this volume covers topics that potentially affect everyone, it will surely be one of the most frequently consulted volumes in the *Health Reference Series.*" *—Rettig on Reference, Nov '97*

■

Ethnic Diseases Sourcebook

Basic Consumer Health Information for Ethnic and Racial Minority Groups in the United States, Including General Health Indicators and Behaviors, Ethnic Diseases, Genetic Testing, the Impact of Chronic Diseases, Women's Health, Mental Health Issues, and Preventive Health Care Services

Along with a Glossary and a Listing of Additional Resources

Edited by Joyce Brennfleck Shannon. 664 pages. 2001. 0-7808-0336-1. $78.

"Recommended for health sciences libraries where public health programs are a priority."
—E-Streams, Jan '02

"Not many books have been written on this topic to date, and the *Ethnic Diseases Sourcebook* is a strong addition to the list. It will be an important introductory resource for health consumers, students, health care personnel, and social scientists. It is recommended for public, academic, and large hospital libraries."
—American Reference Books Annual 2002

"Recommended reference source."
—Booklist, American Library Association, Oct '01

"Will prove valuable to any library seeking to maintain a current, comprehensive reference collection of health resources. . . . An excellent source of health information about genetic disorders which affect particular ethnic and racial minorities in the U.S."
—The Bookwatch, Aug '01

■

Family Planning Sourcebook

Basic Consumer Health Information about Planning for Pregnancy and Contraception, Including Traditional Methods, Barrier Methods, Hormonal Methods, Permanent Methods, Future Methods, Emergency Contraception, and Birth Control Choices for Women at Each Stage of Life

Along with Statistics, a Glossary, and Sources of Additional Information

Edited by Amy Marcaccio Keyzer. 520 pages. 2001. 0-7808-0379-5. $78.

"Recommended for public, health, and undergraduate libraries as part of the circulating collection."
—E-Streams, Mar '02

"Information is presented in an unbiased, readable manner, and the sourcebook will certainly be a necessary addition to those public and high school libraries where Internet access is restricted or otherwise problematic." *—American Reference Books Annual 2002*

"Recommended reference source."
—Booklist, American Library Association, Oct '01

"Will prove valuable to any library seeking to maintain a current, comprehensive reference collection of health resources. . . . Excellent reference."
—The Bookwatch, Aug '01

SEE ALSO Pregnancy & Birth Sourcebook

■

Fitness & Exercise Sourcebook, 1st Edition

Basic Information on Fitness and Exercise, Including Fitness Activities for Specific Age Groups, Exercise for People with Specific Medical Conditions, How to Begin a Fitness Program in Running, Walking, Swimming, Cycling, and Other Athletic Activities, and Recent Research in Fitness and Exercise

Edited by Dan R. Harris. 663 pages. 1996. 0-7808-0186-5. $78.

"A good resource for general readers." — *Choice, Association of College and Research Libraries, Nov '97*

"The perennial popularity of the topic . . . make this an appealing selection for public libraries."
— *Rettig on Reference, Jun/Jul '97*

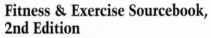

Fitness & Exercise Sourcebook, 2nd Edition

Basic Consumer Health Information about the Fundamentals of Fitness and Exercise, Including How to Begin and Maintain a Fitness Program, Fitness as a Lifestyle, the Link between Fitness and Diet, Advice for Specific Groups of People, Exercise as It Relates to Specific Medical Conditions, and Recent Research in Fitness and Exercise

Along with a Glossary of Important Terms and Resources for Additional Help and Information

Edited by Kristen M. Gledhill. 646 pages. 2001. 0-7808-0334-5. $78.

"This work is recommended for all general reference collections."
— *American Reference Books Annual 2002*

"Highly recommended for public, consumer, and school grades fourth through college."
— *E-Streams, Nov '01*

"Recommended reference source." — *Booklist, American Library Association, Oct '01*

"The information appears quite comprehensive and is considered reliable. . . . This second edition is a welcomed addition to the series."
— *Doody's Review Service, Sep '01*

"This reference is a valuable choice for those who desire a broad source of information on exercise, fitness, and chronic-disease prevention through a healthy lifestyle." — *American Medical Writers Association Journal, Fall '01*

"Will prove valuable to any library seeking to maintain a current, comprehensive reference collection of health resources. . . . Excellent reference."
— *The Bookwatch, Aug '01*

Food & Animal Borne Diseases Sourcebook

Basic Information about Diseases That Can Be Spread to Humans through the Ingestion of Contaminated Food or Water or by Contact with Infected Animals and Insects, Such as Botulism, E. Coli, Hepatitis A, Trichinosis, Lyme Disease, and Rabies

Along with Information Regarding Prevention and Treatment Methods, and Including a Special Section for International Travelers Describing Diseases Such as Cholera, Malaria, Travelers' Diarrhea, and Yellow Fever, and Offering Recommendations for Avoiding Illness

Edited by Karen Bellenir and Peter D. Dresser. 535 pages. 1995. 0-7808-0033-8. $78.

"Targeting general readers and providing them with a single, comprehensive source of information on selected topics, this book continues, with the excellent caliber of its predecessors, to catalog topical information on health matters of general interest. Readable and thorough, this valuable resource is highly recommended for all libraries."
— *Academic Library Book Review, Summer '96*

"A comprehensive collection of authoritative information." — *Emergency Medical Services, Oct '95*

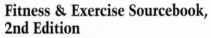

Food Safety Sourcebook

Basic Consumer Health Information about the Safe Handling of Meat, Poultry, Seafood, Eggs, Fruit Juices, and Other Food Items, and Facts about Pesticides, Drinking Water, Food Safety Overseas, and the Onset, Duration, and Symptoms of Foodborne Illnesses, Including Types of Pathogenic Bacteria, Parasitic Protozoa, Worms, Viruses, and Natural Toxins

Along with the Role of the Consumer, the Food Handler, and the Government in Food Safety; a Glossary, and Resources for Additional Help and Information

Edited by Dawn D. Matthews. 339 pages. 1999. 0-7808-0326-4. $78.

"This book is recommended for public libraries and universities with home economic and food science programs." — *E-Streams, Nov '00*

"Recommended reference source."
— *Booklist, American Library Association, May '00*

"This book takes the complex issues of food safety and foodborne pathogens and presents them in an easily understood manner. [It does] an excellent job of covering a large and often confusing topic."
— *American Reference Books Annual, 2000*

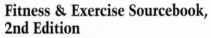

Forensic Medicine Sourcebook

Basic Consumer Information for the Layperson about Forensic Medicine, Including Crime Scene Investigation, Evidence Collection and Analysis, Expert Testimony, Computer-Aided Criminal Identification, Digital Imaging in the Courtroom, DNA Profiling, Accident Reconstruction, Autopsies, Ballistics, Drugs and Explosives Detection, Latent Fingerprints, Product Tampering, and Questioned Document Examination

Along with Statistical Data, a Glossary of Forensics Terminology, and Listings of Sources for Further Help and Information

Edited by Annemarie S. Muth. 574 pages. 1999. 0-7808-0232-2. $78.

"Given the expected widespread interest in its content and its easy to read style, this book is recommended for most public and all college and university libraries."
— *E-Streams, Feb '01*

"Recommended for public libraries."
— *Reference & User Services Quarterly, American Library Association, Spring 2000*

"Recommended reference source."
—*Booklist, American Library Association, Feb '00*

"A wealth of information, useful statistics, references are up-to-date and extremely complete. This wonderful collection of data will help students who are interested in a career in any type of forensic field. It is a great resource for attorneys who need information about types of expert witnesses needed in a particular case. It also offers useful information for fiction and nonfiction writers whose work involves a crime. A fascinating compilation. All levels." —*Choice, Association of College and Research Libraries, Jan 2000*

"There are several items that make this book attractive to consumers who are seeking certain forensic data.... This is a useful current source for those seeking general forensic medical answers."
—*American Reference Books Annual, 2000*

Gastrointestinal Diseases & Disorders Sourcebook

Basic Information about Gastroesophageal Reflux Disease (Heartburn), Ulcers, Diverticulosis, Irritable Bowel Syndrome, Crohn's Disease, Ulcerative Colitis, Diarrhea, Constipation, Lactose Intolerance, Hemorrhoids, Hepatitis, Cirrhosis, and Other Digestive Problems, Featuring Statistics, Descriptions of Symptoms, and Current Treatment Methods of Interest for Persons Living with Upper and Lower Gastrointestinal Maladies

Edited by Linda M. Ross. 413 pages. 1996. 0-7808-0078-8. $78.

"... very readable form. The successful editorial work that brought this material together into a useful and understandable reference makes accessible to all readers information that can help them more effectively understand and obtain help for digestive tract problems."
—*Choice, Association of College & Research Libraries, Feb '97*

SEE ALSO *Diet & Nutrition Sourcebook, 1st and 2nd Editions, Digestive Diseases & Disorders*

Genetic Disorders Sourcebook, 1st Edition

Basic Information about Heritable Diseases and Disorders Such as Down Syndrome, PKU, Hemophilia, Von Willebrand Disease, Gaucher Disease, Tay-Sachs Disease, and Sickle-Cell Disease, Along with Information about Genetic Screening, Gene Therapy, Home Care, and Including Source Listings for Further Help and Information on More Than 300 Disorders

Edited by Karen Bellenir. 642 pages. 1996. 0-7808-0034-6. $78.

"Recommended for undergraduate libraries or libraries that serve the public."
—*Science & Technology Libraries, Vol. 18, No. 1, '99*

"Provides essential medical information to both the general public and those diagnosed with a serious or fatal genetic disease or disorder." —*Choice, Association of College and Research Libraries, Jan '97*

"Geared toward the lay public. It would be well placed in all public libraries and in those hospital and medical libraries in which access to genetic references is limited." —*Doody's Health Sciences Book Review, Oct '96*

Genetic Disorders Sourcebook, 2nd Edition

Basic Consumer Health Information about Hereditary Diseases and Disorders, Including Cystic Fibrosis, Down Syndrome, Hemophilia, Huntington's Disease, Sickle Cell Anemia, and More; Facts about Genes, Gene Research and Therapy, Genetic Screening, Ethics of Gene Testing, Genetic Counseling, and Advice on Coping and Caring

Along with a Glossary of Genetic Terminology and a Resource List for Help, Support, and Further Information

Edited by Kathy Massimini. 768 pages. 2001. 0-7808-0241-1. $78.

"Recommended for public libraries and medical and hospital libraries with consumer health collections."
—*E-Streams, May '01*

"Recommended reference source."
—*Booklist, American Library Association, Apr '01*

"Important pick for college-level health reference libraries." —*The Bookwatch, Mar '01*

Head Trauma Sourcebook

Basic Information for the Layperson about Open-Head and Closed-Head Injuries, Treatment Advances, Recovery, and Rehabilitation

Along with Reports on Current Research Initiatives

Edited by Karen Bellenir. 414 pages. 1997. 0-7808-0208-X. $78.

Headache Sourcebook

Basic Consumer Health Information about Migraine, Tension, Cluster, Rebound and Other Types of Headaches, with Facts about the Cause and Prevention of Headaches, the Effects of Stress and the Environment, Headaches during Pregnancy and Menopause, and Childhood Headaches

Along with a Glossary and Other Resources for Additional Help and Information

Edited by Dawn D. Matthews. 362 pages. 2002. 0-7808-0337-X. $78.

Health Insurance Sourcebook

Basic Information about Managed Care Organizations, Traditional Fee-for-Service Insurance, Insurance Portability and Pre-Existing Conditions Clauses, Medicare, Medicaid, Social Security, and Military Health Care

Along with Information about Insurance Fraud

Edited by Wendy Wilcox. 530 pages. 1997. 0-7808-0222-5. $78.

"Particularly useful because it brings much of this information together in one volume. This book will be a handy reference source in the health sciences library, hospital library, college and university library, and medium to large public library."
— *Medical Reference Services Quarterly, Fall '98*

Awarded "Books of the Year Award"
— *American Journal of Nursing, 1997*

"The layout of the book is particularly helpful as it provides easy access to reference material. A most useful addition to the vast amount of information about health insurance. The use of data from U.S. government agencies is most commendable. Useful in a library or learning center for healthcare professional students."
— *Doody's Health Sciences Book Reviews, Nov '97*

Health Reference Series Cumulative Index 1999

A Comprehensive Index to the Individual Volumes of the Health Reference Series, Including a Subject Index, Name Index, Organization Index, and Publication Index

Along with a Master List of Acronyms and Abbreviations

Edited by Edward J. Prucha, Anne Holmes, and Robert Rudnick. 990 pages. 2000. 0-7808-0382-5. $78.

"This volume will be most helpful in libraries that have a relatively complete collection of the Health Reference Series." — *American Reference Books Annual, 2001*

"Essential for collections that hold any of the numerous *Health Reference Series* titles."
— *Choice, Association of College and Research Libraries, Nov '00*

Healthy Aging Sourcebook

Basic Consumer Health Information about Maintaining Health through the Aging Process, Including Advice on Nutrition, Exercise, and Sleep, Help in Making Decisions about Midlife Issues and Retirement, and Guidance Concerning Practical and Informed Choices in Health Consumerism

Along with Data Concerning the Theories of Aging, Different Experiences in Aging by Minority Groups, and Facts about Aging Now and Aging in the Future; and Featuring a Glossary, a Guide to Consumer Help, Additional Suggested Reading, and Practical Resource Directory

Edited by Jenifer Swanson. 536 pages. 1999. 0-7808-0390-6. $78.

"Recommended reference source."
— *Booklist, American Library Association, Feb '00*

SEE ALSO Physical & Mental Issues in Aging Sourcebook

Healthy Heart Sourcebook for Women

Basic Consumer Health Information about Cardiac Issues Specific to Women, Including Facts about Major Risk Factors and Prevention, Treatment and Control Strategies, and Important Dietary Issues

Along with a Special Section Regarding the Pros and Cons of Hormone Replacement Therapy and Its Impact on Heart Health, and Additional Help, Including Recipes, a Glossary, and a Directory of Resources

Edited by Dawn D. Matthews. 336 pages. 2000. 0-7808-0329-9. $78.

"A good reference source and recommended for all public, academic, medical, and hospital libraries."
— *Medical Reference Services Quarterly, Summer '01*

"Because of the lack of information specific to women on this topic, this book is recommended for public libraries and consumer libraries."
— *American Reference Books Annual, 2001*

"Contains very important information about coronary artery disease that all women should know. The information is current and presented in an easy-to-read format. The book will make a good addition to any library." — *American Medical Writers Association Journal, Summer '00*

"Important, basic reference."
— *Reviewer's Bookwatch, Jul '00*

SEE ALSO Cardiovascular Diseases & Disorders Sourcebook, 1st Edition, Heart Diseases & Disorders Sourcebook, 2nd Edition, Women's Health Concerns Sourcebook

Heart Diseases & Disorders Sourcebook, 2nd Edition

Basic Consumer Health Information about Heart Attacks, Angina, Rhythm Disorders, Heart Failure, Valve Disease, Congenital Heart Disorders, and More, Including Descriptions of Surgical Procedures and Other Interventions, Medications, Cardiac Rehabilitation, Risk Identification, and Prevention Tips

Along with Statistical Data, Reports on Current Research Initiatives, a Glossary of Cardiovascular Terms, and Resource Directory

Edited by Karen Bellenir. 612 pages. 2000. 0-7808-0238-1. $78.

"This work stands out as an imminently accessible resource for the general public. It is recommended for the reference and circulating shelves of school, public, and academic libraries."
— *American Reference Books Annual, 2001*

"Recommended reference source."
— *Booklist, American Library Association, Dec '00*

"Provides comprehensive coverage of matters related to the heart. This title is recommended for health sciences and public libraries with consumer health collections."
—*E-Streams, Oct '00*

SEE ALSO *Cardiovascular Diseases & Disorders Sourcebook, 1st Edition; Healthy Heart Sourcebook for Women*

∎

Household Safety Sourcebook

Basic Consumer Health Information about Household Safety, Including Information about Poisons, Chemicals, Fire, and Water Hazards in the Home

Along with Advice about the Safe Use of Home Maintenance Equipment, Choosing Toys and Nursery Furniture, Holiday and Recreation Safety, a Glossary, and Resources for Further Help and Information

Edited by Dawn D. Matthews. 606 pages. 2002. 0-7808-0338-8. $78.

∎

Immune System Disorders Sourcebook

Basic Information about Lupus, Multiple Sclerosis, Guillain-Barré Syndrome, Chronic Granulomatous Disease, and More

Along with Statistical and Demographic Data and Reports on Current Research Initiatives

Edited by Allan R. Cook. 608 pages. 1997. 0-7808-0209-8. $78.

∎

Infant & Toddler Health Sourcebook

Basic Consumer Health Information about the Physical and Mental Development of Newborns, Infants, and Toddlers, Including Neonatal Concerns, Nutrition Recommendations, Immunization Schedules, Common Pediatric Disorders, Assessments and Milestones, Safety Tips, and Advice for Parents and Other Caregivers

Along with a Glossary of Terms and Resource Listings for Additional Help

Edited by Jenifer Swanson. 585 pages. 2000. 0-7808-0246-2. $78.

"As a reference for the general public, this would be useful in any library." —*E-Streams, May '01*

"Recommended reference source."
—*Booklist, American Library Association, Feb '01*

"This is a good source for general use."
—*American Reference Books Annual, 2001*

Injury & Trauma Sourcebook

Basic Consumer Health Information about the Impact of Injury, the Diagnosis and Treatment of Common and Traumatic Injuries, Emergency Care, and Specific Injuries Related to Home, Community, Workplace, Transportation, and Recreation

Along with Guidelines for Injury Prevention, a Glossary, and a Directory of Additional Resources

Edited by Joyce Brennfleck Shannon. 696 pages. 2002. 0-7808-0421-X. $78.

∎

Kidney & Urinary Tract Diseases & Disorders Sourcebook

Basic Information about Kidney Stones, Urinary Incontinence, Bladder Disease, End Stage Renal Disease, Dialysis, and More

Along with Statistical and Demographic Data and Reports on Current Research Initiatives

Edited by Linda M. Ross. 602 pages. 1997. 0-7808-0079-6. $78.

∎

Learning Disabilities Sourcebook

Basic Information about Disorders Such as Dyslexia, Visual and Auditory Processing Deficits, Attention Deficit/Hyperactivity Disorder, and Autism

Along with Statistical and Demographic Data, Reports on Current Research Initiatives, an Explanation of the Assessment Process, and a Special Section for Adults with Learning Disabilities

Edited by Linda M. Shin. 579 pages. 1998. 0-7808-0210-1. $78.

Named "Outstanding Reference Book of 1999."
—*New York Public Library, Feb 2000*

"An excellent candidate for inclusion in a public library reference section. It's a great source of information. Teachers will also find the book useful. Definitely worth reading."
—*Journal of Adolescent & Adult Literacy, Feb 2000*

"Readable . . . provides a solid base of information regarding successful techniques used with individuals who have learning disabilities, as well as practical suggestions for educators and family members. Clear language, concise descriptions, and pertinent information for contacting multiple resources add to the strength of this book as a useful tool." —*Choice, Association of College and Research Libraries, Feb '99*

"Recommended reference source."
—*Booklist, American Library Association, Sep '98*

"A useful resource for libraries and for those who don't have the time to identify and locate the individual publications." —*Disability Resources Monthly, Sep '98*

Liver Disorders Sourcebook

Basic Consumer Health Information about the Liver and How It Works; Liver Diseases, Including Cancer, Cirrhosis, Hepatitis, and Toxic and Drug Related Diseases; Tips for Maintaining a Healthy Liver; Laboratory Tests, Radiology Tests, and Facts about Liver Transplantation

Along with a Section on Support Groups, a Glossary, and Resource Listings

Edited by Joyce Brennfleck Shannon. 591 pages. 2000. 0-7808-0383-3. $78.

"A valuable resource."
—American Reference Books Annual, 2001

"This title is recommended for health sciences and public libraries with consumer health collections."
—E-Streams, Oct '00

"Recommended reference source."
—Booklist, American Library Association, Jun '00

■

Lung Disorders Sourcebook

Basic Consumer Health Information about Emphysema, Pneumonia, Tuberculosis, Asthma, Cystic Fibrosis, and Other Lung Disorders, Including Facts about Diagnostic Procedures, Treatment Strategies, Disease Prevention Efforts, and Such Risk Factors as Smoking, Air Pollution, and Exposure to Asbestos, Radon, and Other Agents

Along with a Glossary and Resources for Additional Help and Information

Edited by Dawn D. Matthews. 678 pages. 2002. 0-7808-0339-6. $78.

■

Medical Tests Sourcebook

Basic Consumer Health Information about Medical Tests, Including Periodic Health Exams, General Screening Tests, Tests You Can Do at Home, Findings of the U.S. Preventive Services Task Force, X-ray and Radiology Tests, Electrical Tests, Tests of Blood and Other Body Fluids and Tissues, Scope Tests, Lung Tests, Genetic Tests, Pregnancy Tests, Newborn Screening Tests, Sexually Transmitted Disease Tests, and Computer Aided Diagnoses

Along with a Section on Paying for Medical Tests, a Glossary, and Resource Listings

Edited by Joyce Brennfleck Shannon. 691 pages. 1999. 0-7808-0243-8. $78.

"Recommended for hospital and health sciences libraries with consumer health collections."
—E-Streams, Mar '00

"This is an overall excellent reference with a wealth of general knowledge that may aid those who are reluctant to get vital tests performed."
—Today's Librarian, Jan 2000

"A valuable reference guide."
—American Reference Books Annual, 2000

Men's Health Concerns Sourcebook

Basic Information about Health Issues That Affect Men, Featuring Facts about the Top Causes of Death in Men, Including Heart Disease, Stroke, Cancers, Prostate Disorders, Chronic Obstructive Pulmonary Disease, Pneumonia and Influenza, Human Immunodeficiency Virus and Acquired Immune Deficiency Syndrome, Diabetes Mellitus, Stress, Suicide, Accidents and Homicides; and Facts about Common Concerns for Men, Including Impotence, Contraception, Circumcision, Sleep Disorders, Snoring, Hair Loss, Diet, Nutrition, Exercise, Kidney and Urological Disorders, and Backaches

Edited by Allan R. Cook. 738 pages. 1998. 0-7808-0212-8. $78.

"This comprehensive resource and the series are highly recommended."
—American Reference Books Annual, 2000

"Recommended reference source."
—Booklist, American Library Association, Dec '98

■

Mental Health Disorders Sourcebook, 1st Edition

Basic Information about Schizophrenia, Depression, Bipolar Disorder, Panic Disorder, Obsessive-Compulsive Disorder, Phobias and Other Anxiety Disorders, Paranoia and Other Personality Disorders, Eating Disorders, and Sleep Disorders

Along with Information about Treatment and Therapies

Edited by Karen Bellenir. 548 pages. 1995. 0-7808-0040-0. $78.

"This is an excellent new book . . . written in easy-to-understand language."
—Booklist Health Sciences Supplement, American Library Association, Oct '97

". . . useful for public and academic libraries and consumer health collections."
—Medical Reference Services Quarterly, Spring '97

"The great strengths of the book are its readability and its inclusion of places to find more information. Especially recommended."
—Reference Quarterly, American Library Association, Winter '96

". . . a good resource for a consumer health library."
—Bulletin of the Medical Library Association, Oct '96

"The information is data-based and couched in brief, concise language that avoids jargon. . . . a useful reference source."
—Readings, Sep '96

"The text is well organized and adequately written for its target audience."
—Choice, Association of College and Research Libraries, Jun '96

". . . provides information on a wide range of mental disorders, presented in nontechnical language."
—Exceptional Child Education Resources, Spring '96

"Recommended for public and academic libraries."
—Reference Book Review, 1996

Mental Health Disorders Sourcebook, 2nd Edition

Basic Consumer Health Information about Anxiety Disorders, Depression and Other Mood Disorders, Eating Disorders, Personality Disorders, Schizophrenia, and More, Including Disease Descriptions, Treatment Options, and Reports on Current Research Initiatives

Along with Statistical Data, Tips for Maintaining Mental Health, a Glossary, and Directory of Sources for Additional Help and Information

Edited by Karen Bellenir. 605 pages. 2000. 0-7808-0240-3. $78.

"Well organized and well written."
—American Reference Books Annual, 2001

"Recommended reference source."
—Booklist, American Library Association, Jun '00

■

Mental Retardation Sourcebook

Basic Consumer Health Information about Mental Retardation and Its Causes, Including Down Syndrome, Fetal Alcohol Syndrome, Fragile X Syndrome, Genetic Conditions, Injury, and Environmental Sources

Along with Preventive Strategies, Parenting Issues, Educational Implications, Health Care Needs, Employment and Economic Matters, Legal Issues, a Glossary, and a Resource Listing for Additional Help and Information

Edited by Joyce Brennfleck Shannon. 642 pages. 2000. 0-7808-0377-9. $78.

"Public libraries will find the book useful for reference and as a beginning research point for students, parents, and caregivers."
—American Reference Books Annual, 2001

"The strength of this work is that it compiles many basic fact sheets and addresses for further information in one volume. It is intended and suitable for the general public. This sourcebook is relevant to any collection providing health information to the general public."
— E-Streams, Nov '00

"From preventing retardation to parenting and family challenges, this covers health, social and legal issues and will prove an invaluable overview."
— Reviewer's Bookwatch, Jul '00

■

Obesity Sourcebook

Basic Consumer Health Information about Diseases and Other Problems Associated with Obesity, and Including Facts about Risk Factors, Prevention Issues, and Management Approaches

Along with Statistical and Demographic Data, Information about Special Populations, Research Updates, a Glossary, and Source Listings for Further Help and Information

Edited by Wilma Caldwell and Chad T. Kimball. 376 pages. 2001. 0-7808-0333-7. $78.

"The book synthesizes the reliable medical literature on obesity into one easy-to-read and useful resource for the general public."
—American Reference Books Annual 2002

"This is a very useful resource book for the lay public."
—Doody's Review Service, Nov '01

"Well suited for the health reference collection of a public library or an academic health science library that serves the general population." *—E-Streams, Sep '01*

"Recommended reference source."
—Booklist, American Library Association, Apr '01

" Recommended pick both for specialty health library collections and any general consumer health reference collection." *— The Bookwatch, Apr '01*

■

Ophthalmic Disorders Sourcebook

Basic Information about Glaucoma, Cataracts, Macular Degeneration, Strabismus, Refractive Disorders, and More

Along with Statistical and Demographic Data and Reports on Current Research Initiatives

Edited by Linda M. Ross. 631 pages. 1996. 0-7808-0081-8. $78.

■

Oral Health Sourcebook

Basic Information about Diseases and Conditions Affecting Oral Health, Including Cavities, Gum Disease, Dry Mouth, Oral Cancers, Fever Blisters, Canker Sores, Oral Thrush, Bad Breath, Temporomandibular Disorders, and other Craniofacial Syndromes

Along with Statistical Data on the Oral Health of Americans, Oral Hygiene, Emergency First Aid, Information on Treatment Procedures and Methods of Replacing Lost Teeth

Edited by Allan R. Cook. 558 pages. 1997. 0-7808-0082-6. $78.

"Unique source which will fill a gap in dental sources for patients and the lay public. A valuable reference tool even in a library with thousands of books on dentistry. Comprehensive, clear, inexpensive, and easy to read and use. It fills an enormous gap in the health care literature." *— Reference and User Services Quarterly, American Library Association, Summer '98*

"Recommended reference source."
— Booklist, American Library Association, Dec '97

■

Osteoporosis Sourcebook

Basic Consumer Health Information about Primary and Secondary Osteoporosis and Juvenile Osteoporosis and Related Conditions, Including Fibrous Dysplasia, Gaucher Disease, Hyperthyroidism, Hypophosphatasia, Myeloma, Osteopetrosis, Osteogenesis Imperfecta, and Paget's Disease

Along with Information about Risk Factors, Treatments, Traditional and Non-Traditional Pain Management, a Glossary of Related Terms, and a Directory of Resources

Edited by Allan R. Cook. 584 pages. 2001. 0-7808-0239-X. $78.

"This would be a book to be kept in a staff or patient library. The targeted audience is the layperson, but the therapist who needs a quick bit of information on a particular topic will also find the book useful."
—*Physical Therapy, Jan '02*

"This resource is recommended as a great reference source for public, health, and academic libraries, and is another triumph for the editors of Omnigraphics."
—*American Reference Books Annual 2002*

"Recommended for all public libraries and general health collections, especially those supporting patient education or consumer health programs."
—*E-Streams, Nov '01*

"Will prove valuable to any library seeking to maintain a current, comprehensive reference collection of health resources. . . . From prevention to treatment and associated conditions, this provides an excellent survey."
—*The Bookwatch, Aug '01*

"Recommended reference source."
—*Booklist, American Library Association, July '01*

SEE ALSO Women's Health Concerns Sourcebook

■

Pain Sourcebook, 1st Edition

Basic Information about Specific Forms of Acute and Chronic Pain, Including Headaches, Back Pain, Muscular Pain, Neuralgia, Surgical Pain, and Cancer Pain

Along with Pain Relief Options Such as Analgesics, Narcotics, Nerve Blocks, Transcutaneous Nerve Stimulation, and Alternative Forms of Pain Control, Including Biofeedback, Imaging, Behavior Modification, and Relaxation Techniques

Edited by Allan R. Cook. 667 pages. 1997. 0-7808-0213-6. $78.

"The text is readable, easily understood, and well indexed. This excellent volume belongs in all patient education libraries, consumer health sections of public libraries, and many personal collections."
—*American Reference Books Annual, 1999*

"A beneficial reference." —*Booklist Health Sciences Supplement, American Library Association, Oct '98*

"The information is basic in terms of scholarship and is appropriate for general readers. Written in journalistic style . . . intended for non-professionals. Quite thorough in its coverage of different pain conditions and summarizes the latest clinical information regarding pain treatment." —*Choice, Association of College and Research Libraries, Jun '98*

"Recommended reference source."
—*Booklist, American Library Association, Mar '98*

Pain Sourcebook, 2nd Edition

Basic Consumer Health Information about Specific Forms of Acute and Chronic Pain, Including Muscle and Skeletal Pain, Nerve Pain, Cancer Pain, and Disorders Characterized by Pain, Such as Fibromyalgia, Shingles, Angina, Arthritis, and Headaches

Along with Information about Pain Medications and Management Techniques, Complementary and Alternative Pain Relief Options, Tips for People Living with Chronic Pain, a Glossary, and a Directory of Sources for Further Information

Edited by Karen Bellenir. 670 pages. 2002. 0-7808-0612-3. $78.

■

Pediatric Cancer Sourcebook

Basic Consumer Health Information about Leukemias, Brain Tumors, Sarcomas, Lymphomas, and Other Cancers in Infants, Children, and Adolescents, Including Descriptions of Cancers, Treatments, and Coping Strategies

Along with Suggestions for Parents, Caregivers, and Concerned Relatives, a Glossary of Cancer Terms, and Resource Listings

Edited by Edward J. Prucha. 587 pages. 1999. 0-7808-0245-4. $78.

"An excellent source of information. Recommended for public, hospital, and health science libraries with consumer health collections." —*E-Streams, Jun '00*

"Recommended reference source."
—*Booklist, American Library Association, Feb '00*

"A valuable addition to all libraries specializing in health services and many public libraries."
—*American Reference Books Annual, 2000*

■

Physical & Mental Issues in Aging Sourcebook

Basic Consumer Health Information on Physical and Mental Disorders Associated with the Aging Process, Including Concerns about Cardiovascular Disease, Pulmonary Disease, Oral Health, Digestive Disorders, Musculoskeletal and Skin Disorders, Metabolic Changes, Sexual and Reproductive Issues, and Changes in Vision, Hearing, and Other Senses

Along with Data about Longevity and Causes of Death, Information on Acute and Chronic Pain, Descriptions of Mental Concerns, a Glossary of Terms, and Resource Listings for Additional Help

Edited by Jenifer Swanson. 660 pages. 1999. 0-7808-0233-0. $78.

"This is a treasure of health information for the layperson." — *Choice Health Sciences Supplement, Association of College & Research Libraries, May 2000*

"Recommended for public libraries."
—*American Reference Books Annual, 2000*

"Recommended reference source."
—*Booklist, American Library Association, Oct '99*

SEE ALSO Healthy Aging Sourcebook

Podiatry Sourcebook

Basic Consumer Health Information about Foot Conditions, Diseases, and Injuries, Including Bunions, Corns, Calluses, Athlete's Foot, Plantar Warts, Hammertoes and Clawtoes, Clubfoot, Heel Pain, Gout, and More

Along with Facts about Foot Care, Disease Prevention, Foot Safety, Choosing a Foot Care Specialist, a Glossary of Terms, and Resource Listings for Additional Information

Edited by M. Lisa Weatherford. 380 pages. 2001. 0-7808-0215-2. $78.

"Recommended reference source."
  — Booklist, American Library Association, Feb '02

"There is a lot of information presented here on a topic that is usually only covered sparingly in most larger comprehensive medical encyclopedias."
  — American Reference Books Annual 2002

Pregnancy & Birth Sourcebook

Basic Information about Planning for Pregnancy, Maternal Health, Fetal Growth and Development, Labor and Delivery, Postpartum and Perinatal Care, Pregnancy in Mothers with Special Concerns, and Disorders of Pregnancy, Including Genetic Counseling, Nutrition and Exercise, Obstetrical Tests, Pregnancy Discomfort, Multiple Births, Cesarean Sections, Medical Testing of Newborns, Breastfeeding, Gestational Diabetes, and Ectopic Pregnancy

Edited by Heather E. Aldred. 737 pages. 1997. 0-7808-0216-0. $78.

"A well-organized handbook. Recommended."
  — Choice, Association of College and Research Libraries, Apr '98

"Recommended reference source."
  — Booklist, American Library Association, Mar '98

"Recommended for public libraries."
  — American Reference Books Annual, 1998

SEE ALSO *Congenital Disorders Sourcebook, Family Planning Sourcebook*

Prostate Cancer Sourcebook

Basic Consumer Health Information about Prostate Cancer, Including Information about the Associated Risk Factors, Detection, Diagnosis, and Treatment of Prostate Cancer

Along with Information on Non-Malignant Prostate Conditions, and Featuring a Section Listing Support and Treatment Centers and a Glossary of Related Terms

Edited by Dawn D. Matthews. 358 pages. 2001. 0-7808-0324-8. $78.

"Recommended reference source."
  —Booklist, American Library Association, Jan '02

"A valuable resource for health care consumers seeking information on the subject....All text is written in a clear, easy-to-understand language that avoids technical jargon. Any library that collects consumer health resources would strengthen their collection with the addition of the *Prostate Cancer Sourcebook.*"
  — American Reference Books Annual 2002

Public Health Sourcebook

Basic Information about Government Health Agencies, Including National Health Statistics and Trends, Healthy People 2000 Program Goals and Objectives, the Centers for Disease Control and Prevention, the Food and Drug Administration, and the National Institutes of Health

Along with Full Contact Information for Each Agency

Edited by Wendy Wilcox. 698 pages. 1998. 0-7808-0220-9. $78.

"Recommended reference source."
  — Booklist, American Library Association, Sep '98

"This consumer guide provides welcome assistance in navigating the maze of federal health agencies and their data on public health concerns."
  — SciTech Book News, Sep '98

Reconstructive & Cosmetic Surgery Sourcebook

Basic Consumer Health Information on Cosmetic and Reconstructive Plastic Surgery, Including Statistical Information about Different Surgical Procedures, Things to Consider Prior to Surgery, Plastic Surgery Techniques and Tools, Emotional and Psychological Considerations, and Procedure-Specific Information

Along with a Glossary of Terms and a Listing of Resources for Additional Help and Information

Edited by M. Lisa Weatherford. 374 pages. 2001. 0-7808-0214-4. $78.

"An excellent reference that addresses cosmetic and medically necessary reconstructive surgeries. . . . The style of the prose is calm and reassuring, discussing the many positive outcomes now available due to advances in surgical techniques."
  — American Reference Books Annual 2002

"Recommended for health science libraries that are open to the public, as well as hospital libraries that are open to the patients. This book is a good resource for the consumer interested in plastic surgery."
  —E-Streams, Dec '01

"Recommended reference source."
  —Booklist, American Library Association, July '01

Rehabilitation Sourcebook

Basic Consumer Health Information about Rehabilitation for People Recovering from Heart Surgery, Spinal Cord Injury, Stroke, Orthopedic Impairments, Amputation, Pulmonary Impairments, Traumatic Injury, and More, Including Physical Therapy, Occupa-

tional Therapy, Speech/ Language Therapy, Massage Therapy, Dance Therapy, Art Therapy, and Recreational Therapy

Along with Information on Assistive and Adaptive Devices, a Glossary, and Resources for Additional Help and Information

Edited by Dawn D. Matthews. 531 pages. 1999. 0-7808-0236-5. $78.

"This is an excellent resource for public library reference and health collections."
— *American Reference Books Annual, 2001*

"Recommended reference source."
— *Booklist, American Library Association, May '00*

Respiratory Diseases & Disorders Sourcebook

Basic Information about Respiratory Diseases and Disorders, Including Asthma, Cystic Fibrosis, Pneumonia, the Common Cold, Influenza, and Others, Featuring Facts about the Respiratory System, Statistical and Demographic Data, Treatments, Self-Help Management Suggestions, and Current Research Initiatives

Edited by Allan R. Cook and Peter D. Dresser. 771 pages. 1995. 0-7808-0037-0. $78.

"Designed for the layperson and for patients and their families coping with respiratory illness. . . . an extensive array of information on diagnosis, treatment, management, and prevention of respiratory illnesses for the general reader." — *Choice, Association of College and Research Libraries, Jun '96*

"A highly recommended text for all collections. It is a comforting reminder of the power of knowledge that good books carry between their covers."
— *Academic Library Book Review, Spring '96*

"A comprehensive collection of authoritative information presented in a nontechnical, humanitarian style for patients, families, and caregivers."
— *Association of Operating Room Nurses, Sep/Oct '95*

Sexually Transmitted Diseases Sourcebook, 1st Edition

Basic Information about Herpes, Chlamydia, Gonorrhea, Hepatitis, Nongonoccocal Urethritis, Pelvic Inflammatory Disease, Syphilis, AIDS, and More

Along with Current Data on Treatments and Preventions

Edited by Linda M. Ross. 550 pages. 1997. 0-7808-0217-9. $78.

Sexually Transmitted Diseases Sourcebook, 2nd Edition

Basic Consumer Health Information about Sexually Transmitted Diseases, Including Information on the Diagnosis and Treatment of Chlamydia, Gonorrhea, Hepatitis, Herpes, HIV, Mononucleosis, Syphilis, and Others

Along with Information on Prevention, Such as Condom Use, Vaccines, and STD Education; And Featuring a Section on Issues Related to Youth and Adolescents, a Glossary, and Resources for Additional Help and Information

Edited by Dawn D. Matthews. 538 pages. 2001. 0-7808-0249-7. $78.

"Recommended for consumer health collections in public libraries, and secondary school and community college libraries."
— *American Reference Books Annual 2002*

"Every school and public library should have a copy of this comprehensive and user-friendly reference book."
— *Choice, Association of College & Research Libraries, Sep '01*

"This is a highly recommended book. This is an especially important book for all school and public libraries." — *AIDS Book Review Journal, Jul-Aug '01*

"Recommended reference source."
— *Booklist, American Library Association, Apr '01*

"Recommended pick both for specialty health library collections and any general consumer health reference collection." — *The Bookwatch, Apr '01*

Skin Disorders Sourcebook

Basic Information about Common Skin and Scalp Conditions Caused by Aging, Allergies, Immune Reactions, Sun Exposure, Infectious Organisms, Parasites, Cosmetics, and Skin Traumas, Including Abrasions, Cuts, and Pressure Sores

Along with Information on Prevention and Treatment

Edited by Allan R. Cook. 647 pages. 1997. 0-7808-0080-X. $78.

". . . comprehensive, easily read reference book."
— *Doody's Health Sciences Book Reviews, Oct '97*

SEE ALSO *Burns Sourcebook*

Sleep Disorders Sourcebook

Basic Consumer Health Information about Sleep and Its Disorders, Including Insomnia, Sleepwalking, Sleep Apnea, Restless Leg Syndrome, and Narcolepsy

Along with Data about Shiftwork and Its Effects, Information on the Societal Costs of Sleep Deprivation, Descriptions of Treatment Options, a Glossary of Terms, and Resource Listings for Additional Help

Edited by Jenifer Swanson. 439 pages. 1998. 0-7808-0234-9. $78.

"This text will complement any home or medical library. It is user-friendly and ideal for the adult reader."
— *American Reference Books Annual, 2000*

"A useful resource that provides accurate, relevant, and accessible information on sleep to the general public. Health care providers who deal with sleep disorders patients may also find it helpful in being prepared to answer some of the questions patients ask."
— *Respiratory Care, Jul '99*

"Recommended reference source."
— *Booklist, American Library Association, Feb '99*

■

Sports Injuries Sourcebook, First Edition

Basic Consumer Health Information about Common Sports Injuries, Prevention of Injury in Specific Sports, Tips for Training, and Rehabilitation from Injury

Along with Information about Special Concerns for Children, Young Girls in Athletic Training Programs, Senior Athletes, and Women Athletes, and a Directory of Resources for Further Help and Information

Edited by Heather E. Aldred. 624 pages. 1999. 0-7808-0218-7. $78.

"While this easy-to-read book is recommended for all libraries, it should prove to be especially useful for public, high school, and academic libraries; certainly it should be on the bookshelf of every school gymnasium."
— *E-Streams, Mar '00*

"Public libraries and undergraduate academic libraries will find this book useful for its nontechnical language."
— *American Reference Books Annual, 2000*

■

Sports Injuries Sourcebook, Second Edition

Basic Consumer Health Information about the Diagnosis, Treatment, and Rehabilitation of Common Sports-Related Injuries in Children and Adults

Along with Suggestions for Conditioning and Training, Information and Prevention Tips for Injuries Frequently Associated with Specific Sports and Special Populations, a Glossary, and a Directory of Additional Resources

Edited by Joyce Brennfleck Shannon. 614 pages. 2002. 0-7808-0604-2. $78.

■

Stress-Related Disorders Sourcebook

Basic Consumer Health Information about Stress and Stress-Related Disorders, Including Stress Origins and Signals, Environmental Stress at Work and Home, Mental and Emotional Stress Associated with Depression, Post-Traumatic Stress Disorder, Panic Disorder, Suicide, and the Physical Effects of Stress on the Cardiovascular, Immune, and Nervous Systems

Along with Stress Management Techniques, a Glossary, and a Listing of Additional Resources

Edited by Joyce Brennfleck Shannon. 610 pages. 2002. 0-7808-0560-7. $78.

Substance Abuse Sourcebook

Basic Health-Related Information about the Abuse of Legal and Illegal Substances Such as Alcohol, Tobacco, Prescription Drugs, Marijuana, Cocaine, and Heroin; and Including Facts about Substance Abuse Prevention Strategies, Intervention Methods, Treatment and Recovery Programs, and a Section Addressing the Special Problems Related to Substance Abuse during Pregnancy

Edited by Karen Bellenir. 573 pages. 1996. 0-7808-0038-9. $78.

"A valuable addition to any health reference section. Highly recommended."
— *The Book Report, Mar/Apr '97*

". . . a comprehensive collection of substance abuse information that's both highly readable and compact. Families and caregivers of substance abusers will find the information enlightening and helpful, while teachers, social workers and journalists should benefit from the concise format. Recommended."
— *Drug Abuse Update, Winter '96/'97*

SEE ALSO Alcoholism Sourcebook, Drug Abuse Sourcebook

■

Surgery Sourcebook

Basic Consumer Health Information about Inpatient and Outpatient Surgeries, Including Cardiac, Vascular, Orthopedic, Ocular, Reconstructive, Cosmetic, Gynecologic, and Ear, Nose, and Throat Procedures and More

Along with Information about Operating Room Policies and Instruments, Laser Surgery Techniques, Hospital Errors, Statistical Data, a Glossary, and Listings of Sources for Further Help and Information

Edited by Annemarie S. Muth and Karen Bellenir. 600 pages. 2002. 0-7808-0380-9. $78.

■

Transplantation Sourcebook

Basic Consumer Health Information about Organ and Tissue Transplantation, Including Physical and Financial Preparations, Procedures and Issues Relating to Specific Solid Organ and Tissue Transplants, Rehabilitation, Pediatric Transplant Information, the Future of Transplantation, and Organ and Tissue Donation

Along with a Glossary and Listings of Additional Resources

Edited by Joyce Brennfleck Shannon. 628 pages. 2002. 0-7808-0322-1. $78.

Traveler's Health Sourcebook

Basic Consumer Health Information for Travelers, Including Physical and Medical Preparations, Transportation Health and Safety, Essential Information about Food and Water, Sun Exposure, Insect and Snake Bites, Camping and Wilderness Medicine, and Travel with Physical or Medical Disabilities

Along with International Travel Tips, Vaccination Recommendations, Geographical Health Issues, Disease Risks, a Glossary, and a Listing of Additional Resources

Edited by Joyce Brennfleck Shannon. 613 pages. 2000. 0-7808-0384-1. $78.

"Recommended reference source."
   — Booklist, American Library Association, Feb '01

"This book is recommended for any public library, any travel collection, and especially any collection for the physically disabled."
   —American Reference Books Annual, 2001

■

Vegetarian Sourcebook

Basic Consumer Health Information about Vegetarian Diets, Lifestyle, and Philosophy, Including Definitions of Vegetarianism and Veganism, Tips about Adopting Vegetarianism, Creating a Vegetarian Pantry, and Meeting Nutritional Needs of Vegetarians, with Facts Regarding Vegetarianism's Effect on Pregnant and Lactating Women, Children, Athletes, and Senior Citizens

Along with a Glossary of Commonly Used Vegetarian Terms and Resources for Additional Help and Information

Edited byChad T. Kimball. 375 pages. 2002. 0-7808-0439-2. $78.

■

Women's Health Concerns Sourcebook

Basic Information about Health Issues That Affect Women, Featuring Facts about Menstruation and Other Gynecological Concerns, Including Endometriosis, Fibroids, Menopause, and Vaginitis; Reproductive Concerns, Including Birth Control, Infertility, and Abortion; and Facts about Additional Physical, Emotional, and Mental Health Concerns Prevalent among Women Such as Osteoporosis, Urinary Tract Disorders, Eating Disorders, and Depression

Along with Tips for Maintaining a Healthy Lifestyle

Edited by Heather E. Aldred. 567 pages. 1997. 0-7808-0219-5. $78.

"Handy compilation. There is an impressive range of diseases, devices, disorders, procedures, and other physical and emotional issues covered . . . well organized, illustrated, and indexed." *— Choice, Association of College and Research Libraries, Jan '98*

SEE ALSO *Breast Cancer Sourcebook, Cancer Sourcebook for Women, 1st and 2nd Editions, Healthy Heart Sourcebook for Women, Osteoporosis Sourcebook*

Workplace Health & Safety Sourcebook

Basic Consumer Health Information about Workplace Health and Safety, Including the Effect of Workplace Hazards on the Lungs, Skin, Heart, Ears, Eyes, Brain, Reproductive Organs, Musculoskeletal System, and Other Organs and Body Parts

Along with Information about Occupational Cancer, Personal Protective Equipment, Toxic and Hazardous Chemicals, Child Labor, Stress, and Workplace Violence

Edited by Chad T. Kimball. 626 pages. 2000. 0-7808-0231-4. $78.

"As a reference for the general public, this would be useful in any library."   *—E-Streams, Jun '01*

"Provides helpful information for primary care physicians and other caregivers interested in occupational medicine. . . . General readers; professionals."
   — Choice, Association of College & Research Libraries, May '01

"Recommended reference source."
   — Booklist, American Library Association, Feb '01

"Highly recommended."   *— The Bookwatch, Jan '01*

■

Worldwide Health Sourcebook

Basic Information about Global Health Issues, Including Malnutrition, Reproductive Health, Disease Dispersion and Prevention, Emerging Diseases, Risky Health Behaviors, and the Leading Causes of Death

Along with Global Health Concerns for Children, Women, and the Elderly, Mental Health Issues, Research and Technology Advancements, and Economic, Environmental, and Political Health Implications, a Glossary, and a Resource Listing for Additional Help and Information

Edited by Joyce Brennfleck Shannon. 614 pages. 2001. 0-7808-0330-2. $78.

"Named an Outstanding Academic Title."
   —Choice, Association of College & Research Libraries, Jan '02

"Yet another handy but also unique compilation in the extensive Health Reference Series, this is a useful work because many of the international publications reprinted or excerpted are not readily available. Highly recommended."
   —Choice, Association of College & Research Libraries, Nov '01

"Recommended reference source."
   —Booklist, American Library Association, Oct '01

Teen Health Series

Helping Young Adults Understand, Manage, and Avoid Serious Illness

Diet Information for Teens
Health Tips about Diet and Nutrition

Including Facts about Nutrients, Dietary Guidelines, Breakfasts, School Lunches, Snacks, Party Food, Weight Control, Eating Disorders, and More

Edited by Karen Bellenir. 399 pages. 2001. 0-7808-0441-4. $58.

"Full of helpful insights and facts throughout the book. . . . An excellent resource to be placed in public libraries or even in personal collections."
—*American Reference Books Annual 2002*

"Recommended for middle and high school libraries and media centers as well as academic libraries that educate future teachers of teenagers. It is also a suitable addition to health science libraries that serve patrons who are interested in teen health promotion and education." —*E-Streams, Oct '01*

"This comprehensive book would be beneficial to collections that need information about nutrition, dietary guidelines, meal planning, and weight control. . . . This reference is so easy to use that its purchase is recommended." —*The Book Report, Sep-Oct '01*

"This book is written in an easy to understand format describing issues that many teens face every day, and then provides thoughtful explanations so that teens can make informed decisions. This is an interesting book that provides important facts and information for today's teens." —*Doody's Health Sciences Book Review Journal, Jul-Aug '01*

"A comprehensive compendium of diet and nutrition. The information is presented in a straightforward, plain-spoken manner. This title will be useful to those working on reports on a variety of topics, as well as to general readers concerned about their dietary health."
—*School Library Journal, Jun '01*

Drug Information for Teens
Health Tips about the Physical and Mental Effects of Substance Abuse

Including Facts about Alcohol, Anabolic Steroids, Club Drugs, Cocaine, Depressants, Hallucinogens, Herbal Products, Inhalants, Marijuana, Narcotics, Stimulants, Tobacco, and More

Edited by Karen Bellenir. 472 pages. 2002. 0-7808-0444-9. $58.

Mental Health Information for Teens
Health Tips about Mental Health and Mental Illness

Including Facts about Anxiety, Depression, Suicide, Eating Disorders, Obsessive-Compulsive Disorders, Panic Attacks, Phobias, Schizophrenia, and More

Edited by Karen Bellenir. 406 pages. 2001. 0-7808-0442-2. $58.

"In both language and approach, this user-friendly entry in the *Teen Health Series* is on target for teens needing information on mental health concerns." —*Booklist, American Library Association, Jan '02*

"Readers will find the material accessible and informative, with the shaded notes, facts, and embedded glossary insets adding appropriately to the already interesting and succinct presentation."
—*School Library Journal, Jan '02*

"This title is highly recommended for any library that serves adolescents and parents/caregivers of adolescents." —*E-Streams, Jan '02*

"Recommended for high school libraries and young adult collections in public libraries. Both health professionals and teenagers will find this book useful."
—*American Reference Books Annual 2002*

"This is a nice book written to enlighten the society, primarily teenagers, about common teen mental health issues. It is highly recommended to teachers and parents as well as adolescents."
—*Doody's Review Service, Dec '01*

Sexual Health Information for Teens
Health Tips about Sexual Development, Human Reproduction, and Sexually Transmitted Diseases

Including Facts about Puberty, Reproductive Health, Chlamydia, Human Papillomavirus, Pelvic Inflammatory Disease, Herpes, AIDS, Contraception, Pregnancy, and More

Edited by Deborah A. Stanley. 400 pages. 2002. 0-7808-0445-7. $58.